Therapeutic Chair Massage

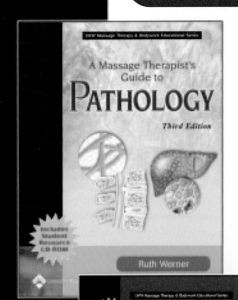
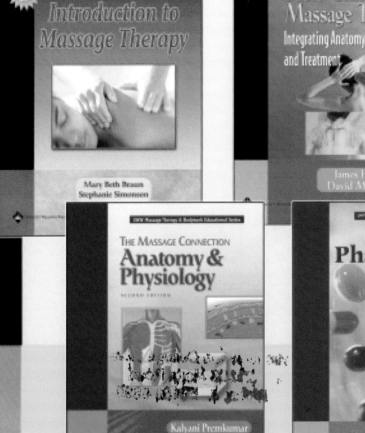
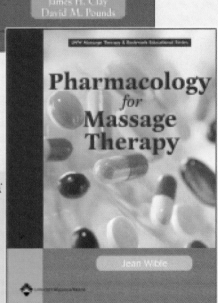
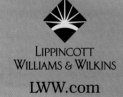

Therapeutic Chair Massage

Ralph R. Stephens

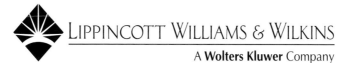

LIPPINCOTT WILLIAMS & WILKINS

A **Wolters Kluwer** Company

Philadelphia • Baltimore • New York • London
Buenos Aires • Hong Kong • Sydney • Tokyo

Executive Acquisitions Editor: Pete Darcy
Developmental Editor: David Payne
Senior Marketing Manager: Christen DeMarco
Production Editor: Kevin Johnson
Designer: Doug Smock
Photography: Fisheye
Illustration Planner: Wayne Hubbel
Typesetter: Maryland Composition
Printer: RR Donnelly and Sons

351 West Camden Street
Baltimore, Maryland 21201-2436 USA

530 Walnut Street
Philadelphia, Pennsylvania 19106 USA

Printed in the United States of America

Library of Congress Cataloging-in-Publication Data

Stephens, Ralph, 1948–
    Therapeutic chair massage / Ralph Stephens.—1st ed.
      p. ; cm.
    Includes index.
    ISBN 0-7817-4234-X
  1. Massage therapy.   2. Chairs.   3. Massage therapy—Equipment and supplies.
    I. Title.
    [DNLM: 1. Massage—methods.   WB 537 S835t 2006]
RM721.S75 2006
615.8′22—dc22

                                                                    2005009803

To purchase additional copies of this book, call our customer service department at **(800) 638-3030** or fax orders to **(301) 824-7390.** For other book services, including chapter reprints and large quantity sales, ask for the Special Sales department.

For all other calls originating outside of the United States, please call **(301)714-2324.**

Visit Lippincott Williams & Wilkins on the Internet: **http://www.lww.com**. Lippincott Williams & Wilkins customer service representatives are available from 8:30 am to 6:00 pm, EST, Monday through Friday, for telephone access.

00 01 02 03 04
1 2 3 4 5 6 7 8 9 1

Mom—for having me, encouraging me, and believing in me.

Debra L. Brooks—the catalyst for this project, whose love, help, and talent are most appreciated.

Aaron Mattes—for his selfless service to people in pain. His mentoring, support, friendship, and encouragement to learn and to share his work have been an inspiration.

To you the readers, may this book help you help more people.

Preface

When I began this project, there was no textbook available on seated massage. School owners and participants in my Seated Therapeutic Massage Seminars were all requesting such a text. In addition, I desired a textbook to use in teaching continuing education seminars on seated therapeutic massage as a supplement to my *Seated Therapeutic Massage* video series. I set out to fill this need for a textbook that could be used in either a short, entry level seated massage course or in a comprehensive, advanced course. This book is intended to be an educational resource on seated massage that will captivate and inspire beginning students as well as motivate and stimulate practicing therapists to grow to their fullest potential.

GOALS

This textbook accomplishes three primary goals. First and foremost, it provides core knowledge for students in entry-level massage training programs and possibly even for lay people who want to learn how to give a basic seated massage. The easy-to-follow writing style and the review of massage basics such as hygiene, body mechanics, and strokes makes this text accessible for beginners. The relaxation routine presented in Chapter 9 can be easily learned and effectively performed by beginning students of massage.

Second, this book provides continuing education information in advanced chair massage techniques for practicing professionals or advanced students in schools, seminars, and home study programs. The comprehensive coverage of common upper body musculoskeletal complaints and injuries such as frozen shoulder, carpal tunnel syndrome, and tennis and golfer's elbow in the therapeutic routines presented in Chapters 10–12, along with the inclusion of a chapter on business promotion, will meet the needs of advanced students and practicing therapists.

Third, it provides valuable supplementary information on fascia, body mechanics, and the neurological effects of massage strokes and stretching techniques, which are missing in many entry-level textbooks. In addition to using this text to teach seated massage, schools can use this additional information to supplement their current curriculum materials on these other subjects, enabling them to provide a more complete educational program. Practicing therapists will find this information to be useful in both their chair and table practices as it will give them a more complete understanding of how the nervous system, fascia, and muscles respond to massage and stretching techniques than has been typically taught in entry level programs. The body mechanics presented in Chapter 6 and reinforced throughout the techniques chapters will help protect both beginning and advanced therapists from massage-related injuries.

ORGANIZATION

The chapters of the book are organized progressively in four sections. The first provides the background information a therapist needs to know before performing seated massage. It covers the history and applications of seated massage, as well as equipment and techniques, hygiene, safety, contraindications, client-therapist communications, assessment methods for seated massage, and ways to develop treatment plans.

The second section presents the actual hands-on techniques. It begins with a chapter on body mechanics, and then details massage techniques used in seated massage in two separate chapters, one on massage strokes and one on stretching techniques.

The third section includes both basic relaxation and advanced therapeutic techniques, organized in easy-to-follow, thorough routines.

The fourth section consists of an in-depth chapter on business and marketing which will help the therapist become successful in establishing a chair massage business and reaching the public. The principles of this chapter apply to marketing both chair and table practices.

UNIQUE CONTENT FEATURES

The content features unique to this textbook are the massage routines and the concepts presented to support them at both the intellectual and physical levels. Seated massage therapists need to know more than just how to do a seated massage, they also need to know why they are doing each technique, how each technique affects the client's nervous system, and how to minimize the chance of massage-related injury to themselves. The best trained therapist may not be successful if she does not have marketing skills; therefore an extensive section is dedicated to marketing. Promotional tips and ideas are also included throughout the textbook.

Each of these features is described below.

Relaxation Routine

Most entry-level massage and bodywork programs just teach a basic relaxation routine in the seated position, often spending only 4 to 6 hours on the subject. Chapter 9, "Relaxation Routine," provides exactly what these programs need. This foundational routine will teach students how to perform an effective chair massage in 10 to 15 minutes. It is a complete upper body routine, including the arms, that will allow even the beginning therapist to predictably create a significant relaxation response. This routine can be taught in 4 to 6 hours and will enable the student to participate in outreach events, post-event sports massage, student clinics, and to begin a chair massage practice. It is the foundation that all the advanced techniques are built upon.

Therapeutic Routine

For practicing therapists and advanced students near the end of their school programs, this text presents specific, therapeutic techniques in Chapters 10–12 to take their seated massage practice from relaxation to restorative/therapeutic levels. Techniques are clearly explained and illustrated for addressing most common soft-tissue complaints of the back, neck, forearm, wrist, hand, and shoulder. Combined with the stretching techniques presented in Chapter 8, the therapist will be able to "create" a unique massage to address the needs of each individual client. This greatly expands the potential market for chair massage beyond stress relief to injury prevention, performance enhancement, and rehabilitation and restorative applications. Therapeutic chair massage can be integrated into healthcare and rehabilitation clinics, sports medicine, chiropractic offices, and workplaces with high exposure to upper body soft tissue injuries. Learning these therapeutic techniques will improve the "marketability" of any therapist and increase the likelihood of him having a successful career.

Neurological Effects of Massage and Fascia

There is a lack of good information on the neurological effects of massage strokes and stretching in entry-level massage texts. There is also a lack of clear, practical, easily understood and applied information on the fascia. This book fills that void by providing that information in Chapters 7 and 8, making it a valuable supplement to general, entry-level textbooks and useful for both basic and advanced techniques classes.

Injury Prevention

Because injury prevention is critical to a successful practice, body mechanics, stretching, and strengthening are covered in this book. Body mechanics (correct use of hands and posture) is presented in Chapter 6 and emphasized throughout the techniques chapters. It is vitally important that hands-on practitioners use proper body mechanics; otherwise their careers may be compromised by injury, fatigue, or "burn-out." Stretching and strengthening programs to help prevent massage-induced injuries to therapists are also included.

Business Promotion

Marketing skills are often lacking in many massage therapists' training and life experiences. A therapist can seldom eat well on massage skills alone. Successful promotion of a massage practice or of one's own abilities to be an employee is essential for success. The ultimate goal of this book is to train therapists to be able to help more people. Being able to communicate in ways that effectively promote their business is just as much an essential part of helping people as knowing how to massage someone's shoulder. Chapter 13, "Business Promotion," guides students through both a self analysis and a market analysis to help them determine the best ways for them to develop their business. It then shares methods that have been proven to work by successful chair practitioners to promote various types of professional chair massage practices.

PEDAGOGIC FEATURES

In addition to a wealth of color photos and illustrations, this book includes a number of features to aid the reader in learning the concepts presented. Features include:

- **Objectives** provide the clear goals to ensure mastery of the content presented in the chapter.
- **Experiential Exercises** create a deeper understanding of content through hands-on exercises that allow students to "feel" an anatomical structure or massage technique in their own bodies or a partner's.
- **Clinical Tips** provide practical application and problem solving hints that are only learned through years of clinical experience.
- **Contraindications** identify general and specific contraindications to seated massage techniques.
- **Special Interest Boxes** contain additional information on related and interesting topics.
- **Case Studies** emphasize the practical application of content, using critical thinking questions and situations to help the practitioner adapt the information and techniques presented to specific clients.
- **Chapter Summaries** "wrap-up" each chapter by briefly summarizing the major chapter content.

FINAL NOTE

This textbook is intended to be accessible, enjoyable, and easy to use. I have tried to write in a comfortable, conversational style and to illustrate the techniques and anatomy in a way that facilitates learning. Furthermore, the content provides all of the basics needed by beginners as well as detailed coverage of advanced concepts required by experienced practitioners. I hope this resource serves the teachers and students of chair massage well. Most importantly, I hope it helps bring the healing power of human touch to ever increasing numbers of people through the medium of chair massage. May our collective efforts bring about a healthier and more peaceful world.

Acknowledgments

SPECIAL ACKNOWLEDGMENTS

David Palmer, for starting this whole chair massage thing.

Debra Brooks, who directed an acquisitions editor from LWW my way at an AMTA convention and later assisted with the photos and illustrations.

Pete Darcy, who picked up the file, got me to submit a proposal, and has generously allowed this project to grow as needed.

David Payne, my developmental editor (DEs are the unsung heroes of textbook publishing), who stepped into the project at its lowest ebb, organized, gently prodded, coached, put up with me, pulled together the photo shoot, and did everything an editor should—and more. Thanks David—you saved the day.

Ben Benjamin and Judith DeLany, for their brilliant and concise contribution on referred pain—thanks so much!

Lindy Fox, who served as beta-tester, proofreader, and editor for my preliminary drafts of each chapter, and as my lead therapist model in both the scratch and final photos. As a therapist, she helped keep me together. Her help has been invaluable.

John Fanuzzi, who asked me to make a video with his chair. Thanks for asking!

Golden Ratio Woodworks, for their help, support, and encouragement, especially Denis Ouellette for graphics support and Jodie Jensen for logistics.

The LWW staff—Thanks for everything. It's in your hands now!

To my daughter and grandson, you mean more to me than you will ever know, more than I can ever show.

PRODUCTION ACKNOWLEDGMENTS

Massage Chairs provided by Golden Ratio Woodworks, www.goldenratio.com (800-345-1590).

Massage tools provided by Scrip, Inc., www.scrip-inc.com (800-747-3488).

Therapist's shirts for photo shoot provided by Karen Duprey, www.massageclothing.com (800-562-1944).

Photographic efforts and service above and beyond the call of duty by John Thomas at Fisheye, Hiawatha, IA.

Other photos provided by Body Support Systems, Custom Craftworks, Golden Ratio Woodworks, The Himalayan Institute & Yoga International, and David Palmer.

HEARTFELT THANKS TO

Models: Debra Brooks, Lindy Fox, Genavive Johanson, Jen McCluskey, David Payne, Gary Rowray, Trang.

Reviewers—you really helped.

Kimberly Battista, for her illustrations on a moment's notice.

James Clay and David Pounds for use of their illustrations.

Beth Anderson for data entry, research assistance, and for keeping me organized, in spite of myself.

Pandit Rajmani Tiguniat and The Himalayan Institute staff—Sandy Anderson, Mary Cardinal, Darlene Clark, Shelly Craigo, Deborah Willoughby, and all.

Robert K. King, for his ongoing advice, support, inspiration, and humor.

Dr. Jason Cupp, DC—Family Chiropractic Center, Iowa City, IA—for keeping "computer back" at bay.

David Kent, for on the spot consulting.

Dr. Gregory T. Lawton, BS, DN, DC, for encouragement, inspiration, and for sharing information on pain and prosperity.

American Medical Massage Association for resources and information from their website (www.americanmedicalmassage.com).

Body Support Systems, Bio-Safe, Bio-Tone, Custom CraftWorks, PDI.

Kirk Nelson, and MassageWorks of Weston.

Tiffany Field, Touch Research Institute.

Lynda Solien-Wolfe.

Synergy Health & Healing Center, Cedar Rapids, IA.

Serenity, Inc. Yoga Center and Jen Smith, Cedar Rapids, IA.

Reviewers

Diane Charmley, RN, BS, LMT
Virginia Mason Medical Center
Seattle, Washington

Sara Corkery, BA, BFA, LMT
Communications and Marketing
Chicago School of Massage Therapy
Villa Park, Illinois

Mary Duquin, PhD
Associate Professor
Department of Health and Physical Activity
University of Pittsburgh
Pittsburgh, Pennsylvania

Richard M. Gold, PhD, LAc
Professor and Practitioner
Pacific College of Oriental Medicine
International Professional School of Bodywork
Certified Instructor of AOBTA (American
    Organization of Body Therapies of Asia)
San Diego, California

Richard Greely, BA, MEd
Assistant Professor
Columbus State Community College
Columbus, Ohio

Matthew Nolan, BSc, CPT, RMT, MTI
Owner/Director
The Center for Life Enrichment
Richardson, Texas

Contents

Therapeutic Chair Massage

CHAPTER 1

Introduction to Seated Massage

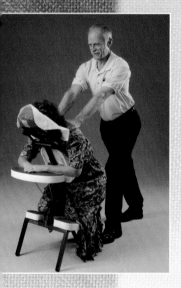

"The beauty of Chair Massage is its simple message that massage can make you feel better—whatever that means to you—any time you want. You don't have to be sick or enlightened or wealthy to appreciate its benefits. It is truly massage for the masses."

DAVID PALMER

Objectives

■ Define concisely "seated massage."

■ Summarize briefly the history of seated massage.

■ Identify the benefits unique to seated massage compared with table massage.

■ Identify the body regions that seated massage is most effective in treating.

■ Identify several complaints and conditions that seated massage is effective in treating.

■ List potential locations where seated massage might be performed and occupations that might likely benefit from seated massage.

Key Terms

Body mechanics: the proper use of posture, movement and joint alignment to perform massage therapy efficiently and with minimum stress and trauma to the practitioner. The use of correct body mechanics reduces the chance of injury to the practitioner and improves the quality of touch to the recipient. Also called *biomechanics.*

Paradigm: a pattern or model for something, especially one that forms the basis of a methodology or theory.

Parasympathetic response: the response by the parasympathetic division of the autonomic nervous system, which conserves body resources and brings about body calmness; generally antagonistic to the sympathetic division.

Sympathetic response: The response by the sympathetic division of the autonomic nervous system which spends body resources and prepares the body for emergency situations; it is the "fight or flight" response to perceived stress or threats.

Spasm: an involuntary contraction of one or more muscle groups, which cannot be stopped by voluntary relaxation, ranging from increased tension causing discomfort and restricted movement to cramps causing pain and sudden, uncontrolled movement or distortion.

Tonus: a state of continuous, partial contraction of muscle tissue, creating a normal, continuous tension by virtue of which the parts are kept in shape, alert, and ready to response to stimulus. Excessive tonus (hypertonus) causes discomfort, restricts range of motion, and wastes body energy.

W hat exactly is seated massage? How is it different from table massage? Can it be used for more than just "relaxation"? As students or practitioners considering seated massage as a career or as a supplement to your current practice, these are questions you likely have. It is the goal of this introductory chapter to answer these questions and provide you with an overview of seated massage.

Simply put, seated massage is massage performed on a person who is sitting erect. He or she may be seated on the ground or on almost any supportive device, such as a chair, stool, or specifically designed massage chair. The term "chair massage" is often used instead of "seated massage" to distinguish massage performed on a massage table from massage performed on a massage chair. In this book, however, the terms are used interchangeably because all the basic concepts, principles and techniques presented apply to all seated massage, whether it is done with or without a massage chair.

Building on this definition, the remainder of this chapter provides an historical context for seated massage, distinguishes it from table massage, presents the body regions to which it is most effectively applied, identifies common conditions that may be treated by it, and explores common practice settings in which it may be used.

HISTORY OF SEATED MASSAGE

"H istory helps us understand change and how the society we live in came to be. The past causes the present, and so the future. Only through studying history can we grasp how things change, and only through history can we understand what elements of an institution or a society persist despite change."

PETER N. STERNS, American Historical Association

Beginnings

Massage is one of the things that has persisted in society for centuries. It has evolved into many different styles, yet still retains its recognizable form. Historical records indicate that seated massage has been practiced for millennia. Egyptian hieroglyphics dated from 2,500 BC show people sitting on the ground massaging each others' feet and hands. Centuries-old Japanese block prints show people receiving massage while seated on low stools. The roots of the modern movement of seated massage, however, lie in the twentieth century. In the United States during the late 1970s and early 1980s (the "renaissance" of massage), therapists were performing seated massage, usually with the client on a stool. Russian sports massage therapists have long used the seated position for treating the posterior neck and shoulders. The athlete is seated on a chair or stool and leans against a cushion that is resting on a table. Some Japanese methods, such as *Amma*, require a portion of each session, usually at the beginning or end, to be performed with the client seated.

David Palmer and the Advent of the Massage Chair

The founder of modern seated massage is generally acknowledged to be David Palmer, a visionary massage practitioner and massage school owner who was inspired to adapt *Amma* techniques and create acupressure-based massage routines for the seated position. Through his efforts and remarkable promotional skills, seated massage as we know it today came into being. Palmer did not invent seated massage; however, he did shine the public spotlight on chair massage in a way that highlighted its unique features. His goal was to make massage as accepted and accessible as a haircut.

David Palmer began teaching the first training program in seated massage in 1982 while director of The Amma Institute of Traditional Japanese Massage in San Francisco, California (Fig. 1-1). He recognized that for massage to become popular, it would have to avoid its association with adult entertainment, while becoming convenient, affordable, and accessible to the masses. The seated format he developed and taught accomplished all these things.

The following year, he and Stephen Pizzella began a seated massage business employing practitioners trained in his program. In 1984, Palmer and Pizzella signed their first major corporate customer, Apple Computer, which eventually paid to have seven practitioners provide 350 seated massages per week for its employees.

Also in 1984, Palmer enlisted the help of French cabinetmaker Serge Bouyssou to design a portable chair that would comfortably support the client's whole body and allow easy access by a massage practitioner. In 1986, Living Earth Crafts introduced the first production version of the Palmer-Bouysson massage chair. It weighed 26 pounds and was made primarily of wood. This chair put a face to seated massage and became the model for client positioning in virtually all subsequent massage chairs (Fig. 1-2).

Palmer founded the TouchPro Institute in 1986 to teach chair massage as continuing education classes.

He coined the term "chair massage" to describe massage done using a special massage chair and the term "on-site massage" for massage performed at the client's site.

In 1989, Golden Ratio Woodworks introduced the Quicklite Massage Chair. Conceptualized by Scott Breyer, a student of David Palmer, and developed by John Fanuzzi, it was the first metal-framed, lightweight massage chair. It weighed only 14 pounds and featured quick and simple adjustments (Fig. 1-3).

Influence of Sports Massage

Sports massage has played a significant role in the growth of the public's awareness of the massage profession in general and, more specifically, chair massage. In the early 1980s, event sports massage performed by "sports massage teams" became popular and served as the primary outreach tool in the promotion of the emerging profession at that time. The first such team to work a major event was organized by Gayle Davidson, Steve Kitts, and James

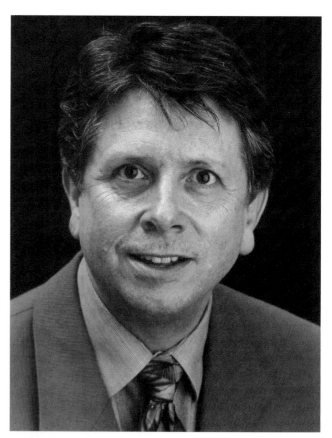

Figure 1–1 David Palmer. (Photo courtesy of www.touchpro.com)

No longer were the organization, coordination, and participation of many therapists in a sports massage team necessary to bring massage out in the open. No longer was the exposure for massage limited to athletes and their fans. With the advent of the massage chair, one or many therapists could easily go to a business, public place, or event and demonstrate their work. This allowed individual therapists to introduce massage to any demographic segment of the public. Sports massage teams and the massage chair can be given a great deal of credit for the dramatic growth of the massage profession, which began in the last half of the 1980s. They both continue to be effective promotional strategies today, but for the reasons discussed above, the massage chair has become the most popular and widely used.

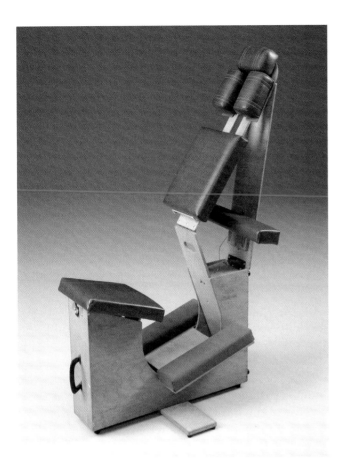

Figure 1–2   The first commercial massage chair, 1986. Designed by David Palmer and Serge Bouyssou; made and marketed by Living Earth Crafts.

Hackett to work the Boston Marathon in 1984. However, this early event sports massage was limited by two things. First, it takes quite a bit of organization and the volunteer efforts of many therapists to get a team together to work an event. Second, most communities have a limited number of high-profile sporting events suitable for a sports massage team. Still, event sports massage was effective in bringing therapists and their tables out of private rooms and into the light of day, where the public could watch professional massage in a non-threatening environment and observe athletes stand in line to receive it. This endorsement by athletes through their participation rapidly increased the acceptance of massage by the general public. It also generated a great deal of positive media coverage.

Thus, sports massage helped pave the way for chair massage, so that when the massage chair came into being in 1986, the public was more prepared to embrace this new type of massage. Also, the chair expanded the accessibility and efficiency of massage.

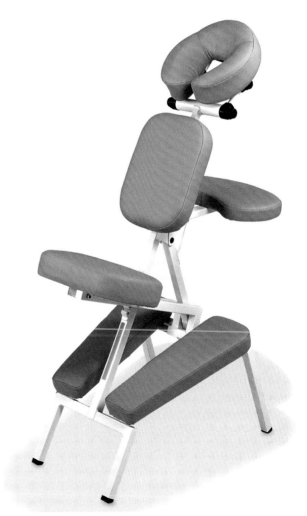

Figure 1–3   The Quicklite massage chair, 1989. The first metal-framed, lightweight massage chair. Designed by Scott Breyer and John Fanuzzi; made and marketed by Golden Ratio Woodworks. (Photo courtesy of Golden Ratio Woodworks, Inc., Emigrant, MT. www.goldenratio.com)

Beyond Relaxation: Therapeutic Chair Massage

Palmer described the intention of his chair massage routine(s) as being a simple relaxation service rather than a "treatment" or "therapy." As the concept of chair massage became accepted, it evolved beyond just relaxation. In 1989, Raymond Blaylock joined with the AVEDA Corporation to introduce aromatherapy and spa applications for chair massage. In 1995, this author introduced therapeutic concepts to chair massage, adapting specific massage and stretching techniques to address common soft tissue injuries and complaints. Chair massage techniques and equipment will most likely continue to evolve and reach more segments of the population as the public's acceptance of massage increases.

The benefits of chair massage have been documented by scientific research. In 1996, the Touch Research Institute at the University of Miami School of Medicine, under the direction of Dr. Tiffany Field, PhD, published research demonstrating that chair massage "reduces anxiety and enhances EEG pattern[s] of alertness and math computations." This landmark double-blind study validated chair massage as a valuable wellness program in the workplace. In the group receiving chair massage, speed and accuracy of math computations improved, while anxiety levels, depression scores, and job stress scores were lower (1).

SEATED VERSUS TABLE MASSAGE

As indicated in the previous section, seated massage has come into its own as an approach that has distinct advantages over table massage in many situations. Probably the most obvious benefit of seated massage over table massage is that it is more portable and requires less space than table massage, facilitating on-site work. Massage chairs, especially the new metal-framed massage chairs, are easier to carry, quicker to set up, and have a much smaller footprint than any massage table. Chair massage provides a much more practical, convenient, and efficient format with which to take massage to the client.

In office or clinic massage practices, salons, and spas, chair massage can be done in smaller rooms than are required for table massage. Chair massage can be done without a private room in many situations, giving high visibility to potential clients in such places as waiting rooms, merchandise areas, and workout rooms, to name a few.

Probably the biggest advantage seated massage offers over table massage is that seated massage does not require the client to disrobe. With a client in the seated position, fully clothed, the association of massage with adult entertainment is virtually eliminated. People feel safe trying massage in this format, which is not threatening or suggestive and which keeps the client in control of the situation. If at any time a client feels uncomfortable, she knows she can stand up and walk away, unlike most table massage situations in which the client is lying down, at least partially disrobed, and in a small private room. Also, with no disrobing, less time is spent between clients, allowing therapists to better utilize their time.

Since the client is fully clothed during seated massage, lubricants (oils, lotions, crèmes, etc.) are not used. This is appealing to many people, especially those who have skin allergies or who object to the greasy feeling after a massage. It also reduces the therapist's supply expenses.

Two of the biggest obstacles to table massage are the time commitment required for the client and the price. Table massage sessions are seldom less than 30 minutes and often as long as 90 minutes. It is not unusual for an hour massage to be over $70.00. Add to this the time to get to a therapist's office and back to home or work, and a massage can become a half-day project. Many people cannot allocate this amount of time and financial resources. Seated massage eliminates this obstacle. A very effective seated massage can be done in as little as 10 minutes. The ideal session is between 15 and 20 minutes. Seated massage comes to the client in on-site situations, or is easily accessible at airports, malls, storefronts, or other handy venues. At this writing, seated massage typically costs a dollar a minute. Most people will take 15 to 30 minutes total to do something beneficial for themselves. Fifteen dollars is seldom a hardship for most people. They can get a chair massage on their lunch hour and still have time for lunch! We live in an era where convenience is required for most products and services to be successful. Seated massage is the most convenient and economical format for presenting massage to the public, especially as a wellness service.

The reasons presented above enable seated massage to become as affordable and commonplace as a haircut. They comprise the marketing concept behind seated massage. However, there are also

Box 1-1

Think About This

The body usually functions in the erect position. Most people gain relief from their discomfort when they lie down a while. If we provide therapy with the client in the supine and prone positions (table massage), we may not get an accurate assessment of the effectiveness of the massage. Of course they feel better, they have been lying down for 30–90 minutes in a relaxing environment. In seated massage we do not have this working for us. Therefore, if they feel better after a seated massage, isn't it logical to believe that they really *are* better, not just relieved by lying down?

To take this thought further, might the body be able to integrate therapy (and the resulting changes from the therapy) better when in the more erect, seated position than when supine-prone?

some very good technical reasons to use the seated position for massage. Some clients, especially those with "bad backs," have difficulty getting on and off a massage table. These clients can usually get onto a massage chair with little problem, and if you learn therapeutic techniques such as those presented in Chapter 10, you can effectively address many painful low back conditions with the client in a massage chair. The seated position provides better access to some muscles than table massage positions, and different access to others. More stretching can be done for the cervical and shoulder regions with the client in the seated position than when they are prone or supine. Of course, the seated position has its limitations, too. There are some areas of the body that cannot be effectively addressed with the client seated. These will be discussed in the next section.

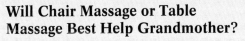

CASE STUDY

Will Chair Massage or Table Massage Best Help Grandmother?

You receive a call from the daughter of a 70-year-old woman. The 70-year-old mother has pain in her right shoulder that is limiting her range of motion—she cannot reach up to get her tea out of the cupboard. The mother's doctor told her that it was frozen shoulder and prescribed a muscle relaxant. The daughter is urging her to try massage and got your number from a colleague who is a patient of yours. The daughter wants to know if you can make a house call. She is also concerned that her mother will not want to take off her clothes to receive a massage and wonders if there is any way you can work through her clothes. You have both a portable massage table and a massage chair.

1. Would a massage chair or a massage table be a better support system for this situation?
2. Will you be better able to perform stretches and range of motion exercises on the grandmother's shoulder if she is on a massage table or on a massage chair?
3. Which support system will be easier for an elderly woman to get onto and off of?
4. Which support system will most likely avoid any boundary issues with the grandmother and possibly make her more receptive to the therapy?
5. Are there any advantages to using a massage table in this situation?

BODY REGIONS TREATABLE WITH SEATED MASSAGE

Seated massage support systems, especially a good massage chair, allow at least some access to every region of the body. However, access is limited and relatively ineffective in some places. The chair is most practical for addressing the upper body when giving either relaxation or therapeutic massages. It gives the therapist excellent access to the client's entire back, shoulders, posterior neck, forearms, wrists, and hands. Although you can access some of the hips and the lower extremities, it is not practical. The hips, thighs, legs, and feet are so low to the ground when the client is in the seated position that your **body mechanics** would be extremely compromised if you tried to work on these areas. For instance, if you were to maintain the lunge position, your feet would be so far apart that your legs would very rapidly become tired. If you were to bend over at the waist, you would risk injuring your lower back. If you were to sit or kneel, you would have to work from your back, shoulders, and arms, which could cause fatigue and possible injury unless you have been trained to work from your "center" when sitting or kneeling, as when doing Shiatsu on a mat on the floor. It is the recommendation of this author that you try to avoid performing any significant amount of massage on the lower body with the client in a massage chair. If they really need lower body massage therapy, they need to receive table massage and should be advised to make an appointment with you or another therapist. If you feel you must do something on the lower body during a relaxation treatment to "tie the body together," be brief and superficial, using tapotment, vibration, and light effleurage.

Furthermore, even if you are willing to risk injuring yourself to address the lower body, realize that the massage will likely not be effective for the client. The client's gluteal and quadriceps muscles are stretched so tight when in the seated position that it is difficult to penetrate the tissues. Additionally, the client's clothes are stretched tight at the hip and at the knees, with the clothes adding another layer of resistance. This combination will prevent effective treatment of the tissue and could injure you. Although you can have the client straighten his or her knee, either by removing the client's legs from the leg pads or having the client turn backwards in the chair, it is still a clumsy and ineffective position to address the knee and thigh. You cannot effectively access the hamstrings no matter how the client sits, nor can you address the lower part of the hip because the client is sitting on it.

If you are trained in foot reflexology, you can use this method by having the client sit backwards in the chair and you sit facing him or her. The client can put the foot being massaged on your thigh, allowing you to provide reasonably good treatment. However, sitting backwards in most massage chairs is not comfortable for long, and a common chair (particularly a recliner) would work just as well if not better.

CLINICAL TIP

Adapting Table Massage for Your Chair Massage Client

If you recommend table massage to your client for some condition that cannot be treated effectively in a massage chair, mention that he or she will not be required to undress. Also indicate that since only lower extremity work (for example) is required, possibly only one knee or ankle, the session can still be 15–30 minutes and priced similarly to seated, on-site massage. This should reassure your client, who may be reluctant to undress or to pay more than they are used to for a session. Of course, if the client agrees, full body massage for 60–90 minutes could be performed with them disrobed.

Many other conditions could also be treated, depending on your level of expertise and creativity. Some of these conditions are covered in Chapters 10–12.

As previously mentioned, the seated position is excellent for most upper body complaints. These can be divided into five areas: the lumbar region (low back), the thoracic region (mid-back), the shoulder region, the posterior cervical region (neck), and the upper extremity (arm, wrist, and hand).

The upper body areas that are not practical to address in the seated position include the abdomen, the anterior thoracic region, and the anterior cervical region. These areas are inaccessible due to their position against the chair. Although an experienced therapist might be able to treat these areas by having the client sit backwards in the chair, table massage in a clinical setting would be a more appropriate way of treating these regions. The anterior cervical and thoracic regions will be addressed in this textbook using stretching techniques shown in Chapter 8: Stretching Techniques for Seated Massage. Some major conditions that can be addressed with the client in a massage chair are included in Table 1-1.

In addressing these soft tissue complaints, some of which may be considered medical conditions, you must keep in mind the scope of practice of a massage therapist. This varies from state to state, so be familiar with the legal limitations of your state. If any information or techniques given in this textbook conflicts with the laws of your area, disregard this textbook on that issue and obey the law.

However, at this writing, every state allows massage therapists to practice massage. Massage consists of manually examining tissue and relaxing muscle contractions (**spasms**). Stretching techniques have historically been recognized as a part of the practice of massage therapy, as they help relax muscle contractions that restrict normal range of motion. Massage is appropriate for most minor musculotendinous complaints ("minor" meaning that surgical

Table 1-1 Major Conditions Treatable by Chair Massage, by Body Region

Lumbar	Thoracic	Shoulder	Upper Extremity	Cervical
Low back pain and tension	Pain between the shoulders	Rotator cuff injuries	Carpal tunnel syndrome	Whiplash
Low back strains and sprains	Lack of range of motion of the scapula	Stiffness and lack of flexibility (ROM)	Lateral epicondylitis (Tennis elbow) and medial epicondylitis (Golfer's elbow)	Headaches
Muscle spasm related to disc injuries, lifting, accidents, falls, and other trauma	Postural distortion	Impingement	Tension, pain, tingling, and numbness in forearm, wrist, or hand	ROM restrictions
Acute onset low back pain	Pain on deep breath	Acromioclavicular joint pain	ROM limitations	Stiffness, pain, and ache in the neck
Lack of flexibility		Strains and sprains Frozen shoulder Aches and pains in the shoulder	Postural distortions Some types of arthritis (consult with their physician) Postural distortions Wrist, finger, and thumb pain Strains and sprains pain	Athletic injuries Postural distortion

intervention is not required). Therefore, assess the client to determine what their complaint is and what massage and stretching techniques are safe and appropriate for them. Contracted tissues will be tender when touched with moderate to firm pressure. Find the tender, abnormally contracted tissues; then massage and stretch them until they are normal or at least better. You will find that if you normalize the soft tissue, restore normal range of motion, and relax the client, most of the above conditions will improve or disappear. You did not treat a medical condition, you just did massage and stretching to normalize tissue **tonus.** Isn't the power of structured touch and movement amazing?

THERAPEUTIC APPLICATIONS

There are two major paradigms of massage, relaxation and therapeutic. Both attempt to invoke a relaxation response from the client's nervous system. The relaxation **paradigm** uses non-specific techniques and routines to create a general, systemic relaxation. The therapeutic paradigm uses muscle or region-specific routines to create localized relaxation in individual muscles or tissue groups, which also contributes to an overall systemic relaxation. The therapeutic paradigm begins with general techniques to warm and soothe tissues, just like the relaxation paradigm does. But it continues beyond to examine and treat tissues specifically, attempting to elicit a significant change in a particular spot or area. A relaxation therapist may discover a tender point and address it, but that is not the intent of the treatment. Usually a relaxation massage stays general. A therapeutic therapist will tend to begin with general techniques, then switch to specific techniques, examining tissue, treating abnormal tissues, and then finishing with additional general techniques. In addition to eliciting the general relaxation response, the therapeutic therapist is trying to facilitate changes in the client's body to reduce pain, change posture, increase range of motion, or some other specific treatment goal, usually in response to the client's complaint(s).

The original chair massage routines, as developed by David Palmer, were choreographed routines that were only to provide relaxation and stress relief. They were not intended to be therapy or a treatment, but a service. The routines were general and were not structured to address any particular complaint, pain, or injury.

Learning a relaxation routine is a great way to learn chair massage, just like learning a full-body Swedish relaxation routine is a great way to learn table massage. The relaxation routine is the foundation for therapeutic techniques. It is important that you learn a general relaxation routine before attempting therapeutic techniques. Relaxation is one of the most important results of massage. The primary soft tissue problem is muscle spasm—too much muscle tonus—which means too many fibers in a muscle are held "on" or contracted by the nervous system. This hypertonicity exists both generally (systemically) and specifically (locally). A relaxation routine addresses the systemic tension by inducing a generalized state of relaxation. This is sometimes referred to as the **parasympathetic response.** It can be argued that eliciting the overall parasympathetic response is one of, if not the most powerful healing methods, as it is during the parasympathetic response that immune function, digestion, and other physiological body processes are facilitated, helping healing to occur. The **sympathetic response** is our reaction to any perceived threat or stress (our "fight or flight mechanism") and causes increased muscle tonus, heart rate, respiratory rate, blood pressure, perspiration, adrenal activity, and decreased immune and digestive functions. Pain is usually perceived as a stressor by the nervous system and elicits the sympathetic response, although, depending on the cause and degree of pain, it may be only a localized response. Multiple local responses, or even a single significant response, contribute to a systemic response. A severe low back pain can cause the entire body to tense up, as can a significant headache. Most painful complaints are local—a specific tissue or muscle or maybe even just a small part of one muscle.

Reducing overall systemic tension with a relaxation massage will not usually change local tension significantly. Once the client becomes active after the massage, the local tension (pain) will usually be experienced again and re-facilitate the systemic tension with the sympathetic response to the pain. The beneficial parasympathetic response from a general massage is lost very quickly if the local dysfunctional tissues are not addressed and changed. Unfortunately, just reducing a local source of tension will only lower its contribution to the overall systemic

tension. The overall sympathetic response it and all other local irritations caused still needs to be addressed. Therefore, to obtain the best results for the client, both systemic and local tension should be reduced. Reducing pain complaints, improving posture, and increasing flexibility is an excellent and long-lasting way to reduce stress and create relaxation. This is why the format of working from general to specific to general is recommended in therapeutic work. By treating the client's specific complaints that contribute to their overall stress, along with treating their systemic tension, you achieve a much deeper and longer-lasting parasympathetic (relaxation) response. This is the primary reason for incorporating therapeutic massage and stretching techniques into chair massage.

Massage therapists who set out to do only relaxation chair massage usually find that many of their clients ask about specific aches and pains. If the therapist has not learned therapeutic protocols for the massage chair, she cannot address the specific needs of her clients. Of course, there is nothing wrong with just giving general relaxation therapy. Some therapists are very happy doing this, and it is a great service to provide to humanity.

However, many therapists get bored after a while, and some "burn out" doing virtually the same routine on every client. Therapeutic techniques are never boring; they are challenging, exciting, and rewarding, as each massage, like each client, is different. Besides, a patterned routine, a "one size fits all" treatment designed only for relaxation, sells the potential of seated massage short and limits its potential market, not to mention its potential benefit to the client.

Most people have specific, unique, painful complaints above and beyond the need to relax. More people will pay to get out of pain and discomfort than will pay for "stress reduction" and relaxation. Relaxation is a luxury that people will pay for only when they have the spare time and money. If a person believes you can help them get rid of their pain they will make the time and find the money. Pain relief is a necessity for most people. You will find many more opportunities to provide massage when you can also do therapeutic treatments. There are many people who need specific soft tissue care who will not participate in clinical massage at an office practice, due to their belief systems and resources as previously discussed. They are more likely to receive the care they need when it is available to them in the seated massage format.

This textbook provides a general relaxation routine in Chapter 9. This routine will serve you well in all situations where general relaxation is the primary goal. If you desire to learn more, stretching and therapeutic massage techniques are presented in Chapters 8, 10, 11, and 12. These build on the relaxation routine and take you into the exciting realm of therapy, where opportunities are unlimited because there are innumerable people in pain.

PRACTICE SETTINGS

The beauty of seated massage is that it can be done almost anywhere. Virtually everyone can benefit from seated massage, but so many people do not know that yet. You must recognize the opportunities in your community and do the necessary education (marketing) to create your practice.

Box 1-2 lists places, A to Z, where you might consider practicing massage, such as a salon, clinic, or airport, as well as places that have potential for occasional or regular on-site visits such as accounting offices and factories. Also included are professions and occupations that need massage and are potentially receptive, such as dentists, musicians, and sales people, who might provide on-site opportunities or might come to your fixed location (at the mall, for example) if they knew about your practice there (Fig. 1-4).

CASE STUDY

Defining Your Target Population

To help you begin to develop your vision for your seated massage practice, answer the following questions. Write your answers down and save them. See if they have changed when you get to Chapter 11 and begin to develop your business plan and marketing strategies.

1. Knowing what you do about seated massage, do you think you want to provide relaxation services only, or do you want to also provide therapy?
2. Write down at least three and no more than five specific populations you would prefer to provide seated massage for. (Examples are athletes, senior citizens, and accountants.)
3. For each specific population you have listed, write down three to five places, business locations, or events where you could reach that population.

SUMMARY

Seated massage is massage performed on a person who is sitting erect, on the ground or on some supporting device, most commonly a massage chair. Seated massage has been utilized for centuries, but its current form is credited to David Palmer, who began teaching the first modern training program in seated massage in 1982 and invented the first massage chair in 1986. Palmer's vision for seated massage was as a relaxation, stress reduction service, which he hoped would become as common, accessible, and affordable as a haircut.

The massage chair will never replace the massage table, but it does provide a way to present massage in a more user-friendly, convenient, and economical format. The major advantages to seated massage are:

1. Shorter appointments—the average being 15 minutes.

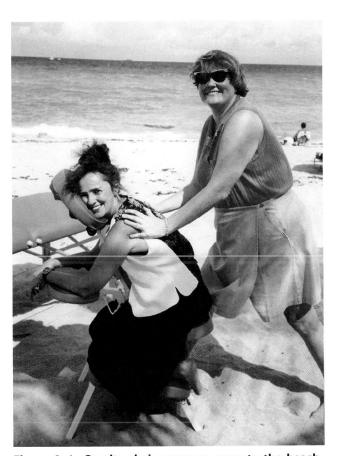

Figure 1–4 On-site chair massage goes to the beach. Lynda Solien-Wolfe, LMT, gives a chair massage to Dr. Tiffany Field, PhD, on a Florida beach. (Photo courtesy of Golden Ratio Woodworks, Inc., Emigrant, MT. www.goldenratio.com)

Box 1-2

Potential Seated Massage Clients and Practice Settings From A to Z

Here are some suggestions to consider as you seek potential clients and practice settings for seated massage. Suggestions marked with asterisks have, historically, been receptive to on-site seated massage.

A airports,* accountants' offices,* abstract offices, acupuncturists, advertising agencies, assisted living facilities, alcohol treatment centers, arcades, amusement parks, architects' offices, art galleries and museums, association offices, athletes,* attorneys' offices, auditoriums, automobile dealerships

B ballet companies and studios, ballrooms, bathrooms, banks,* barber shops, the beach, beauty salons,* behavioral therapists, bingo rooms, blood plasma centers, botanical gardens, bowling alleys, boxing gyms

C campgrounds, charter and private canoe trips, car dealerships, casinos, caterers, certified public accountants, child care facilities, chiropractic offices,* church organizations, church events, consultants, conventions, cruises, colleges

D dance studios, dance companies, dancers, data processing offices, day care facilities, dentists' offices, dentists, dental technicians, designers, detectives, diet centers, dinner theaters, drivers, doctors, drug abuse and treatment centers,* drummers, dude ranches

E e-commerce company offices, educational services, employee programs,* engineers,* exhibits

F factories,* fairgrounds, farmers' markets, festivals, fingernail salons, fire departments, fitness centers,* flea markets, float trips, floats in parades

G golf courses, golf stores, golf practice ranges, golf tours, golfers, girls' clubs, promotions and organizations, grocery stores, gun clubs and ranges

H HIV treatment centers, hair care salons,* health care facilities, health clubs,* health food stores,* herbalists' offices, herb stores, hiking equipment stores, hockey teams, holistic health centers,* homes, house calls, horse race tracks, horse training facilities, hospitals, hospices, hotels, hypnotherapists' offices

I ice skating facilities, income tax services,* infertility treatment centers, interdisciplinary health clinics,* investment offices,* iridologists' offices

J judo centers

K karate centers, kayak clubs, kiosks, kung-fu studios

L laboratories,* lacrosse clubs, landscape architects,* laundromats, libraries, long-term health care facilities

M malls, manicure and pedicure salons, manufacturing facilities,* massage offices,* medical clinics, medical doctors, meeting and banquet facilities,* mental health facilities, modeling agencies, money management consultants,* motels, museums, musicians

N nail care salons, natural food stores,* naturopaths' offices, neighborhood centers, nursery schools, nurses, nursing homes, nutritionists' offices

O office buildings, occupational therapy clinics, organizations, outlet malls

P painters, party planning services, pediatricians offices, physical fitness facilities,* physical therapy clinics, physicians' offices, plasma centers, police departments, political organizations and candidates*

Q quality consultants

R race tracks, racquetball clubs, radio stations, real estate offices, reception halls, rehabilitation services, residential care homes, retreat facilities, riding academies, riverboats, rodeos, rugby teams

S sales contests and incentives, schools, seminars, senior citizens' centers, shopping centers, sleep disorder clinics, snow skiing and snow boarding facilities, ski clubs (snow and water), soccer clubs and teams, special events, sports clubs, sports facilities, substance abuse programs, support groups, surgeons' offices, symphonies

T television stations, tae kwon do studios, tai chi studios, tanning salons, telemarketing offices, telephone companies, tennis clubs, tool and die makers, tourist attractions, tours, trade shows, trade expositions, trade fairs, travel agencies, truck lines, trust companies

U universities, used car dealerships, utility company offices

V vacation attractions, veterans' organizations, veterans' hospitals, veterinarians' offices, volleyball courts

W web site developers, wedding consultants, wedding parties, wellness centers, holistic practitioners' offices, women's organizations

X x-ray clinics

Y yacht clubs, yacht charters, youth organizations

Z zoos

2. Lower cost—the average being a dollar per minute.
3. May be provided either on-site at the client's location, or at a convenient, fixed location such as at a mall, special event, spa, storefront, etc.
4. Clients are not required to disrobe and no massage lubricants are used.
5. Requires less physical space than a massage table.
6. Is lighter and smaller than a table and thus easier to transport.
7. Does not require a private room, usually being performed out in the open, allowing increased visibility.

The seated position provides the therapist access to all regions of the body. However, it is best suited for addressing the back, posterior neck, shoulders, arms, wrists, and hands. The lower extremities, abdomen, chest, and anterior neck are more appropriately treated with table massage.

The therapeutic paradigm can easily be adapted to the seated position and allows the therapist to address common soft tissue complaints such as low back pain, whiplash, headaches, frozen shoulder, rotator cuff injuries, golfer's elbow, tennis elbow, and carpal tunnel syndrome, to name a few. Most people need both general (systemic) relaxation and help with painful, minor musclo-tendinous complaints. Therapists who go beyond the relaxation paradigm of seated massage and learn therapeutic massage and stretching techniques will be able to help more people.

Chair massage can be offered in a variety of settings and can be a full-time practice or used to promote your table massage practice. Virtually everyone can benefit from chair massage. Your biggest challenge will be educating potential clients about the benefits of chair massage. Creativity and the ability to recognize opportunities in your community will help you build a successful chair massage practice.

REFERENCES

1. Field T, Ironson J, Scafidi F, et al. Massage therapy reduces anxiety and enhances EEG pattern of alertness and math computations. *Int J Neurosci* 1996;86:197–205.

CHAPTER 2

Equipment Considerations

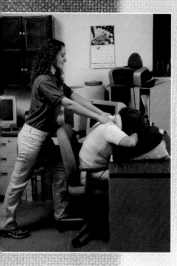

"Massage is an enormously important experience for every human being to undergo. . . ."

ASHLEY MONTAGU (1905–1999)

Objectives

■ List the three types of seated massage support systems appropriate for professional applications.

■ Describe the system that best fulfills the needs of your typical practice setting and clients.

■ List the important parts of a massage chair.

One of the attractive things about seated massage is the relatively low investment in equipment. Even when purchasing professional equipment, the initial investment is considerably less for seated massage than for table massage. A seated massage can be done on anyone who is sitting in a chair, on the floor, or on any other stable surface. All that is needed is a pair of hands. No investment in equipment is required at all when seated massage is done on a casual level. However, if you are going to give seated massages more than just occasionally in a casual setting, it is highly recommended that you have a support system to position the massage recipient. Support systems increase the therapeutic impact of your work and make giving the massage less stressful on your own body. This chapter will look at the types of equipment available and give you guidance as to how to select the best equipment for you to use in your application. There are several general types of seated massage support systems. These are cushion systems, desktop systems, and massage chairs.

CUSHION SYSTEMS

Cushion systems can be as simple as a few pillows placed on the back of a chair, a counter, or a table. They can be as sophisticated as the *bodyCushion*™ system. Pillows are fine for amateurs at home or in a situation where nothing else is available. Pillows are inexpensive and usually are readily available. If a spontaneous opportunity to give a seated massage arises in a care facility, while visiting someone's home, or almost anywhere, pillows can be used to support the recipient in whatever manner makes them comfortable. The disadvantages of depending

on pillows are that there may not be enough of them, they may be of awkward sizes, and doing the laundry for all the pillow cases. Figures 2-1 and 2-2 show examples of pillows being used as the support system.

If you want to utilize a cushion system for your professional practice, you should invest in a well designed, professional package like the *bodyCushion*™ system. The *bodyCushion*™ is a specially designed orthopedic positioner made from sculpted foam covered with vinyl. It has a detachable face cradle, two large cushions that support the body with

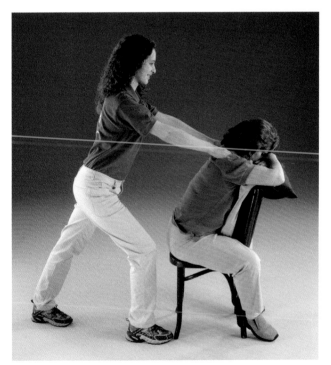

Figure 2-1　Pillows being used on the back of a chair.
Pillows work well in homes and in settings where nothing else is available.

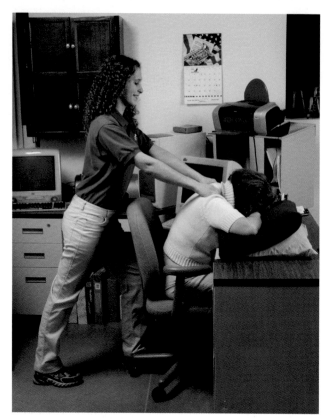

Figure 2–2 Pillows being used for head and arm support on a desk.

cut-outs for the abdomen and breasts, along with a knee/ankle bolster. When used on a massage table, the cushions are laid out flat with one cushion supporting the upper body and the other the lower body. The face cradle supports the face when the client is prone and the bolster supports the ankles when the client is prone and the knees when supine. When used as a seated massage support system, the two large cushions are folded together and placed against the back of a chair with the upper body cushion to-

ward the client, providing cut-outs for the abdomen and breasts. The face cradle is placed at the top of the two cushions for the client to lean forward and rest their face in. (The ankle/knee bolster is not used in seated applications of the *bodyCushion*™.) Figures 2-3 and 2-4 show applications of the *bodyCushion*™ system.

If you only perform seated massage occasionally, in casual settings, or only for special events once in a while, a cushion system may meet your needs. They are quick, simple, lightweight, and provide adequate support for the client. The primary disadvantage to this system is that some clients will have trouble balancing on the front of the chair and there is no support for the arms so you cannot perform any specific massage on the upper extremities. The *bodyCushion*™ can be used in your table massage practice as well, if you have one, so it can be a valuable, multi-use investment.

DESKTOP SYSTEMS

Desktop systems, sometimes called tabletop systems, consist of a face cradle with some type of bracket, clamp, or foot to attach it to or allow it to rest on a desk, table, counter, or shelf. Some even provide an upper chest support. Most desktop systems are made by the same manufacturers that produce massage chairs, and almost always include the same face cradle design the manufacturers use for their massage chair coupled to some system for attaching it to or resting it on the edge of a flat surface.

While desktop systems work fairly well for massaging the neck and shoulders, access to the client's lower back is severely restricted because the client is usually sitting in a regular chair; therefore, the back

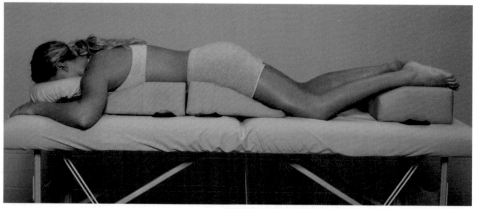

Figure 2–3 The *bodyCushion*™ as used on a massage table. (Photo courtesy of Body Support Systems, Inc., Ashland, OR. www.bodysupport.com)

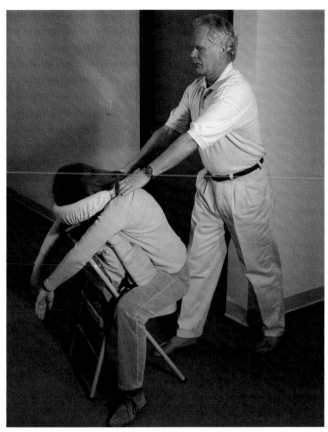

Figure 2–4 **The *bodyCushion*™ being used on an ordinary folding chair.** Note the position of the face cradle for seated massage. (Photo courtesy of Body Support Systems, Inc., Ashland, OR. www.bodysupport.com)

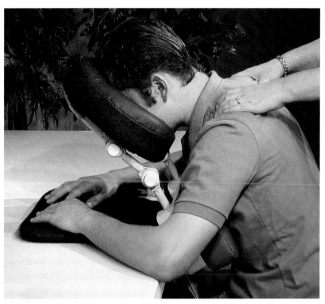

Figure 2–5 **A desktop system provides good support for neck and shoulders massage.** They are inexpensive, small, lightweight, quick, and easy to use. (Photo courtesy of Golden Ratio Woodworks, Inc., Emigrant, MT. www.golden ratio.com)

of the chair is in between you and the client's back. To reach the client's low back you must compromise your body mechanics. It is also difficult to accomplish any significant treatment of the arms, wrists, or hands as no support is provided for them and the desk, table top, or shelf usually prevents you from standing in front of the client.

Desktop systems are relatively inexpensive compared to massage chairs because they are fairly simple devices and do not have to support the entire weight of the client. They are very lightweight and are easy to transport and store. Desktop systems are even less expensive than a *bodyCushion*™ system and, while they do not provide as much comfortable support for the chest, they permit more adjustment of the face cradle and the client has more room to sit on the seat of the chair.

Desktop systems are a good, economical investment if you do seated massage only occasionally, or as a special tool for working with special needs populations like the wheelchair-bound. Unfortunately, they have significant limitations and are probably

not your best choice if you plan on chair massage being a major part of your professional massage practice. A desktop system is shown in use in Figures 2-5 and 2-6.

CLINICAL TIP

Clients in Wheelchairs

One very good application for tabletop systems is for those clients confined to wheelchairs. See Figure 2-6.

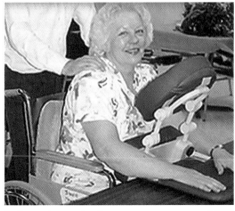

Figure 2–6 **Using a desktop system to provide support for a wheelchair-bound client.** (Photo courtesy of Golden Ratio Woodworks, Inc., Emigrant, MT. www.goldenratio.com)

If you decide to select a desktop system, look for the same features you would look for in the face cradle of a good massage chair. Then consider the way the unit sits on, or attaches to, the supporting desk, table, etc. Is it quick and easy, yet stable? Finally, be sure the chest pad system, if it has one, actually does provide some support for the client and has some adjustability for client comfort. If a travel bag is available, it is a worthwhile investment as it will protect the unit while you carry it around and will keep it clean during periods of storage.

MASSAGE CHAIRS

Massage chairs are the best support systems for massage professionals who intend to do seated massage as a regular part of their practice. Figure 2-7 shows a high-quality massage chair with its parts labeled. There are many designs on the market and prices vary according to the features and quality of the chair. Inexpensive chairs are generally of lower quality, have fewer features, are not as strong, do not provide reliability, and wear out sooner. They also have lower resale value should you decide to sell your chair some day. The good professional chairs are all in the same price range. A high-quality chair will last many years, possibly your entire career. More importantly, your clients deserve the best and the safest equipment available, so if you are going to buy a chair for professional use, buy a high-quality chair. After recovering from "sticker shock," no one ever regrets buying the best.

Features of a High-Quality Massage Chair

A good massage chair provides a comfortable, isolating environment that helps clients relax in the midst of chaos at the office, in an airport, at a mall, in a health club, at an outdoor concert, or wherever you are working. It should be entirely stable as it is difficult for clients to relax when they are sitting on something that is shifting, squeaking, creaking, or feels as if it will fall apart or fall over.

A quality massage chair should be lightweight, as it must be carried around and lifted in and out of vehicles for transport. It should also be quick and easy to set up and adjust. Less time spent adjusting the chair means more time spent serving clients!

The ultimate purpose of a massage chair is to position the client in a position of ease where their

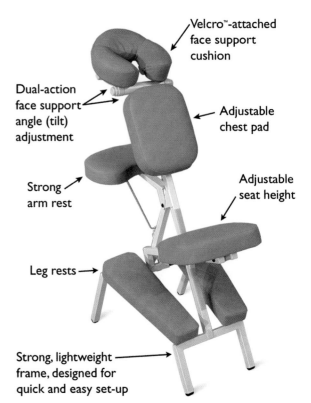

Figure 2–7   Photo of a high-quality massage chair with each major part of the chair labeled. (Photo courtesy of Golden Ratio Woodworks, Inc., Emigrant, MT. www.golden ratio.com)

muscles naturally relax as much as possible. Even while leaning against a chest pad, face cradle, and arm rest, if the person is positioned too far forward or "over-flexed," the erector spinae muscles of the spine and the extensor muscles of the neck will be reactively tensioned by the nervous system to keep the client from "falling farther forward." If the arms are positioned too inferior, too far forward, or even too far medial, so that the client is reaching or hanging anterior in an internally rotated position, the rhomboid, mid-trapezius, latissimus dorsi, infraspinatus, and other external rotator and retractor muscles will be in reactive tension. You will not be able to overcome this muscle tension through massage. Therefore, a massage chair that does not position the client properly can be a hindrance to your work. You will not be able to tell if a muscle is tight from a spasm or if it is tight from the position it is in. Seriously evaluate purchasing chairs that put the client in "the swimming position," which is when the spine is excessively anteriorly flexed and the shoulders internally rotated, arms hanging down, as if the client is swimming through water. Look for the best combination of strength, stability, weight, ease of set-up and adjustment, client comfort, and best positioning of the client for access to their tissues while maintaining proper therapist body mechanics.

Chair Accessories

Very few options or accessories are necessary for massage chairs. The most important one is a **travel bag**. A travel bag protects the chair during transport and during periods of storage. Generally, a chair is easier to transport in a travel bag, as the bags have handles and shoulder straps. There is usually room in the bag to put your face cradle covers, sanitation supplies, schedule book, receipt book, etc.

A **sternum pad** is a small pillow, usually half-round or triangular in shape, that attaches to the chest pad. It is used to provide better comfort and support for pregnant or large-breasted women and for people with large abdomens. A sternum pad is shown in Figure 2-8.

Choice of Vinyl

The vinyls used today by the major manufactures of massage chairs are comfortable and durable. However, some manufacturers offer premium vinyls that are softer and more leather-like in feel. If you have an upscale practice, want to have a comfort edge on most other therapists, or need a bigger tax deduction, you may want to consider this extra cost option. However, it is in no way necessary.

It is best to select a chair produced by a major, recognized manufacturer that has been in business for some time. This generally indicates they will be in business in the future when you need a part or a repair some day. Box 2-1 summarizes the features of a high-quality massage chair.

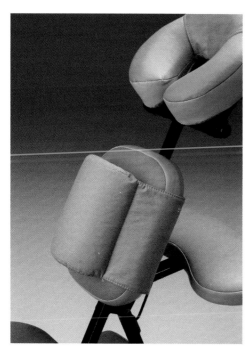

Figure 2–8 A massage chair with the sternum pad accessory. (Photo courtesy of Golden Ratio Woodworks, Inc., Emigrant, MT. www.goldenratio.com)

CASE STUDY

Selecting the Best Seated System for Your Practice

You have been in practice for six months, and your business is growing slowly but steadily. You are asked by some massage therapists in your community to join them in providing seated massages for the firefighters in your town one morning during Massage Therapy Awareness Week. The local paper and TV station have committed to covering the event. You do not have a seated support system of any kind. You have been thinking about getting one, but this is the first time you have had an opportunity to use one. You decide you do not want to develop a significant chair massage practice but would like to be able to join in on events like this one a few times a year for the networking and exposure.

1. Should you buy a massage chair or some other type of seated system, such as a desktop or cushion system, or use pillows for this event?
2. What system could best be utilized in your office between occasional promotional events? (Hint: Consider each option carefully, as a massage chair can be utilized in an office practice for shorter sessions or for clients who have difficulty getting on and off a massage table.)
3. Can you afford to invest in any system at this time without compromising your business's cash flow?
4. Will an investment in seated equipment bring a profitable return in the form of increased clients if you only use it a few times a year?
5. Do you need a tax write-off this year?

Box 2–1

Features of a High Quality Massage Chair

Features to look for in a massage chair include the following:

1. Quick, easy set-up and adjustment

2. Light weight

3. Strength and stability

4. A face cradle that has an *enclosed* adjustment mechanism. Locking cam levers with open gear-like teeth can pinch fingers, catch hair, and wear out more quickly, allowing slippage. Also, the client or therapist can accidentally move the locking lever during the massage, causing the face cradle to fall down.

5. A face-cradle pillow with seams to relieve pressure on the client's eye sockets.

6. An armrest strong and stable enough to be able to support therapeutic work on the forearm, wrist, and hand at a height and width that places the client's arms and shoulders in a position of ease. The armrest must be high enough from the floor to provide proper therapist body mechanics. (Remember, there are many people with forearm, wrist, and hand repetitive-injuries in business and industry who can be helped with chair massage.)

7. Seat height that provides access to the low back muscles while maintaining proper therapist body mechanics.

8. Simple, quick adjustments that do not require a secondary compensating adjustment or require the client to get out of the chair.

SUMMARY

A massage chair is a significant investment for a massage therapist. However, it is a necessary investment if you intend to make seated massage a significant item on your menu of services or plan to use seated massage as an effective promotional strategy on a regular basis. If you only perform seated massage occasionally, a cushion or desktop system may be adequate.

Notes

CHAPTER 3

Sanitation, Personal Hygiene, and Safety

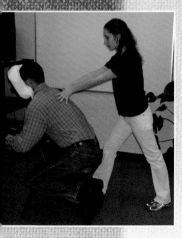

"An education isn't how much you have committed to memory, or even how much you know. It's being able to differentiate between what you do know and what you don't."

ANATOLE FRANCE (1844–1924)

Objectives

▪ List three areas that require protection from microorganisms when performing seated massage.

▪ List the areas of the chair that must be cleaned between clients.

▪ Identify effective products to sanitize the chair and clean the therapist's hands.

▪ Describe how to keep the therapist's skin safe from pathogens and the chemicals in cleaning products.

▪ Describe alternative methods to clean the hands when time or facilities do not allow normal hand-washing before and after each client.

▪ List four types of face cradle covers and the advantages and disadvantages of each.

▪ Describe several measures professional massage therapists take to ensure personal hygiene.

▪ Identify eight safety considerations for seated massage.

Key Terms

Antisepsis: prevention of infection; disinfection.

Microbe: any very minute organism, including both microscopic and ultramicroscopic organisms (spirochetes, bacteria, rickettsiae, and viruses).

Microorganism: a microscopic organism (plant or animal).

OSHA: Occupational Safety and Health Administration of the U.S. Department of Labor; responsible for establishing and enforcing safety and health standards in the workplace.

Pathogen: any virus, microorganism, or other substance causing disease.

Sanitation: use of measures designed to promote health and prevent disease; development and establishment of conditions in the environment favorable to health.

Sanitize: to clean something thoroughly by disinfecting or sterilizing it.

Sterilize: to destroy all microorganisms in or about an object.

Practitioners of seated massage have traditionally ignored the need for **sanitation**. The fact that clients are fully clothed has given massage therapists a false sense of security. Although it is true that most **microbes** cannot thrive on clothes, face cradles are in contact with skin, saliva, nasal mucus, and exhalations. Arm rests are in contact with forearms and hands, which are the primary carriers of *E. coli* and *Salmonella* bacteria and viruses that cause communicable diseases such as colds and flu. In warmer climates, clients wearing shorts will have skin in contact with the leg rests of the chair. It is important for massage professionals to maintain high standards of hygiene in order to protect not only the client but themselves.

To prevent the spread of microbes, massage therapists are taught to wash their hands with hot water and soap before and after working on each client. Unfortunately, in some on-site situations where seated massage is offered, washrooms are not readily available. Furthermore, the brief duration of seated massage makes the before-and-after hand-washing routine impractical. It is not reasonable to spend 5 to 10 minutes going to the restroom twice to wash your hands between clients when only doing 10 to 15 minute treatments. Fortunately, several products are available to help massage professionals ensure sanitation when performing seated massage. These will be described in the first main section of this chapter.

In addition to sanitation, massage therapists must maintain scrupulous personal hygiene and exhibit professionalism. We'll talk about what that means in practical terms later in this chapter. Finally, massage

therapists have an obligation to ensure the safety of their clients. Not only your equipment but your entire work environment must be safe if you are to achieve a therapeutic outcome. Because client safety is so important, we present a thorough discussion of the topic at the close of this chapter.

SANITIZATION

To **sanitize** is to reduce the level of **microorganisms** on inanimate objects so that they are safe for public use. The goal of cleanliness in massage is to decrease the level of microorganisms on your equipment (sanitization) and your hands and forearms (**antisepsis**) to prevent the spread of disease. Table 3-1 illustrates the terms and levels involved in disease control. Three main areas of concern in sanitation when performing seated massage are:

1. The surfaces of the chair
2. The therapist, primarily the hands and forearms
3. The client, primarily the face.

Sanitizing the Surfaces of the Chair or Support System

Any vinyl, metal, plastic, and wood areas of the massage chair that come into contact with skin or breath should be sanitized after each client. This applies to desktop and cushion support systems as well. Various solutions of essential oils, common household cleaning products, and many other products claim to accomplish this, but not all of these cleaners are backed by laboratory research. It is important to use

Table 3-1 Terminology of Infectious Disease

Term	Definition	Example
Antisepsis	Use of a non-toxic chemical to reduce the number of microorganisms on the skin.	A nurse applies rubbing alcohol to an injection site.
Disinfection	A process that destroys most or all disease-causing microorganisms on an object or surface.	Your silverware is disinfected in your dishwasher.
Sanitization	Reduction in the number of microorganisms to a level that meets public health standards.	A restaurant's silverware is sanitized in its dishwasher.
Sterilization	A process that destroys all microorganisms and viruses on an object or surface.	Medical equipment is sterilized using pressurized steam in an autoclave.

products that are clinically proven to provide significant protection against as many pathogens as possible, especially when working in a healthcare facility.

Sanitizing products must be practical to use in the seated massage setting. For example, it is not practical to carry around a 10% solution of chlorine bleach when doing on-site massage.

Professional germicidal wipes are the best sanitizing product currently available. These are not the products found in supermarkets and variety stores. General purpose household-grade products are not effective against many infectious diseases common today. Use professional grade products found at medical supply stores. Look in the Yellow Pages under "medical supply" for a store near you.

As a general rule, if a product is effective against tuberculosis (TB), it is likely to be effective against many other organisms. Tuberculosis is a good "test germ" because it can survive much longer on inanimate objects than most bacteria and viruses. Look for the "tuberculocidal" claim on the label of any product you consider using. However, some products that have been tested to be effective against tuberculosis have not been tested against Hepatitis B virus. Likewise, some products that have been tested and approved against Hepatitis B have not been tested against TB. It is very expensive and takes a long time to put a product through the tests necessary to claim effectiveness against a specific pathogen. Read labels carefully and choose the product that best suits your needs considering the population you are working with.

Professional Disposables International (PDI) makes an excellent line of professional germicidal wipes. The *Sani-Cloth®* brand of germicidal wipes shown in Figure 3-1 are available in low-alcohol and alcohol-free formulas that are more compatible with vinyl than products high in alcohol. The alcohol-free formula, *Sani-Cloth HB®*, is effective against the Hepatitis B virus. All PDI germicidal wipes have been tested against specific organisms that are listed on the label. All PDI germicidal wipes are approved by the U.S. Environmental Protection Agency (EPA) and meet **OSHA** requirements.

A problem with most of these sanitization products is that the solutions that kill the various mi-

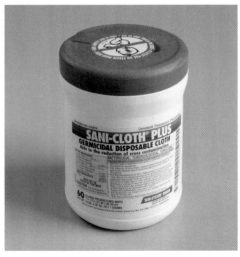

Figure 3-1 Sani-Cloth® wipes manufactured by the PDI Company.

croorganisms are drying to the skin and are somewhat toxic. Since they are absorbed through the skin, direct exposure to them needs to be limited. As professional health workers, massage therapists should be using gloves during product application to avoid direct contact of germicidal wipes to the skin. OSHA guidelines recommend that all healthcare workers wear gloves when performing environmental cleaning as a universal precaution (1).

With gloved hands, use these germicidal wipes to clean the face cradle, chest pad, arm rest, and leg rests after each client. Also clean any other parts of the chair that the client may have been breathing on. Sanitize a desktop unit or a *bodyCushion*™ system, much like you would a massage chair. If using pillows for support, change pillow cases. Also, clean any thumb-saving tools you may have used. There are other sanitizing products available that do not require gloves for use. One of these is a natural product made from grapefruit seed extract. While this product has been shown to be effective against most common bacteria and viruses in laboratory tests, as of this writing it is still in the approval process and, until that process is completed, no specific claims may be made for the product's germicidal effectiveness (2). Look for anti-microbial or germicidal information on the label of any product you are considering.

Your clients will notice and appreciate this attention to their safety. They will be more likely to return to you than to a therapist who does not openly practice proper hygiene. Figure 3-2 shows a massage chair being sanitized.

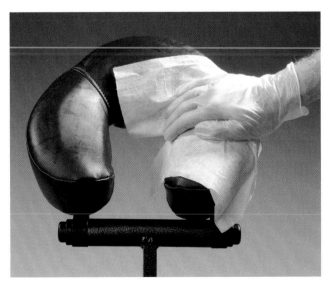

Figure 3–2 **Cleaning a massage chair with Sani-Cloth® wipes.**

When doing seated massage in a non-clinical environment, you should still be aware of contraindications and the Universal Precautions, and follow them appropriately. If the overall level of health in the general U.S. population continues to decline as it has since World War II, you will be facing more and more people in routine, on-site situations who require special precautions. It is important that you take all necessary precautions for your own safety, the safety of the client, and for the next person(s) you will have in your chair.

Be sure to learn and follow the facilities guidelines for Universal Precautions as issued and updated by the Centers for Disease Control (CDC). These are available at the CDC website, www.cdc.gov.

CLINICAL TIP

When should a seated massage therapist wear gloves?

It is unusual for a seated therapist to wear gloves while working on their clients. The following guidelines can help you determine when you should wear gloves.

1. While handling any form of body fluid (blood, mucus, urine, vomit, etc.). This is unlikely in seated massage, but people do have "accidents," especially in healthcare environments.
2. When working with someone who has open skin lesions, forms of dermatitis, psoriasis, eczema, etc.
3. Any time there is a break in your or the client's skin or an infectious skin disease on the forearm(s) or hand(s). If the condition is only at the distal part of one of your digits, a finger cot may be used instead of a full glove. Examples of this situation would be a paper cut, an open cuticle, or a puncture wound.
4. If the client requests you to wear gloves.
5. If you do not feel comfortable without them.
6. If the client has a communicable disease.
7. When using medical-grade anti-microbial wipes to clean your equipment if you are not using a skin-protecting product.

If several of these conditions are present, it warrants double-gloving or rescheduling the appointment to some time after the conditions change.

It is a good idea to always have a few pairs of gloves with you. You never know when a client will get sick and possibly vomit or when you may cut yourself on the way to the worksite. Always be prepared.

Protecting Your Hands and Forearms

It is highly recommended that you use an anti-microbial skin barrier product. Often called *skin protectants*, these products were developed for medical personnel who had to wear surgical gloves for extended periods of time. They prevented contact dermatitis and sensitivities to the powders in the gloves. Later, a safe anti-microbial agent, triclosan, was incorporated to provide protection from **pathogens** as well.

The first product of this type on the market was sold under the name *Pro Tec®*. Another early product was called *Derma-Shield®*. *Bio-Safe®* is a newer product in lotion form and other skin protectants are available as foams, gels, and wipes. All of these products use liquefied polymers which bond to the epidermis of the skin and dry to form a protective glove or barrier that blocks absorption through the skin, while allowing the skin to continue to breathe. Once dry, there is no feeling or sensation that you have the product on. It breaks down naturally in about four hours from the accumulated effect of normal epithelial slough. Since protectants are anti-microbial, they kill most pathogens on contact. They also protect your skin from alcohol and other chemicals, and even poison oak and ivy. Thus, they protect you and your clients from one another, preventing cross contamination. The Clinical Tip below explains how to choose a skin protectant. Figure 3-3 shows several skin protectant products.

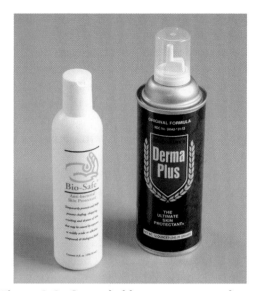

Figure 3–3 Several skin protectant products.

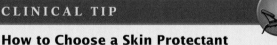

How to Choose a Skin Protectant

Should you wonder if a particular skin protectant product will perform properly, here are the standards a skin protectant should meet:

1. Should be registered with the U.S. Food and Drug Administration (FDA).
2. Should be produced in an FDA-registered and licensed facility in accord with FDA Good Manufacturing Practices (GMPs).
3. A manufacturer of skin protectants needs to be able to provide documentation of clinical, lab, and work site testing to verify claims and, upon customer request, to make these test data available to the customer.
4. At a minimum, the lab tests need to include:
   A. USP Challenge Test
   B. Minimum Inhibitory Concentration effectiveness against "X" number of pathogens. In other words, what pathogens does the product provide effective protection from?
   C. Oral Toxicity
   D. Draize Test
   E. Double-Blind Studies
   F. Dermal Absorption Test Data
   G. Certificates of Analysis
5. Each batch needs to be tested to ensure conformity to specifications. Testing needs to be done in an independent, FDA-registered, state-licensed laboratory, and such test data needs to be available to customers who request it.

Manufacturers, dealers, or sales people of skin protectant products should be able to provide you with this information. If they cannot or will not, you might want to keep shopping (3).

To use a skin protectant, thoroughly wash your hands and forearms with hot water and soap, and dry them. Then apply the skin barrier product according to the label directions and let it dry for four to five minutes. Once dry, it forms an "invisible shield" that helps prevent absorption through the skin for about four hours. During this time, you can wash your hands and use many cleaning and petrochemical products without damaging or drying your skin. The polymer shield can be broken by abrasion, however, so do not use soaps that contain abrasives like pumice in them. After four hours, thoroughly wash your hands and forearms and re-apply the product.

Note that skin protectants will NOT seal open wounds, cuts, abrasions, etc. As long as there is no weeping or bleeding, they tend to provide the same protective coating as they do on intact skin. Unfortunately, this can fail for a variety of reasons; therefore, it is best to supplement protectants with gloves or finger cots in areas of compromised skin. They are not a replacement for gloves when those are necessary or indicated by Universal Precautions. Universal Precautions are explained in the Clinical Tip below.

CLINICAL TIP

Universal Precautions

Universal Precautions were issued by the CDC in 1987 and are updated as necessary. They are guidelines and recommended procedures to prevent the spread of bacterial and viral infections. Their application in seated massage is generally limited to where you may come in contact with skin conditions, body fluids, body waste, or vomit. It is always best to be prepared for anything, wherever you may be working. A few pairs of gloves and some approved germicidal wipes do not take up much space and are very lightweight. Remember that Universal Precautions work both ways: They protect you from the client and the client from you. People with suppressed immune systems can be very susceptible to infection from a therapist with a cold, a skin infection, etc. Always keep in mind the population you are working with and take the appropriate precautions to protect the health and safety of everyone involved.

Update your information on sanitary procedures every six months. The CDC has a voice information system at (404) 332-4555. The website is www.cdc.gov.

Skin protectant products are also useful when cleaning your office or home to protect you from cleaning chemicals. They can protect you from yard and garden chemicals as well as petrochemicals like gasoline, oil, paint, paint thinners, etc. Use them regularly. (Read the instructions on the product label, since each one is a bit different.)

A note on waterless hand sanitizers: some therapists like to use the waterless hand cleaners now available. While these are anti-microbial, they also contain harsh chemicals that can be absorbed through the skin. Therefore, you should apply a skin protectant before beginning work, then use the waterless cleaners between clients if you choose to.

Protecting the Client's Face

After sanitizing the face cradle, it is best to cover it. The sanitizing products used to clean the face cradle can irritate sensitive skin, and skin on vinyl is not very comfortable. Covers provide a softer, safer surface to rest against. Covers also prevent makeup from staining the vinyl. (Makeup can be very difficult to remove and is not very appealing to the next client.) Place a clean cover on your face cradle for each client. Several materials have been used successfully.

Paper Towels

The cheapest and most abundant face cradle covers are paper towels. Tear two sheets off the roll, then tear the two sheets halfway apart. Place them over the face cradle with the seam running vertically and the tear at the bottom, as shown in Figure 3-4.

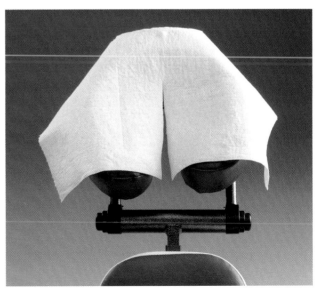

Figure 3–4 Using two paper towels as a face cradle cover.

Bouffant Caps

The plastic bouffant caps used in healthcare settings fit nicely over the face cradle, look more professional than paper towels, and they are relatively inexpensive. You can purchase them from medical supply or beauty supply stores. Unfortunately, they are not very soft and may feel a bit scratchy to some people. They also need to have a hole torn in them to facilitate the client's ability to breathe through them, but they seldom tear neatly so the professional look is quickly lost. See Figure 3-5 for an example of a bouffant cap on a face cradle.

Washable Cloth Covers

Washable cloth covers, as shown in Figure 3-6, are very comfortable and look professional. They are usually 100% cotton with an elasticized perimeter band to snugly fit the cover to the face cradle cushion. Using them requires you to purchase a lot of them (at least a full day's supply) and to be willing to do a load of laundry daily.

Getting makeup out of them is a challenge. The recommended procedure is to fill your washer with hot water, add your regular detergent and then add 1/4 cup of plain (not scented) Cascade® dishwashing detergent. This particular product has been found to be the most effective. Allow this to mix thoroughly, then put in the face cradle covers. This mixture also works well to remove fresh oil from sheets. A lipstick and makeup removal method is to wet the covers and then squeeze in GOOP® hand cleaner. Let it set for a while, then wash in hot water as described above. If you are willing to do the laundry, cloth covers are a

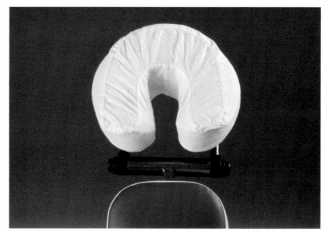

Figure 3–6 A washable cloth face cradle cover on a chair face cradle.

great way to go. They are commonly available from massage supply vendors and equipment manufacturers; they look professional, are easy to use, and are comfortable for clients.

Face Favors®

Face Favors® face cradle covers are specially cut, high-quality paper covers. A *Face Favor®* cover is shown in Figure 3-7. Although a bit more expensive than paper towels, these are superior to either paper towels or bouffant caps. Unlike ordinary paper towels, *Face Favors®* are made from first-quality paper and without air fluffing. Paper towels are made from second-quality papers and are air fluffed so the product looks thicker than it is. *Face Favors®* are 0.014

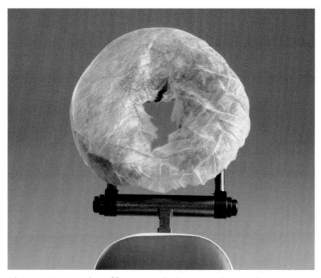

Figure 3–5 A bouffant cap being used as a face cradle cover. Note the tear in the center.

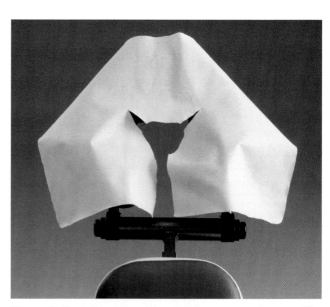

Figure 3–7 A *Face Favor®* cover in use on a face cradle. (*Face Favor®* courtesy of Bio-Tone Professional Products.)

inch thick, compared to a two-ply towel, which is generally 0.08 inch thick. These pre-cut, smooth, absorbent covers fit all face cradles, look professional, are efficient for you to use, and are very comfortable for your clients.

The *Face Favor®* and the washable cloth covers are the most professional, highest-quality face cradle cover products available. Use the one you prefer and believe is the best for your clients. Hopefully, you always want your clients to have the very best and to associate you with providing the very best.

PERSONAL HYGIENE AND PROFESSIONAL DEMEANOR

Above and beyond the rather mechanical procedures discussed so far, there is one more, **very** important area of consideration: YOU. Massage, whether seated or on a table, on-site or in an office, is a healthcare service. To win clients' trust, you need to look and act like a professional healthcare provider.

You are asking individuals to entrust their bodies to you, whether for general relaxation or help with specific problems. You should always be clean, neat, and professional in appearance. This means clean, neatly kept hair and short, clean fingernails. As discussed earlier, clean hands are an essential part of personal hygiene. You should never have body odor, bad breath, or noticeable perfumes, aftershaves, or other scents. Many people are allergic to perfumes and fragrances, and you never know who until it is too late.

Your clothes should be clean, functional, and appropriate for the setting you are working in. Your equipment should be clean, sanitized, in good repair, and well organized.

Professional demeanor is the way you present yourself to the public; your behavior, manner, and appearance reflect your character. It is always best to act in a friendly, professional manner. Show your concern for each client and his or her needs. Be on time and stay on schedule. It is very disrespectful of other people to be late or to make them late. Treat every client as you would want to be treated.

If you want to be accepted and treated as a professional, look like a pro, act like a pro, and talk like a pro. A major factor in your success will be your ability to gain people's trust and respect. First impressions are lasting and are difficult to overcome. No matter how much you know, you must gain a person's trust and respect before they will entrust their body to you, especially for another appointment. Presenting a professional appearance in as many ways as possible is the best way to create a favorable first impression, which is so necessary to gain that trust.

SAFETY

Fortunately, massage is not a hazardous occupation. However, in on-site seated massage there are several important safety issues to keep in mind.

Inspecting Your Chair

Inspect your chair regularly for cracks or damage. Travel is hard on equipment. Keep your chair in perfect working order. It is a great practice to sit in your chair after setting it up, before your first client, to be sure it is properly set up and stable. If a client is injured, not only are you liable, but your reputation as a trustworthy business person is severely damaged.

Moving Your Equipment Safely

Lift and carry your chair and other equipment using proper lifting postures so you do not injure yourself getting to and from the work site. If you have long distances to carry equipment, consider investing in a two-wheeled cart or a bag with wheels. If you use a cart, be sure to secure the chair to the cart with elastic "bungee cords" so it does not fall off while turning corners or traversing rough terrain.

Creating a Safe, Clean, and Comfortable Work Area

Set up your chair in a safe area. Be sure you have clear, unobstructed space on all sides of the chair to allow you to work in proper postures, as shown in Figure 3-8. The lunge position (archer stance) requires a few feet of room on all sides of the chair (more if you are a tall person). Be sure to place your carry bag out of the way of everyone. It should not be within your working space around the chair.

It is especially important that the clients have a clear, unobstructed path to your chair, to avoid injury due to tripping or falling. In everything you do, operate out of genuine concern for the safety and well-being of your clients. Furthermore, if a client is injured, you may be liable and possibly sued.

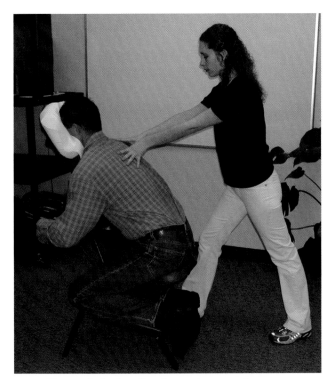

Figure 3–8 A safe, clear, clean work space.

Be sure there are no risk factors for accidents around your chair such as extension cords, slick floors, obstacles, or any equipment that could malfunction and cause a problem. If you cannot eliminate or avoid the dangerous object or situation, for example, a slick floor, be sure to advise clients as they enter the space and assist them as necessary to prevent an accident.

Try to avoid setting up in the direct path of a heating or cooling vent. Having cool or hot air blowing directly on the chair is usually uncomfortable for the client and for you. It is hard for the client to relax in the chair if they are being chilled or roasted. Likewise, do not set up near a window that is drafty or through which the sun is shining directly onto the chair. Direct sun through glass can become uncomfortably warm. However, if you have to set up in a cold room, take advantage of heat vents and sun through windows just like you would of air movement in very warm rooms.

It is important to have the area you are setting up in as clean as possible. If necessary, arrive early enough to get a broom or vacuum and clean the area before clients arrive. If you have to set up in a less than ideal situation (which is often the case in on-site massage), just do the best you can, be adaptable, be pleasant to work with, and do your best to ensure the safety of the client and yourself.

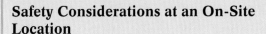

CASE STUDY

Safety Considerations at an On-Site Location

As an employee of a group practice, you go to a small manufacturing plant to provide three hours of chair massage for production workers who have back pain, headaches, and wrist injuries due to overuse. However, when you get to the factory you find the space they have for you to work in is in a dingy corner of the production room. There are power cords lying in standing water only a few feet away and the air quality is very poor. You do not feel safe working in this environment, yet the employees are obviously delighted to see you and your massage chair.

1. What should you do?
2. Whom should you discuss these safety issues with? (The factory representative who showed you to the space, your office or boss, the factory workers you are massaging?)
3. Should you just set up and do the three hours, hoping for the best, and let your boss deal with it before next time, or should you refuse to work in the space provided and walk out?

SUMMARY

Sanitization, hygiene, and safety are all very important aspects of professional seated massage. Universal Precautions are safety guidelines that help prevent the spread of disease. Massage therapists should observe these guidelines at all times.

You should use professional medical-grade cleaning products to sanitize your equipment and your hands. Anti-microbial skin protectants can be used to protect your hands and forearms from gloves, cleaning products, pathogenic microbes, and cross contamination. Gloves should be worn when appropriate.

For client comfort and to protect the vinyl of your face cradle from makeup, place a cover over the face cradle. Change the cover between each client. Suitable face cradle covers include paper towels, bouffant caps, cloth covers, and *Face Favors*®, a high-quality, specially shaped, disposable paper cover.

Present yourself in a clean, neat, appropriately dressed, and professional manner because first impressions are important in establishing client trust and scheduling repeat appointments.

Create a clean, safe area to set up and work in, doing the best you can (considering the situation) to ensure the safety of the client and yourself. Remember to respect each client and always treat them as you would like to be treated.

REFERENCES

1. Newman B. Product Manager, Healthcare, Professional Disposables International, Orangeburg, NY 10962-1376. *Personal communication*, 2004.
2. Perry R. General Manager, Bio/Chem Research, Lakeport, CA 95453. *Personal communication*, 2004.
3. Steward H. President, Bio-Safe Enterprises, Inc., Milwaukee, OR 97222. *Personal communication*, 2004.

CHAPTER 4

Contraindications to Seated Massage

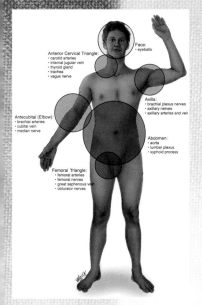

Anterior Cervical Triangle:
• carotid arteries
• internal jugular vein
• thyroid gland
• trachea
• vagus nerve

Face:
• eyeballs

Axilla:
• brachial plexus nerves
• axillary nerves
• axillary arteries and vein

Antecubital (Elbow):
• brachial arteries
• cubital vein
• median nerve

Abdomen:
• aorta
• lumbar plexus
• xyphoid process

Femoral Triangle:
• femoral arteries
• femoral nerves
• great saphenous vein
• obturator nerves

"Whenever a doctor cannot do good, he must be kept from doing harm
Make a habit of two things: to help; or at least to do not harm.
The life so short, the craft so long to learn."

HIPPOCRATES (460–377 BC)

Objectives

▪ Evaluate client conditions and complaints to determine if massage is appropriate or contraindicated.

▪ Determine if massage is totally contraindicated or partially contraindicated.

▪ Explain when clients should be referred to another health care provider.

Key Terms

Absolute contraindication: a condition or circumstance that would make any massage a risk to the client.

Contraindication (kon'trah-in'di-ka'shun): any special symptom or circumstance that renders the use of a remedy or the carrying out of a procedure inadvisable, usually due to risk.

Endangerment points: relatively small, specific areas where massage could potentially cause harm.

Mechanical pain: pain associated with movement or a particular position.

Non-mechanical pain: pain that is relatively constant and not significantly affected by movement or positions.

Partial contraindication: a condition or circumstance that allows massage but restricts it from a particular area or prohibits a particular technique. Also known as local contraindications.

Referral: the act or process of referring somebody to somebody else, especially sending a client to consult with a medical practitioner.

The overall purpose of massage is to help people. Hippocrates, one of the world's great massage therapists, stated that a physician should do no harm. It is the duty of every massage therapist to be sure to determine if massage is appropriate for each individual client and to ensure that massage will not have a detrimental effect. While most people will benefit from massage, contraindications do exist. When in doubt, err on the side of caution. If there is any question as to the appropriateness of massage for a client, consult with his physician or have him do so and obtain permission in writing to do massage. This is especially true for conditions like heart disease, cancer, and diabetes.

A **contraindication** for seated massage is any special symptom, condition, disease, or injury that could possibly be made worse or cause harm if massaged. Massaging these conditions could put the client at risk. The same contraindications that apply to massage also apply to seated massage and should be observed. Refer to your general massage textbook for more specific information and lists of contraindications, universal precautions, and endangerment points.

We should not allow contraindications to cause us to work in a state of fear, but in a state of cautious respect for the well-being of the people who come to us for help. Doing massage is like playing jazz music. Jazz musicians will agree that what you do not play is as important as what you do play. Contraindications help us determine what not to do for an individual. Then we can decide what is best to do for them. This chapter is here to help you make wise choices.

REFERRALS

Referral is a process in which one healthcare provider, such as a massage therapist, recommends that a client see another healthcare professional for diagnosis and treatment of a disease, condition, complaint, or injury. For example, a massage therapist may notice subtle changes in a client's mood and refer the client to a psychotherapist for evaluation. Or a client may bring a condition or injury to a massage therapist that is beyond the scope of the practice of massage, hoping that massage will resolve the problem without the client having to see a physician. It is the therapist's duty to determine if massage (in this case, seated massage) is appropriate for the client's complaint. If not, it becomes the therapist's duty to refer the client to another provider, usually a physician or chiropractor, but possibly a physical therapist, counselor, personal trainer, another massage therapist, or whomever you feel is appropriate. You should note in the client's file that you made a referral. If the referral is for a disease, significant injury, or a condition for which massage is contraindicated, ask the client to get a written statement from the physician that she was seen and that massage may or may not be done, along with any special instructions. Keep that statement in the client's file as you continue to work with her. Specific conditions that indicate a referral include the following:

- Severe pain
  - If constant and worse at night (tumors, infections, and significant inflammation are often worse at night).

- If the client has intense local pain that developed after a recent, significant trauma (this could be a bone fracture or a joint injury).
  - If the client cannot be positioned somewhat comfortably in the chair, it is best for them to be evaluated before you treat them (1).
  - If you determine it is appropriate to treat someone in severe pain, be cautious and conservative.
- Significant fatigue
- Inflammation
- Lumps and tissue changes
- Rashes and changes in the skin
- Edema
- Mood alterations (e.g., depression, anxiety, hysteria)
- Infection, local or general
- Bleeding or bruising
- Nausea, vomiting, or diarrhea
- Temperature (fever), high or low

When these symptoms present with no logical explanation, it is best to refer. Logical explanations vary. For example, clients who have been working long hours, traveling, or have been up late may present with fatigue and probably need a massage, not a referral. A trigger point may cause pain, and it is perfectly appropriate for a massage therapist to address the pain. Seated massage can help people with depression as long as they are under a physician's care. Use good sense. Be practical. These are guidelines, not absolutes. Your concern should be to promote the safety and well-being of each unique client.

CASE STUDY

Client with Varicose Veins

A male client, 50 years of age, comes to your office for stress reduction massage. On his client intake form he relates that he has severe varicose veins. When you ask him about this, he pulls up his trouser legs and you see that he has numerous, severe varicose veins, such that you cannot imagine how you could massage his legs.

1. Since he seeks stress reduction and has no pain complaints, would chair massage be a good option to suggest?
2. What areas, if any, are contraindicated by this condition?

As seated massage becomes more accepted, it will be increasingly used in clinical and medical settings to address musculo-tendinous complaints involved in a variety of severe medical conditions and diseases. In these settings the massage therapist needs to be very aware of massage contraindications and work closely with the medical staff, especially the managing physician of the case, so as to provide appropriate, safe care for the client and observe scope of practice boundaries.

ABSOLUTE CONTRAINDICATIONS

Conditions in which massage may be generally harmful and is not advised are known as **absolute contraindications** (sometimes called *general contraindications*). This means that no massage may be given to the individual. It is rare that a physician would recommend massage for a client with these conditions, but some exceptions occur. A physician's written clearance is advised for clients with absolute contraindications. Fortunately, there are very few situations in which massage is completely contraindicated. These few situations are listed in the accompanying Box 4-1.

There are many contraindications to be concerned with in massage. Written medical authorization not only protects clients from injury, but also protects you in the event of a lawsuit. If you work on someone who has a recognized contraindication and his condition worsens in the next few weeks, it is possible that the client, some family member, one of the client's doctors, or even the government could charge you with malpractice and seek damages. If taken to court, you would be vulnerable to such charges unless you could present evidence such as a written prescription or recommendation of the client's physician authorizing massage treatment. You would then be partially protected, at least. Do not work in fear, work smart.

PARTIAL CONTRAINDICATIONS AND ENDANGERMENT POINTS

Most contraindications are **partial** (or local) **contraindications.** These require caution and possibly some adaptation to ensure the safety and comfort of the client. Most of the time, a contraindication will just be for a localized area. Massage may

Box 4–1

Absolute Contraindications

- Active state (acute or flare-up) of contagious diseases
- Acute skin conditions and diseases (chickenpox, measles, widespread contact dermatitis, ringworm, scleroderma, widespread rashes)
- Autoimmune diseases or acute inflammatory processes during exacerbation or flare-up period
- Cancer without physician's approval
- Cardiac arrest
- Diabetes (if severe), without physician's approval
- Embolism (stroke)
- Fever
- General acute inflammatory and infectious processes
- Hepatitis (during acute phase)
- Lice
- Recent significant injury (wait 72 hours or until physician's approval is obtained)
- Recent surgery (wait until managing physician's approval is given or client is released from physician's care)
- Rheumatoid arthritis (during flare-up)
- Anyone who will not disclose basic medical history or answer questions
- Anyone under the influence of intoxicating substances
- Anyone on drugs that inhibit or distort their ability to give accurate feedback regarding discomfort or pain (2)

be administered in other places. Examples of relative contraindications are listed in Box 4-2.

In seated massage, many of these conditions will be covered by clothing. If the client does not report them during the intake interview, you will not know

Box 4–2

Examples of Partial Contraindications

For these conditions, avoid the affected area(s). If condition is widespread, it may be an absolute contraindication for massage (see Box 4-1), in which case the client should be referred to a physician for authorization to receive massage.

- Abnormal lumps
- Acne vulgaris
- Blister
- Bruise (if less than 72 hours old)
- Cysts
- Herpes simplex outbreak
- Local inflammation
- Open wounds
- Shingles outbreak
- Skin rashes limited to a small area
- Spina bifida
- Swollen lymph glands
- Unhealed burns and abrasions
- Warts

about them prior to beginning the massage. You may discover them as you massage, feeling the texture of the tissues or when the client suddenly flinches when you touch a particular area. Immediately ask the client about her reaction or what you feel. If she explains it is one of the above, avoid that area until it heals. Boxes 4-3 and 4-4 compare indications and contraindications for conditions affecting the shoulder and neck.

Endangerment points or sites are areas in the body where delicate anatomical structures that are easily injured are superficial and relatively unprotected (Fig. 4-1). These areas merit caution during a massage. Typical endangerment points are nerves, blood vessels, organs, small or prominent bony projections, and any abnormal findings such as lumps, masses, moles, or cysts. Caution should be exercised at these sites. Work slowly, lightly, and carefully when in or around these sites. Endangerment points from the hips up include the following:

Posterior:
  Kidney area (lower back) with heavy tapotement
  Floating ribs with heavy pressure or tapotement
  Spinous processes
  Radial and ulnar nerves in the elbow
  Posterior cervical triangle
  Brachial plexus
  Styloid process
  External jugular vein
  Subclavian artery

Box 4-3

Indications/Contraindications Affecting the Shoulder

Indications	Contraindications
Pain in the shoulder	Inflammation*
Limited range of motion	Bursitis
Subacute injuries	Acute injuries
Poor posture	Bad bruising
Headaches	Broken bones
Carpal tunnel syndrome	Dislocated joint
Fatigue in the arms and hands (5)	

Anterior:
  Anterior cervical triangle
    Carotid arteries
    Internal jugular vein
  Axilla (armpit): brachial plexus nerves, arteries, and veins
  Abdomen (rarely addressed in seated massage)
    Aorta
    Lumbar plexus
    Xiphoid process (2)

Note: In the unlikely event you are working a lower extremity in the seated position, avoid the femoral triangle (medial, proximal thigh) and the popliteal area (posterior knee).

2. What factors related to the past surgery could complicate the massage? (Hint: Were lymph nodes removed?)
3. What other major upper body area is probably involved?
4. If you have training in posture analysis, should you invest time in posture analysis for this person?

A major reason massage is contraindicated in many conditions is the circulatory nature of Swedish massage, primarily from the effleurage stroke. Effleurage is seldom used in seated massage. Even then, it is not usually done to move fluids, but to soothe and sedate. It is difficult to accomplish effective effleurage through the clothes, and the areas typically treated in seated massage do not have large blood vessels close to the surface. This means that the normal seated massage in which the back, neck, shoulders, and forearms are the primary areas addressed is very safe. Therefore, after consulting with the client's physician, you will sometimes be authorized to perform seated massage when typical table Swedish massage would not be advisable.

At all times respect the client. Be grateful for the opportunity to serve them. Do so with the highest concern, care, and integrity.

CASE STUDY

Client with Mastectomy

You are working at a chair massage concession at the airport. A middle-aged woman comes up and asks for a massage. Her intake form relates that she had a mastectomy as a result of breast cancer two years ago, on her right side, but the cancer is now in remission. She has pain and tingling in her right arm and restriction of movement in her right shoulder. Carrying her briefcase has become painful, and she wonders if you can do anything to help her.

1. Is chair massage appropriate for this individual?

Box 4-4

Indications/Contraindications for Conditions Affecting the Neck

Indications	Contraindications
Stiff neck	Severe trauma
Pain/numbness in arm	Fever
Pain in neck/shoulders	Skin disorders
Whiplash	Recent injury/surgery
Tension in throat	Severe hypertension
Postural deviations (5)	

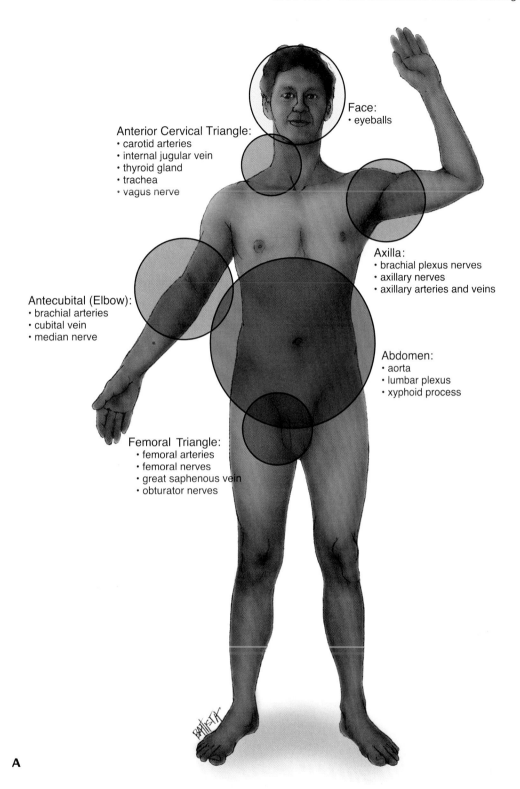

Face:
• eyeballs

Anterior Cervical Triangle:
• carotid arteries
• internal jugular vein
• thyroid gland
• trachea
• vagus nerve

Axilla:
• brachial plexus nerves
• axillary nerves
• axillary arteries and veins

Antecubital (Elbow):
• brachial arteries
• cubital vein
• median nerve

Abdomen:
• aorta
• lumbar plexus
• xyphoid process

Femoral Triangle:
• femoral arteries
• femoral nerves
• great saphenous vein
• obturator nerves

A

Figure 4–1   **Endangerment points. (A)** Anterior.

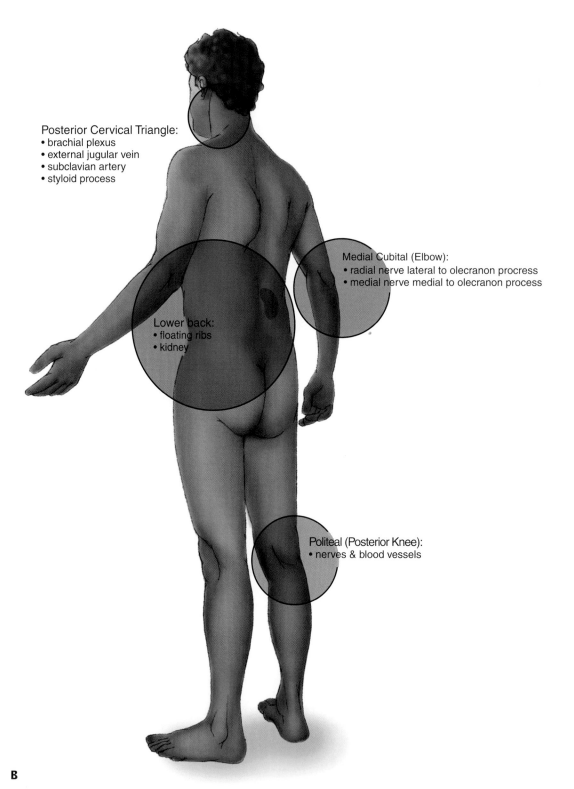

Posterior Cervical Triangle:
• brachial plexus
• external jugular vein
• subclavian artery
• styloid process

Medial Cubital (Elbow):
• radial nerve lateral to olecranon procress
• medial nerve medial to olecranon process

Lower back:
• floating ribs
• kidney

Politeal (Posterior Knee):
• nerves & blood vessels

B

Figure 4–1 *Continued* **(B)** Posterior.

CONTRAINDICATIONS FOR PEOPLE WITH SEVERE PAIN

People who are experiencing severe pain do not usually seek out a seated massage therapist. However, as the awareness of massage grows, more people will be bringing more conditions to seated therapists, so it is best to be prepared.

Mechanical versus Non-mechanical Pain

There are two kinds of pain, mechanical pain and non-mechanical pain. **Mechanical pain** is related to movement, activity, and posture. Moving or changing positions changes the pain experience. An example of mechanical pain would be a client who comes to you and says, "I have this pain right here and it hurts more when I move like this." Massage therapy is usually very effective in reducing mechanical pain.

Non-mechanical pain is usually constant, does not correlate with movement, and typically cannot be identified or isolated by palpation of muscles and tendons. An example of non-mechanical pain would be a client who comes to you and says, "I have this pain deep in my back that gets worse at night and nothing seems to make it better."

Massage will seldom change non-mechanical pain and even if it does, the pain returns to pre-massage levels soon after the massage. This is a good sign the cause of pain may be visceral or pathological. Visceral problems with the esophagus, kidneys, gall bladder, intestinal tract, other organs and glands, tumors, and cancer can cause non-mechanical pain in the low back, for instance. A client whose pain complaint seems to be non-mechanical should be referred to a medical provider for a diagnosis.

he just read an article on massage and wants to try it.

1. What could the blank spaces on the intake form mean?
2. What, if anything, should you say to the client about the incompleteness of the intake form?

If a person in significant pain comes to you for help, you must quickly determine if the person has a pathologic condition (non-mechanical pain) for which massage could be contraindicated, or if they have benign, non-pathogenic (mechanical) pain that would benefit from seated massage. The following history questions can help you make this determination:

1. Do you have constant pain that is worse at night and not relieved by any position? (Tumors and infections, as well as significant inflammation, are often worse at night.)
2. Do you have a constant writhing or cramping pain? (If so, rule out tumor and infection before working on them.)
3. Do you have intense local pain that developed after a recent, significant trauma? (If yes, rule out fracture.)
4. Do you have a fever?
5. Do you have a history of cancer or other serious medical problems?
6. Do you have any unintended weight loss? (Often associated with cancer and sometimes diabetes.)
7. Do you have bladder or bowel control problems? (May indicate pressure on spinal cord.)
8. Do you have significant, unexplained tingling, pain, or weakness in either of the upper or lower limbs? (May indicate pressure on spinal cord or significant nerve-root compression.) (1)

CASE STUDY

Incomplete Intake Form

A young man comes to you for a seated massage while you are working on-site at an accountant's office. He only partially fills out the intake form, leaving most questions blank. He tells you orally that he has never had a massage before, but that

CLINICAL TIP

Pain

The most common reason people go to a health care provider is to gain relief from pain. What is pain? Pain is a psychological experience resulting from physical stimuli. It is an emotion, expressed as a feeling. One of the best discussions of pain is found in an article entitled *Basic Concepts in*

Pain Physiology, written by the staff of the American Medical Massage Association and published on their website (3). It is based on systematized pain terminology developed by the International Association for the Study of Pain (4).

If your client has severe pain, answers yes to any of the above questions, and has not been seen by a doctor prior to seeing you, refer that person out for evaluation prior to working with that person.

SUMMARY

Contraindications are guidelines that help you determine what should not be done and what can be safely done to help the people who come to you. In general, massage therapists are most effective in addressing mechanical, soft tissue pain. If you suspect someone has non-mechanical pain, a serious disease, or any condition beyond the scope of practice of massage therapy, you should refer them to a physician for a diagnosis. Do no harm. When in doubt, refer it out.

CASE STUDY

Client in Pain on Medications

An obese middle-aged woman comes to you for a seated massage. She indicates that she has foot pain, knee pain, low back pain, neck pain, and headaches. She is on blood thinners and anti-inflammatory medications.

1. What can you safely do for this person using the format of chair massage?

REFERENCES

1. Hendrickson T. *Massage for Orthopedic Conditions*. Baltimore: Lippincott, Williams & Wilkins, 2003:67–68.
2. Salvo SG. *Massage Therapy: Principles and Practice*, 2nd ed. St. Louis: WB Saunders Company, 2003:96–101.
3. American Manual Medicine Association website, www.americanmedicalmassage.com. Accessed April 12, 2005.
4. International Association for the Study of Pain website, www.iasp-pain.org. Accessed April 12, 2005.
5. Scheuman DW. *The Balanced Body: A Guide to Deep Tissue and Neuromuscular Therapy*, 2nd ed. Baltimore: Lippincott, Williams & Wilkins, 2002:102,200.

Notes

CHAPTER 5

Communication, Assessment, Documentation, and Treatment Plans

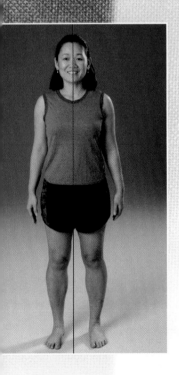

"Love is the communication, by demonstrative acts, through which you communicate to the other your profound involvement in their welfare."

ASHLEY MONTAGUE (1905–1999)

Objectives

- Efficiently and effectively establish communication with clients in the seated massage environment.

- Describe effective communication protocol for client intake.

- Work effectively with clients to properly adjust their chairs for maximum comfort and support.

- Identify four therapeutic communications.

- Describe to the client what to expect after the massage, including post-treatment soreness and homework.

- Perform a basic assessment of the client's complaint or condition.

- List effective strategies to keep client records.

- Develop and communicate a treatment plan.

Key Terms

Anterior: the front of the body or toward the front; for example, the ribs are anterior to the heart.

Assessment: an evaluation of the client's condition based on objective and sometimes subjective findings.

Concentric contraction: the shortening of a muscle during contraction; for example, a bicep curl.

Coronal plane: the vertical plane that divides the body into anterior and posterior sections, running through the ankle, knee, hip, shoulder joints, and ear.

Diagnosis: the determination of the nature of disease or injury causing the client's complaint.

Eccentric contraction: the lengthening of a muscle during contraction; for example, slowly lowering a weight.

Horizontal plane: a plane that runs through the body, parallel to the horizon (level) when in the anatomical position, that divides the body into upper and lower halves or sections. Also known as the transverse plane.

Ischemic: lacking blood in a part or tissue as a result of functional constriction of blood vessels. Ischemic tissue is tender upon palpation and fatigues easily.

Mid-sagittal plane: the vertical plane that divides the body into left and right halves. Also called the median plane.

Posterior: the back of the body or toward the back; for example, the scapula is posterior to the ribs.

Postural distortion: lack of alignment on the mid-sagittal, coronal, and horizontal planes of a person when standing erect and relaxed in the anatomical position; for example, head anterior, high or low shoulder, internally rotated shoulders or arms.

Referred pain: pain or sensation experienced in an area different from the source of the sensation; for example, pain felt in the forearm coming from injury to the shoulder joint.

Soft tissue: body connective tissues other than osseous (bone), cartilaginous, and visceral; in massage, usually considered to be skin, fascia, muscle, tendon, ligament, and sometimes periosteum.

Trigger point: a small, isolated area or spot of abnormal physiology in soft tissue that, when palpated or stressed, is locally tender and causes referred pain or sensation to an area remote (distant) from itself. Sometimes abbreviated TrP.

One of the most important skills of successful massage therapists is their ability to efficiently and effectively communicate with the client. In seated massage, especially when on-site, it is necessary to obtain pertinent information from the client and convey critical information to the client quickly. There is not time for a 20-minute client interview when doing a 15-minute treatment. It is important that you establish and maintain clear communication with the client before, during, and after the massage.

This chapter will help you with the entire communication process. The chapter is divided into four sections: communication, assessment, documentation, and treatment plans. The first section covers general communication with the client, whereas the other three pertain to specific types of communication that relate to the client's case. Communication includes client intake and adjusting the equipment to best support the client's body as well as communication with the client during the massage and after the massage. Assessment helps you determine the client's specific needs, usually when the client has a specific complaint he is seeking help with. Documentation helps you communicate with other providers, possibly the client's physician or insurance company. It also can help you communicate the client's condition to another therapist who may see the client in your absence. Most commonly, however, documentation serves as a record to remind you of your prior treatment techniques, findings, and results. Sample forms for documentation are included in the Appendix. Finally, treatment plans and their applications in chair massage are discussed. Become skilled at communicating with your clients and you will increase your repeat business and referrals.

COMMUNICATION BEFORE THE MASSAGE

Communication with a client during a seated massage can be difficult. We have virtually no eye contact with the client once we begin the massage. Furthermore, high noise levels in settings such as sporting events, concerts, or trade shows can hinder verbal communication. Therefore, communication must be established prior to beginning the massage so it can be continued throughout the treatment.

CASE STUDY

Client on Pain Medication

Let's return to the client from the final case study in Chapter 4: An obese, middle aged woman who is on blood thinners and anti-inflammatory and pain medications.

1. Considering her medications, what communications are extremely important to establish and maintain?

More regular and intense communication is required when doing therapeutic work. Relaxation treatments do not require the level of communication necessary to be effective with specific complaints. Below is a general protocol for communicating with your client.

Greet the Client

Introduce yourself by name and learn the client's name. Speak to her by name from this point on. People appreciate this personal touch and it helps you remember their names in the future. This is also the time to confirm the length of the massage and the price, if it is not posted. Determine if she has ever had a massage before, and particularly if she has ever had a seated massage. If she has never had a seated massage before, you must explain more about massage to her than if she gets massage regularly.

Determine the Client's Needs

Quickly establish the needs of the client. Ask why he has come to you for a massage today. His reason may range from curiosity to stress relief to help with a specific pain complaint or injury. Ask what he hopes to gain from the massage. Establish what his main complaint is, as well as any secondary complaints. (Secondary and main complaints are often related.) Determine if he seeks relief from these complaints. You may determine this from the client's responses on your intake form, from his responses to your questions, or a combination of both. Watch how the client moves and stands. Listen for between-the-lines clues, especially when he is talking. He may not realize that massage can help with a headache, in addition to relieving general stress. In fact, specific massage to the neck and shoulders, relieving the pain, may reduce his headache-induced stress more than a general relaxation massage. If he has a specific pain complaint, for example, "low back pain," have him point to the center of the pain and show you the movement that causes the pain or makes it worse. Once you have determined the client's needs, you can decide if seated massage is appropriate for him.

Decide If Seated Massage is Appropriate for the Client

As indicated in Chapter 1, seated massage is not appropriate for all conditions. For instance, a significant knee injury, or just knee pain, is not a good complaint to attempt to address in the seated position. On the other hand, headaches, low back pain, tightness or pain between the scapulas, tennis elbow, carpal tunnel syndrome, neck and shoulder pain, as well as stress, tension, and the desire to do something positive for one's health are all appropriate complaints to address with seated massage. If the client's complaint is not appropriate for seated massage, you do not have to refuse to work on her. Just explain that although you cannot address her specific complaint in the seated position, you can still provide relaxation massage, barring any contraindications. If you have a table practice, offer to schedule an appointment for table massage if that would be appropriate for her complaint.

Ask Standard Questions

Once you have established what the client's needs are and that seated massage is appropriate for him, you need to gather more information. This is done for the safety of the client and to help you address his needs more effectively. The standard case history questions that you would ask prior to a table massage are appropriate in seated massage. These may be on the client's intake form. It is best to have each client fill in a client intake form and to keep a file with records of each treatment session. Quickly review the form after the client has filled it in and ask additional questions you feel are appropriate. More on intake forms and recordkeeping will be presented later in this chapter.

Be sure to determine whether the client has any injuries, medical conditions he is under medical care for, or past surgery on the neck, shoulder, arm, hand, or low back. Also inquire about medications the client is currently on and their purpose.

Seat the Client

To avoid embarrassment or injury to the client, clearly explain and demonstrate the proper way to sit in the massage chair or other seated support system. If the client has never had a seated massage before, the massage chair will likely seem a strange device to her. Without instruction, the average person is likely to sit incorrectly on the chair and may injure herself by tipping the chair over. People commonly sit in the chair backwards (facing away from the face cradle) if they have not seen chair massage being done before. Less common are those who put a foot on a leg rest and mount the chair like it was a motorcycle. Teaching the client how to sit in the seated system is another aspect of professionalism.

Adjust the Chair to Fit the Client

Every chair adjusts differently. Most have some adjustments that must be made before the client sits on the chair. Make the necessary adjustments before asking the client to sit down. Avoid buying chairs that might require the client to have to get up to make a typical adjustment, such as changing the chest pad or face cradle positions. This is a waste of time and is unprofessional.

Many clients will adjust their bodies to fit the chair. They will slouch down, lean, etc. Always be sure the chair is adjusted to fit each client. Be sure that the distance between the seat and the face cradle is enough so that the client's back is relatively straight (erect) and his chest is naturally against the chest support pad. The arm rest should be low enough that the shoulders are relaxed and not held superior by the humerus. Resist the temptation to overflex the cervical spine by tilting the headrest forward excessively, as this causes extra tension in the neck muscles. Have the cervical spine flexed just enough to allow access to the neck and to ensure the client's

comfort (most clients have head-forward posture, so some anterior flexion is essential for comfort). Overflexion creates more tension in the muscles and they cannot relax as much as if they are in a more neutral position. Once you think you have made the proper adjustments, ask them, "Is there anything you would change or adjust to make the chair more comfortable to you?" Make any suggested changes.

> **CLINICAL TIP**
>
> ### Ask Specific Questions
>
> Do not ask the client a general question about comfort. He may not know how it is supposed to feel to sit in a massage chair. If asked, "Is this comfortable?" or "Does this feel alright?" he will most likely say, "Yes." However, if asked a specific question, such as "Is there anything you would change or adjust to make the chair more comfortable to you?" he will then give you specific, detailed information that you can respond to such as, "I'd raise this face pillow up."

COMMUNICATION DURING THE MASSAGE

Now that the client is comfortably seated in the chair and you are ready to begin the massage, do not let the communication stop. You need to be in touch with the client throughout the massage, getting feedback from him, asking questions about how the massage feels, and giving him directions as necessary. The primary method of getting feedback from the client is what we shall call the four therapeutic communications.

Often, clients are reluctant to communicate feedback to the therapist during massage or are not sure how to communicate this feedback. Thus, it is useful to coach the client on communicating feedback to you. There are four specific areas for which you will need client feedback; these should be established with the client before beginning the treatment, or at least before beginning any specific work. They are explained below.

Tenderness

Normal, healthy **soft tissue** is not tender, even to firm pressure. Tissue with even mild spasm becomes **ischemic**, and ischemic tissue is tender when touched. Ischemic tissue harbors trigger points, fatigues rapidly, and can restrict range of motion. As you massage a client, you are looking for these tender, ischemic areas so you can normalize them. Sometimes you can feel these areas, as they are usually more dense, but they are often difficult to feel when working through clothing. Even when you can feel them, you cannot tell how sensitive they are. The client needs to tell you when you touch a tender area, since it is these tender areas that must be normalized to bring relief from their complaint. Many clients will not tell you unless you have requested them to. Here is a sample dialogue you can use to establish the first therapeutic communication—tenderness:

"Ms./Mr. Client, today I will be thoroughly examining the soft tissues of your shoulders (or back, or neck, or wrist, or whatever combination applies). I will be looking for tight contracted areas of tissues where muscles are in spasm. These areas will be tender to the touch, so when I find a tender place will you tell me?"

It is important to phrase this, and the other therapeutic communications, as a question to them, "Will you tell me?" When the client answers "Yes," she is committing to this communication with you. (It is extremely rare that a client will refuse, in which case you should work very lightly and generally.) If you just tell her to inform you when you find a tender place, she is less likely to do so.

Improvement

Now that you have found a tender place, which is ischemic tissue or possibly a **trigger point**, you should try to normalize it. The most common technique to accomplish this is to apply a sustained pressure to the point for 8 to 12 seconds. During that time, if your pressure is appropriate, the client's nervous system should respond and relax the point. As this happens, it will feel to the client that you are letting up or that the tender area is getting better. If your pressure is too hard, the point will not relax—it will get worse. This will be further discussed in the techniques chapters.

It is important that the client communicate this improvement to you, in addition to the tenderness. This sets up a communication in which the client says, "That's tender" and seconds later says, "That's better." Often, this verbal acknowledgment of the improvement by the client psychologically reinforces the actual improvement.

A sample dialogue for the second therapeutic communication, improvement, is as follows: "When I find a tender place, I will probably stop and hold or compress it for about 10 to 12 seconds. During that time your body will respond and relax the area. That will feel to you like I have let up on my pressure, or that it is getting better, because it is. Will you tell me when a tender spot I am holding gets better?"

CLINICAL TIP

Involve the Client

It is important that clients be actively involved in their own healing process. Notice that the four communications should be posed as questions, requiring the client to respond and participate by giving the therapist feedback such as "That hurts there," and "That's getting better."

The client becomes aware of his body and his pain through this process. The input he provides helps you to work more effectively, which in turn helps the client feel better at the end of the treatment. If they say, "That hurts" and then "That's better" over and over, how will they feel at the end of the treatment? That's right, they will feel better. Isn't that one of the treatment goals?

CASE STUDY

Client with Low Back Pain: Assessment

You are working at a massage center where massages are sold on the basis of a dollar per minute. A young man comes in and tells you that his low back has been hurting for weeks and that for the last week he has also had aching pain between his shoulder blades. His medical doctor examined him, found nothing wrong with him, and told him that he should take Tylenol® to help with the pain. He heard that massage could help back pain, so after walking by your storefront for the last few months on his way to and from work, he decided to stop in and see if you could help.

1. What assessment techniques would help you determine the source of his complaints and give you information to explain to him how massage might help him?

Referred Pain

Referred pain will be discussed in detail later in this book. Briefly, if you touch a point or area on the client's body and she feels a sensation somewhere else, she is experiencing a referred sensation. Referred sensations are most commonly pain but may be tingling or other sensations. An example of this would be if you were massaging the trapezius muscle and the client reported a headache pain in the side of her head. You are a rare individual if you can sense referred sensations. Most likely you will not know they are happening unless the client tells you. It is important to know when a referred sensation is present, as this usually means you have found a trigger point. However, you could be touching a nerve, so always have the client inform you when referred sensations are experienced. A suggested way to communicate this is as follows:

"I may find a very tight band of tissue that, when I massage it, causes you to feel a sensation somewhere besides where I am touching. The sensation may go up, down, or through the body, or radiate out in a bulls-eye-like pattern from where I am pressing. These areas are called trigger points. It is important that I know if I have found a trigger point, and I can only know that if you tell me. So, will you tell me if you feel any sensations anywhere besides right where I am pressing?"

Too Much Pressure

It is essential that you use appropriate pressures when doing massage. The amount of pressure that is appropriate will vary from client to client, and even from one area of the body to another on the same client. Too much pressure can cause excessive pain to the client, reducing the therapeutic benefit of the massage and possibly causing injury. Because some people think they must endure a treatment to get better, they are hesitant to "complain" about pain to the therapist. However, if you regularly use excessive pressure, you are in danger of losing clients and even developing a bad reputation in the community. Therefore, be sure to get clients to agree to tell you if they think you are using too much pressure, and when they do, lighten up, no matter how lightly you may think your are working. If they say it is too hard, it is too hard. An example of how to request this type of communication from a client is as follows:

"If at any time I am working too hard or deep, please let me know right away and I will lighten up. Will you tell me whenever I am working too hard or

deep?" Of course, you can also ask them to tell you if something feels particularly good, too.

Some degree of discomfort is normal. You should work at a level that "hurts so good" when doing therapeutic work. This is often described as between 5 to 7 on a 10-point scale of pain, or 3 to 4 on a 5-point scale. In seated massage, a 5-point scale works better. Have the client raise one hand slightly and hold up the number of fingers to correspond with the level of discomfort they are experiencing on a 5-point scale. As the area you are working on gets better, have them lower their fingers, eventually putting the hand down. They do not need to indicate any sensitivity under a 3.

This same method can be used without the client indicating a specific number; simply have him raise his hand when he experiences significant sensitivity or discomfort and lower it as the tissue gets better. This really works well in noisy areas and does not seem to distract from the relaxation of the treatment.

In addition to these intentional cues provided by the client, you also need to be alert to the client's reflexive response to pain. If they are tensing up, squirming in the chair, pulling away from your touch, "armoring" or otherwise contracting, you are working too hard.

Many people are in denial of their pain and will not tell you when you have found a tender spot, even though they agreed to at the beginning of the treatment. Athletes, for example, are often conditioned to never admit that something hurts. However, the body never lies. When your stimulation reaches too high a level, the body will begin to tense up, either locally or systemically or both. If you ever see or feel this happening in a client's body, you are working too hard. Lighten up, even though the person in the chair may say they can "take it." The point is not to be able to "take it" but to be able to benefit from it. When stimulating a tender area so intensely that the client is tensing up, you are overexciting their nervous system. If this is done for more than a few seconds at a time, you will work them up into a state of response that will leave them in more pain than before you started. It is generally better to err to the side of caution. Precision is usually more effective than just pressure. Remember: You cannot "inflict" relaxation on a client.

COMMUNICATION AFTER THE MASSAGE

Once the massage is over, you should communicate to the client what to expect after the massage and how she can continue to care for her health.

Post-treatment Soreness

It is important to advise the client that after receiving specific massage in tender areas, especially the first few times, she may experience post-treatment soreness in the areas specifically treated. You should mention this in the middle of the massage or near the end. Post-treatment soreness is normal and results from toxins in the tissue, such as lactic acid, being released. However, several things will facilitate the client's recovery from pain. It is important for the client to drink plenty of water after the treatment. Note that it must be water, as opposed to any other beverage, and the purer the better. Vitamin C will also help (as it assists the body in metabolizing lactic acid), as will post-treatment stretching. The post-treatment sensation will be similar to the feeling one has after working out for the first time in a while. It usually begins 4 to 18 hours after the massage and lasts 24 to 48 hours. Be sure to advise the client that this is a normal part of the healing process and that with successive treatments she should experience less and less post-treatment soreness; after several regular treatments, there should be none. If the client is excessively sore and bruised and it lasts for several days, you were using too much pressure on her.

CASE STUDY

Client with Low Back Pain Treatment Plan

Continuing on with the scenario in the last case study, you determine that the client has significant internal rotation at the shoulders and head-forward posture, and you show him this in the mirror. You palpate his quadratus lumborum on the left side, and it reproduces the low back pain he experiences. You tell him that you are now quite confident that you can help him with massage if he will come in regularly for a few weeks. He agrees to get a 20-minute massage as a trial run. As you are examining and treating him, you feel his tissues and note that he is very sensitive in the areas of complaints but not very sensitive in other areas. His tissues respond well and relax under your pressure. At the end of the massage you do the shoulder sequence of Active Isolated Stretching movements explained in Chapter 8. His internal rotators and pectoral muscles are

very tight and range of motion is limited, but he does improve. When he stands, he reports his pain is half of what it was when he came in. You confidently assure him that his pain can be eliminated with regular massage and present the treatment plan you have developed in your mind while working on him.

1. Explain what that treatment plan might be.
2. What would be the frequency of visits and their length?
3. How might you price his future visits to give him added incentive to return as frequently as you have recommended in your plan?
4. Would you offer him a reduced rate if he paid in advance for a number of visits? (This is allowed in company policy and published in the menu of services.)

Client Education

Allow the client to be as involved in his own healing process as possible. Educate him about his condition, his posture, and the work you are doing on him. Use the proper names of the muscles and bones. Assign him stretches to do for "homework" and at the next treatment, check to be sure he has done it. Encourage the client to ask questions, and if you do not know the answer, find out and follow up with him. You will learn a lot from doing this, and your clients will become appreciative supporters of you and your practice.

CLINICAL TIP

Use Client-centered Language

It is much more effective to say, "You need to have a treatment every week" than to say, "I need to see you every week." The client does not care what you need; she cares about herself and her needs. Use client-centered language and you will get more repeat bookings at regular intervals.

ASSESSMENT

An **assessment** is a means of evaluating the client's condition, complaint, or injury to determine whether massage is appropriate for the complaint.

Assessment is not a **diagnosis**. A diagnosis is a statement by a physician of what condition the client has, such as, "He has carpal tunnel syndrome." Massage therapists cannot state that a client has carpal tunnel syndrome, or write that they do in the client's file, if it has not been previously diagnosed by a physician as such. However, a massage therapist can ask questions, examine the tissues, measure range of motion and strength, perform muscle tests if trained to use them, do a posture analysis, and determine that the client has a condition that resembles carpal tunnel syndrome. The condition can then be treated without naming it. Yes, this is a fine line, but it is an important line to stay on the right side of. If you say the client has carpal tunnel syndrome, you have diagnosed and you can be held liable. Not naming the condition, or saying they have a condition that resembles carpal tunnel syndrome and should have it evaluated by a physician, stops just short of diagnosing and keeps you within your scope of practice, which includes assessment. Assessment is done for the safety of the client and to guide you to do the procedures and techniques best suited for his condition. Assessment makes you a more efficient and effective therapist.

If the client is seeking massage for relaxation or stress reduction and reports no specific complaints, there is no specific assessment that needs to be done beyond the intake form and the interview, as described above. Should the client have a specific complaint, such as low-back pain, a headache, carpal tunnel syndrome, or any other significant condition, however, you should perform assessment as part of your intake procedure. Since time is short in seated massage, you should do this efficiently. Assessment is usually done before the massage, such as during the intake procedure or immediately before or after the client is seated on the chair. However, it can be done at any time during the session and may be repeated at the end of a session to assess the effectiveness of the treatment. Below are some assessment considerations.

Physician's Diagnosis

Many people believe they have a condition but have never had it officially diagnosed, and thus could be mistaken. For example, many conditions can cause pain in the wrist besides carpal tunnel syndrome, but many people mistakenly assume that their wrist pain is a result of this well-known syndrome. Ask the client whether she has been to a doctor for her complaint and, if so, what the diagnosis is and what the physician recommends. This will give you an idea of the condition and its severity. Knowing this, you can better decide if massage is appropriate based on contraindications, body region or regions affected by the condition, and your experience.

Be aware that many soft tissue conditions are misdiagnosed, especially if trigger points or other referred pain phenomena are involved, so you may want to be respectfully skeptical of the diagnosis and investigate further. However, you should never argue with or discredit the physician's diagnosis. Do your own assessment and create a massage for the person that is safe and beneficial. If the complaint is reduced, you have done well.

Identification of Painful Region or Movement

An effective assessment technique is to ask the client to point to the area of the pain and to what seems to be its focal point or epicenter. If she cannot reach the area, have her verbally direct you up, down, left, or right until you are touching the center of the pain. If it is a headache, have her outline the painful region on her head with her finger.

Then ask her to demonstrate the movement that causes the pain or that makes the pain worse. Sometimes it only hurts if she moves in a particular way. Other times it hurts all the time, but worse when she moves a certain way. Have her show you the offending movements. This should help you determine which muscles are involved. (Except for headaches, if it hurts all the time and movement causes little change, this is an indication it may not be a soft tissue condition, but a pathological problem that a physician should diagnose as soon as possible.)

This simple assessment technique will give you a lot of information. It tells you where the pain is and is not, what muscles are painful, and what muscles are involved in the condition based on the painful movements. It also gives you and the client a reference point to evaluate the effectiveness of the massage. After the treatment, have her perform the movement again and see how much the discomfort has lessened and movement has improved. The greater your knowledge of anatomy, the more effective this assessment technique becomes.

Find Abnormal Soft Tissue and Normalize It

Remember, our job is to find abnormal soft tissue and then to normalize it and restore its range of motion. We find abnormal tissue by examining it with palpation (massage) and movement. We normalize it with massage treatment techniques and therapeutic stretching techniques such as Active Isolated Stretching and Proprioceptive Neuromuscular Facilitation (PNF). Apply this philosophy, observing contraindications and client pain tolerance, to all soft tissue complaints, regardless of diagnosis. When necessary, work above and below the complaint or on the other side of the body. Eventually, as inflammation subsides, the cast is removed, a surgical incision heals, or swelling goes down, you can begin working on the specific area as the client's sensitivity allows. You will be amazed at how fast dreadful conditions ending in "itis," "osis," and "syndrome" disappear in many clients when you use this approach.

Active Isolated Stretching Routine

The Active Isolated Stretching—Mattes Method routines, which are presented in Chapter 8, can serve as assessment techniques for the neck, shoulder, forearm, wrist, and hand. If the client reports pain in the muscle(s) being elongated or the one(s) contracting, you will know where at least part of her problem exists and can examine and normalize those muscles. If the client exhibits restricted range of motion (even without pain) in any particular stretch, you will know something is too tight and needs to be examined and elongated (massaged and stretched). Go through the entire routine for the area of complaint and make notes as to reported discomfort and lack of range of motion. Note any differences between the left and right sides. Explain to the client what you are finding as you go along. This is one way she can learn about herself and appreciate your knowledge and professionalism. This professional touch will contribute to your client's sense of loyalty to you and the likelihood that she will refer others to you.

In some severe cases, most or every stretching movement is painful and restricted. You should still take the client through the entire routine, but instruct her to stop each movement at the edge of pain. In this case, do not assist her movement; just note how far she can go without pain. Sometimes it will only be a few degrees. This will give you a great deal of information. Since most muscles are restricting movement, your treatment will be to examine and treat each muscle, step by step. Efficient routines for this are given in the therapeutic chapters. Examine each muscle, treat and stretch it without causing her to contract involuntarily from excessive pain. Then repeat the initial stretching routine to assess the effectiveness of your treatment.

Posture Analysis

Another assessment method is posture analysis. The skeleton allows us to resist gravity efficiently and maintain balance if its major joints are aligned properly. To achieve this correct posture the human body should be aligned on the **mid-sagittal**, **coronal**, and **horizontal planes** when standing upright and relaxed. (See Figure 5-1 for an illustration of these planes.) Few people are perfectly aligned. Misalignment is called **postural distortion** and is often a contributing cause to pain and injury. The mid-sagittal plane line runs vertically from the top of the head to the feet, dividing the body exactly in half, left and right. We see this plane in the front and back view of the body, as shown in Figure 5-2A and B.

The coronal plane is seen in the side view, running vertically from head to feet, dividing the body into **anterior** and **posterior** parts. Proper alignment on the coronal plane means that the ear, shoulder, hip joint, knee joint, and ankle joint are directly above or below each other, as in Figure 5-3A and B.

The horizontal planes are perpendicular to the mid-sagittal plane and align bilateral structures of the body horizontally. The eyes, shoulders, arms, hips, knees, and ankles should be the same height on the left as on the right, and the hands should rest at the side of the thighs (where the pant seam would be) with the thumb and first finger facing anterior, as in Figure 5-4.

When a person's body is aligned on the mid-sagittal and coronal plane lines, the skeleton is supporting the weight of the body and the muscles are just balancing it and providing movement or stability. This is the most efficient posture. When some part of the body moves off of these planes, the bones no longer support the weight completely and the muscles must take over that job. If forced to do so

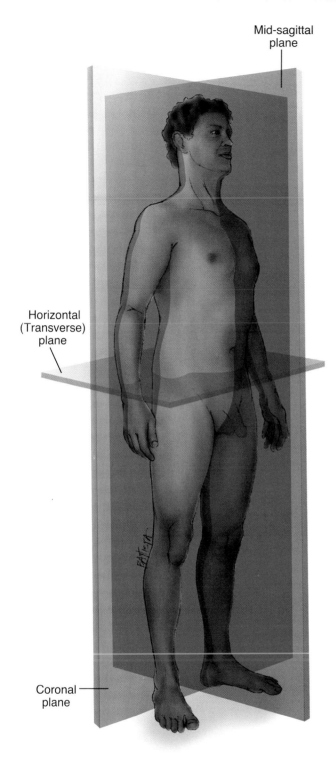

Mid-sagittal plane

Horizontal (Transverse) plane

Coronal plane

Figure 5–1 The major planes of the body. The mid-sagittal plane is the front view and back view of the body. The coronal plane is the side view. The horizontal planes are perpendicular to the other two, parallel to the floor.

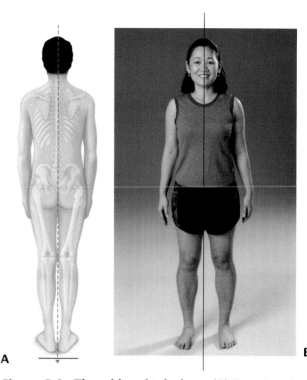

A B

Figure 5–2 The mid-sagittal plane. (A) Posterior view, showing underlying skeleton. **(B)** Anterior view, showing good posture.

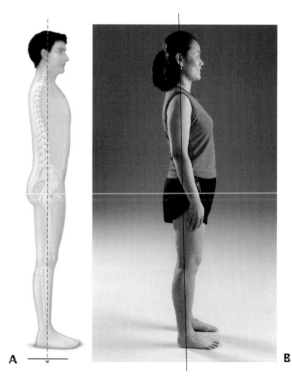

A B

Figure 5–3 The coronal plane. (A) Showing underlying skeleton. **(B)** Showing good posture. Note subject has excellent alignment of ankle, shoulder and ear; however, hips and knees are slightly anterior.

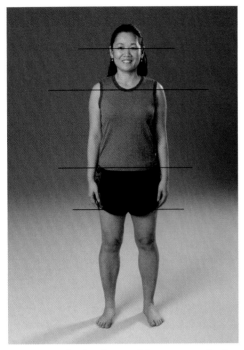

Figure 5–4   The horizontal (transverse) planes.

Davis' Law

"If muscle ends are brought closer together, then the pull of tonus increases, thereby shortening the muscle, which may even cause hypertrophy. If muscle ends are separated beyond normal, then tonus is lessened or lost, thereby 'weakening' the muscle."

Davis' Law was called to the attention of the massage community by Paul St. John, who applied it in his method of neuromuscular therapy. This is a law which describes the condition of postural distortion. A muscle on one side of a joint shortens and becomes stronger (hypertrophies) and the opposite muscle (the antagonist) is lengthened and thus becomes weaker.

While this occurs with every movement, it is not problematic until the muscles are repeatedly held in a shortened or elongated position for extended periods of time, such as regularly holding a phone to the ear by shrugging the shoulder and bending the neck laterally. Another common position is sitting slouched in a chair, head forward and one arm extended to operate a mouse for hours at a time. Eventually, the body accepts this distorted position as "normal" and it becomes locked into the imbalanced posture. This puts extra pressure on the affected joint and fatigues the long, weak, eccentrically contracted muscle. Both muscles will be tender to the touch as both become **ischemic** from the constant, abnormal contraction restricting blood flow through the muscle tissues. However, pain is more often experienced in the long, weak, muscle because it fatigues from holding the load against gravity.

To correct such an imbalance, the short, strong muscle must be relaxed and lengthened using massage and stretching. The lengthened, weak muscle must be relaxed and shortened using massage and strength-building exercises. Active Isolated Stretching is very effective for postural correction, as the long muscle is contracted (exercised) as the short muscle is relaxed (stretched).

for very long, muscles become exhausted, ischemic, and painful. This also puts stress on the bones and joints, contributing to pain, possible injury, or premature failure. Therefore, we should maintain good bone alignment as much as possible. We should also have the muscle strength to support ourselves when we are in positions where the bones are not aligned. Muscles not only cause movement, but they hold us in whatever erect position we assume. If the head is forward of the coronal plane, it is the muscles in the front of the neck that are pulling it forward and the muscles in the back of the neck that keep it from going any farther. The anterior muscles are shortened, tight, and **concentrically contracted**. The posterior muscles are lengthened, taut, and **eccentrically contracted**. The shortened, stronger muscles are the problem, but usually the client will report their pain in the lengthened, weaker muscles. (See Box 5-1 for Davis' Law, which provides a neurological explanation.) This is because the lengthened muscle(s), in this case the posterior cervical muscles, are holding the cranium from falling farther forward and become fatigued, often developing trigger points. The head-forward posture contributes to pain in the back of the neck. If you massage the posterior muscles and relax them, the client will feel better at the moment, but the relaxation will likely allow the tight anterior muscles to pull the head farther forward, creating even more load on the posterior muscles, causing the pain to

return soon after the massage and possibly with additional intensity. This same pattern can exist in the shoulders, pulling them forward, and in the arms, rotating them internally. See Figure 5-5 and for an example of the head-forward, internally rotated posture. Internally rotated, rounded shoulders contribute to pain between the scapulas and sometimes to shoulder and rotator cuff injuries. As we are pulled off the planes of posture, muscles on the side of the

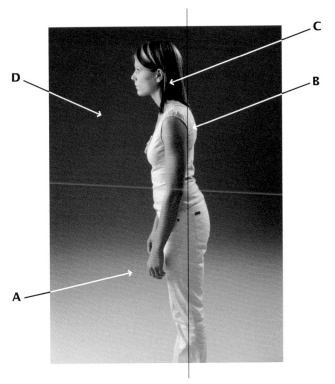

Figure 5–5 Example of the internally rotated, head-forward posture. Note position of the following: (A) Hands, back (dorsal) side facing forward; (B) Excessive thoracic (kyphotic) spinal curvature; (C) Loss of cervical curve (military neck) and extension at the occiput-C-1 level of the neck to keep the eyes looking forward instead of down; (D) Entire upper body, which is leaning anterior.

someone's posture and determine which muscles are short and which are long.

Observe someone's profile when they are standing. The ear, shoulder, hip joint, knee, and ankle should be in a straight, vertical line as shown in Figure 5-3A. If some part is anterior or posterior, a muscle imbalance exists. Looking at her from the front; her hands should be at her sides and you should see her thumbs and first fingers, as in Figure 5-2B, not the backs of her hands. Shoulders should be the same height, head should be straight, and eyes and ears should be level.

Lower body postural distortions are not practical to address in the seated position. Some upper body distortions originate in the lower body from distortions such as over-pronation of a foot, sometimes called a "flat foot." The iliums can rotate anteriorly, causing hyper-lordosis, or posterior, causing a flat back. Both distortions result in a head-forward posture. Iliums can get stuck, or "fixate," in a position of unequal rotation, more on one side than the other. This can contribute to a functionally long leg or to scoliosis, usually both. If you feel lower body misalignments need to be corrected to resolve the client's complaint, you should suggest table massage by a therapist who is trained to address such conditions, or possibly chiropractic treatment.

distortion are shortened, concentrically contracted, strong and tight. Muscles on the opposite side of the distortion are lengthened, eccentrically contracted, weak and taut. Lengthened, taut muscles are often painful and develop trigger points. Shortened, tight muscles need to be relaxed and stretched to allow the person to move back into proper alignment.

Poor posture can result from a number of improper alignments and causes muscular stress. People who do work of any kind in poor posture and alignment are more likely to be in pain. Golfers who do not maintain proper wrist alignment are more likely to suffer from elbow injuries. Athletes with overpronation of the feet are more likely to tear the anterior cruciate ligaments (ACLs). Poor posture contributes to pain, injuries, and poor performance.

Sometimes the postural distortion is in the horizontal plane, such as one shoulder being higher than the other, as shown in Figure 5-6. The body should be symmetrical. Both sides should be the same. If you become observant you will be able to quickly assess

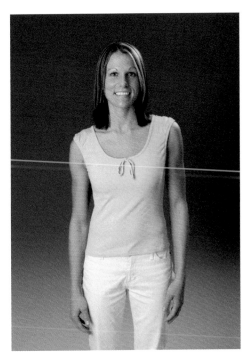

Figure 5–6 An individual with a high left shoulder. This condition can contribute to neck and shoulder pain, as well as headaches.

Some massage disciplines such as neuromuscular therapy, medical massage, and Rolfing use posture analysis as a primary assessment method and spend 15 to 30 minutes of the first appointment performing a very complete postural analysis. In seated massage, due to time constraints and the limitation to primarily upper body treatments, postural analysis can be done quickly, observing front and each side, noting any obvious deviation from vertical and horizontal, and then correlating it with the client's upper body complaint.

Assess your client's posture during your intake procedure and help him become aware of his posture and how it relates to his condition (if it does). Arrange your treatment to address his distortions as well as his pain complaints. Massage and stretch the short, contracted muscles two to four times as much as the long ones. The long muscles need to be massaged and lightly stretched because they are ischemic and, due to the constant overload, often harbor trigger points. They are usually the muscles the client feels their pain in. Massage and stretch them to restore circulation and eliminate any trigger points. This brings the client relief and they have the sense you are attending to their complaint. However, in doing this you are just addressing the symptoms, not the cause of their problem. To address the cause and bring them longer-lasting relief, you should address the short, contracted muscles on the other side of the joint and work to relax and lengthen them. If you treat both sides of the joint equally, you will not change the relative position of the joint or the tone of the muscles. You will just relax both sides. Once the client stands up, they will be in their same posture as before you started and possibly, by relaxing the already long muscles, you will allow the short, tight muscles to pull them farther into their distortion. This is why it is recommended to treat the shortened muscles two to four times as much as the long muscles, significantly relaxing and lengthening the short muscles, allowing the client to stand up into a more correct posture.

Massage techniques alone will relax the muscles, but will not lengthen them. Therefore, massage alone is not enough. You must stretch the short muscles. The reciprocal inhibition types of PNF stretching and all the Active Isolated Stretching—Mattes Method stretches discussed in Chapter 8 not only lengthen the short muscles but strengthen the long muscles at the same time.

This applies to correcting your own posture as well as to when you are treating a client. Once this head-forward, internally rotated posture becomes habit, it typically progresses and eventually leads to the hyper-kyphosis seen in senior citizens. In this posture, the person is falling forward with every step and only catches themselves by getting the front foot down in front of them with each step. Balance in this posture is very poor and any unexpected or unseen change in terrain causes falls. The tendency to form the head-forward, internally rotated posture must be resisted and counterbalanced with exercises which lengthen the habitually shortened muscles and strengthen the habitually long, weak muscles. See Figure 5-7 for the three-step exercise for postural correction. This is an excellent exercise for clients and massage therapists to do regularly to improve upper body posture or to help maintain good posture.

Some common examples of postural distortion include:

- Internally rotated arms and shoulders, contributing to carpal tunnel syndrome and to pain between the scapulas.
- A high shoulder or low shoulder, often contributing to neck and upper thoracic pain, sometimes contributing to headaches.
- The head-forward posture, usually associated with pain in the back of the neck and sometimes with headaches.

To review: When you have determined that a client has a postural distortion and it can be correlated to their complaint, the general rule is to massage the muscles on both sides of the involved joint(s), working two to four times longer on the shortened side. Stretch the shortened muscles, creating length to allow the body part to move back toward alignment. Teach the client one or two stretches to continue lengthening the shortened muscles between appointments. They must maintain what you gain.

Other Assessment Methods

In addition to the techniques discussed above, there are many other systems of soft tissue assessment. Orthopedic physicians have developed an extensive series of tests for assessing muscles, tendons, ligaments, and joints, usually called "Orthopedic Assessment Tests." Physical therapists, most notably Henry and Florence Kendall, have developed a comprehensive system of muscle testing. These systems are a bit involved for the typical seated massage situation, but might be useful if you are working in a medical or clinical environment, a sports massage practice, or a pain clinic. For more information on these methods, see the "Suggested Readings" list.

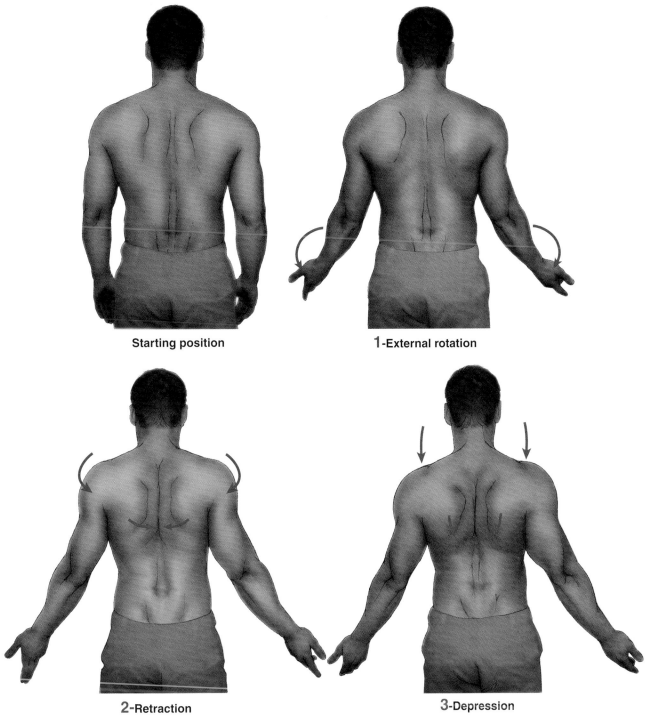

Figure 5-7 **3-Step Posture Exercise.** Starting position: Stand or sit up straight, with arms hanging relaxed at your sides; back of neck long. Step 1: Externally rotate hands/arms ("roll thumbs out"), contracting infraspinatus, teres minor, and deltoid. Step 2: Retract scapulas ("pull shoulder blades together") contracting rhomboids and mid-trapezius. Step 3: Depress scapulas ("pull shoulder blades down"), contracting lower trapezius. Hold for 2 to 5 seconds. Relax and return to starting position. Repeat. Start with five repetitions twice a day and work up to 15 repetitions three times per day.

DOCUMENTATION

It has become absolutely necessary for therapists to keep records of every massage session they perform. Good records help protect both the client and the therapist. There are two types of records that you will need to keep for each treatment you perform: accounting records and client records.

Accounting Records

There are three things you need to do to ensure orderly accounting records: keep a regular appointment schedule book, save receipts and other financial documents, and choose and implement an accounting system that works for you. First, you should record every appointment you make with a client in a schedule book or a Personal Digital Assistant, including those that are missed or canceled (which you should identify as such). Not only can a schedule book be helpful to you when you file your taxes or in the event you are audited, but it can also serve as a backup to your client records. At the end of the year, save your schedule book with your other tax records so that it will be easy to find when you do your taxes. If you are nationally certified through the National Certification Board for Therapeutic Massage and Bodywork, you may need to document the number of hours of massage you performed in the last four years to recertify. Be sure to file your schedule books for the last four years in a place where you can find them. It is also a good idea to record other business appointments that you make, such as doctor's appointments; visits to your accountant, lawyer, or business consultant; presentations that you make to businesses or organizations, vacations, continuing education events; and any other appointments that are at all related to your business, so that you can analyze your use of time and backup business expenses claimed on your taxes. Note: Always keep your schedule book in pencil; it changes regularly and becomes an illegible mess if done in ink. If you use a Personal Digital Assistant or other electronic device, keep regular backups and save paper or media copies of them just as you would a paper schedule book.

Second, you should make it a habit of keeping copies of all receipts for product sales, client services provided, and items that you purchase for business use (of course, you should provide all your clients with receipts for their own records, as well). In other words, keep every receipt for every business transaction, both for income and expenses. Keep the receipts for each month in an envelope or file folder. You might divide them into categories such as income and expenses. You could further break down income into categories of on-site income, office income, merchandise sales, sales tax collected, and so on. Receipts for expenses could be broken down into general categories like credit card receipts, cash receipts, and receipts paid for with checks, or into tax related categories like massage supplies, advertising, printing and copying, continuing education, phone, computer expenses, etc.

Each day's income should be recorded. This can be done from your deposit receipts, as you should deposit each day's income at the end of the day, but be sure to keep your business income deposits separate from personal or other income. It is best to have a separate bank account for your massage business. The IRS frowns upon co-mingling of personal and business funds.

For issuing client receipts, you may use one of any number of receipt systems that are available on the market. These range from simple duplicate receipt books available at any office supply store to computer programs. The computer programs for client receipts are not very practical for seated massage if you are working on-site. It is difficult to set up your computer (even a laptop) and printer everywhere you go. However, advancing technology may change this. At this time, some type of paper duplicate receipt book is easiest for client receipts when you are doing on-site massage. Of course, you may transfer the information to your computer once you are back at your office or home. In addition to receipts, you should also keep mileage logs of business travel, check stubs, copies of cancelled checks, deposit slips, and anything else that might be helpful in documenting your business activity.

Third, you need to choose an accounting system that you can maintain in a timely and efficient manner. If you are technologically savvy, a Personal Digital Assistant and a notebook computer that interface with each other may be the best way for you to handle all your scheduling and accounting. Quickbooks® is an excellent, user-friendly accounting program for your computer that is supported by most accounting and tax preparation offices. It manages your checkbook(s), other bank accounts, income, expenses, and generates receipts, statements, and all the reports necessary for business analysis and tax preparation. There are several other brands of accounting programs available. Check with your tax preparation service to be sure they support the program you choose.

If you prefer a more low-tech approach, consider a paper system. Although less commonly used now as computer programs become more user-friendly and less expensive, paper systems are still a viable alternative. A paper system must have four sections: pages to record income and categorize its sources (on-site massage, office massage, merchandise sold, tips, sales tax collected, etc.); pages to record expenses and to categorize each expense (advertising, postage, massage supplies, continuing education, dues, insurance, etc.); a receipt book to make client receipts and which keeps a duplicate copy of each receipt issued for your records; and pages for summaries. Columnar pads, sold at office supply stores, are inexpensive and work well for income and expense records. Consult with your tax preparation service, if you use one, as you set up your bookkeeping system so that it will interface with their systems at the end of each tax period. The goal is to choose the system that will be the easiest and most efficient for you to use, whether is it paper or electronic.

Client Records

The second set of records that must be kept are client records, often called charts. Client records are kept, most importantly, for the safety of the client, as well as to allow you to provide the client with better, more professional service. Good records also help document the progress of the client over time. This is especially helpful when working with clients with chronic pain who become discouraged and sometimes blame the therapy or the therapist for their continued pain. You can encourage them by showing them how they have increased their range of motion, for example, or how they originally reported pain in the back, neck, and shoulders and how it is now only in the neck. This can be a good "pep talk" for them when they are discouraged or have a minor setback. Of course, their records may show that after some time they are not improving, in which case you must change what you are doing for them or refer them to another therapist who may be better able to help them. There are two popular systems for keeping client records: S.O.A.P. and HxTxCx (1).

S.O.A.P. Charting

The best and most complete system of client charting is called S.O.A.P. Notes. This stands for Subjective,

Objective, Assessment, Plan. This system assists practitioners in solving client medical problems. It is extensive and time-consuming. However, it is well worth the required effort when working with clients who have injuries or medical conditions and you are dealing with insurance companies, either for your reimbursement or for the client's. If you are working with people who have specific complaints, problems, and injuries and you are addressing those conditions in your treatment, it is best to use S.O.A.P. charting. This system is also recommended if you are using the therapeutic routines in this book to help with specific complaints.

S.O.A.P. charting presents special challenges in seated massage, though, especially when doing on-site appointments. Because of the brevity of a standard session, there is typically not time to do a full S.O.A.P. writeup before and after each client. However, clients with ongoing complaints and conditions are generally willing to pay more and spend more time for specific, therapeutic treatments—they will do whatever it takes to get out of pain. Therefore, you can schedule specific sessions with enough time to accomplish the necessary charting. Your compensation for this extra time spent on individuals with specific complaints can come from keeping your standard time and simply charging more per minute for your massage session. Alternatively, you can charge for your actual time spent on client intake, assessment, and charting. Keep in mind that charting is a part of your professional service and is valuable; it does benefit the client and, thus, you should be compensated for it. If you are going to do a full intake using the S.O.A.P. format, inform the client that the first visit will be longer and will cost more. Be clear that followup sessions will be shorter and cost less. Explain that therapeutic work involving charting, insurance billing, extra client education, and teaching them homework (stretches, exercises, etc.) is more extensive and thus more expensive than a general relaxation routine. Most people are delighted to pay for more or better service, especially when it helps them manage or recover from their condition. The scheduling of time is still a bit problematic, as some clients take longer than others, but after a few weeks of full S.O.A.P. charting you will be able to decide how much time to allow between clients and adjust your schedule and fees accordingly. You may use S.O.A.P. charting on some clients and not on others, depending on their needs.

In addition to the S.O.A.P. chart itself, a health information form is used as a client intake form for any client for whom you are going to be doing S.O.A.P. charting. This form is to be filled out by the client before his first massage. He can complete it once he arrives at your location or it can be mailed to him to complete and bring with him.

S.O.A.P. charting is the subject of an entire book that you may want to study if you are doing clinical-type treatments as a regular part of your seated massage practice. The book is *Hands Heal: Communication, Documentation and Insurance Billing for Manual Therapists*, Second Edition, by Diana L. Thompson (1). Sample S.O.A.P. forms from *Hands Heal* are included in Appendix A at the back of this book. However, the full explanation of the S.O.A.P. procedure is beyond the scope of this book. *Hands Heal* will also help you with insurance billing, should you want to become involved with that process.

HxTxCx Charting

A simple and quick way of documenting treatments on relatively healthy people is the HxTxCx charting system. This stands for History (Hx), Treatment (Tx), and Comments (Cx). HxTxCx charts contain a brief intake questionnaire that gathers health history and conditions and provides space for recording treatment provided and any comments you may wish to record. Comments may relate to the client's sensitivity, his personal preferences, variations from a routine, tender areas, progress, and anything else you feel appropriate. The form also includes a consent statement for the client to sign. A sample HxTxCx chart for seated massage is provided in Appendix A at the back of this book. It can be modified to suit your particular situation.

If there is no involvement with insurance reimbursement or physician referral, the HxTxCx system of charting is adequate when doing seated massage for most clients. While full S.O.A.P. charting is the best method, even significant complaints can be handled with the HxTxCx system as long as you make enough notes to know what you did at each treatment and how the person is reacting to the therapy.

Readability and Completeness

An important part of charting is readability. Will you be the only therapist seeing the charts? If so, you can use any abbreviations, slang, or drawings as long as you can read it and know what you

recorded. However, if you work in a setting where other therapists may see your client occasionally or where the client may see a different therapist each time they come in, then recordkeeping must be such that everyone on the staff can understand it. You will have to develop "charting language" with your colleagues. It does not have to make sense outside of your organization, but should be clear to everyone on your staff.

In addition to legibility, it is also important that client charts be as complete as possible. In the worst case, should you (or your supervisor or colleague) ever have to testify for or against a particular client, you may need to be able to explain your treatment for a client from years ago, or even a colleague's treatment of the client. In the best case, you should be able to pick up a client's chart from the office files and identify the following:

1. What his complaint(s) were at his last appointment.
2. What treatment or techniques were performed on him.
3. Any areas of ischemic tissue or trigger points that were found.
4. Any range of motion restrictions noted.
5. What homework was given to the client.
6. Any peculiarities about this client, for example: unusual sensitivity, inability to perform hyperextension movements, preference to not have the face cradle tipped very far forward, etc.
7. How he responded to the treatment and what improvement was reported or observed.

If you can obtain this information from any client in your group practice, your group is recording excellent notes! If there is something you cannot understand or read on a client's chart, be sure to ask the client about it before you begin working on him.

TREATMENT PLANS

People seek massage for a variety of reasons. They may just want a "treat" or relaxation for themselves. In this case, no treatment plan is needed. The relaxation treatment presented in Chapter 9 is its own plan and is self-contained. For those who seek relief from chronic pain or an acute injury, however, treatment plans are necessary. There are two primary reasons for treatment plans. The first is to organize and guide the therapist. The second is to educate the client and hopefully get her to commit to a series of regular treatments.

Types of Treatment Plans

A treatment plan can be as simple as how you are going to structure the treatment that you are about to do. This is done mentally, "on the fly," based on your client intake form and interview. You may decide to do a general relaxation routine or to focus on the client's right arm and wrist for the entire session.

On the other hand, a treatment plan may be quite in-depth if you are working regularly with a client who has a chronic condition or significant injury. Treatment plans may be generic or client-specific. For example, one generic plan might be a pattern used to help most people with low back pain. You might call it the "low back routine" and indicate it as such in your client's records, along with any unusual findings or procedures you may have done that are outside of the routine. The "low back routine" could have a plan of four weeks, one to three treatments per week. At the end of the four weeks, re-evaluate the client and either continue or change to a different routine as indicated by his symptoms. If no improvement has occurred, you better try something different or you will soon lose the client.

A client-specific plan would address the particular complaints of an individual person. It would be muscle- and movement-specific for that person based on their intake information. For example, Mr. Z. indicates on his intake form that he has everyday headaches and cannot turn his head to the right without pain. A quick check of his standing posture shows that his arms are internally rotated 45 degrees, his shoulders are rounded forward, and his ear is 2 inches anterior of his shoulder joint. He can only turn his head 45 degrees to the right but can turn almost 90 degrees to the left. He has no other complaints at this time, no known medical conditions, surgeries, or recent accidents, and is not on any medications. A client-specific plan would specifically outline how you will address these exact complaints for Mr. Z. The plan should list the goals to be achieved (most likely relief of headaches and normal range of motion to the right), along with the techniques you will use, the recommended frequency of treatments, length of treatments, and homework to be assigned.

Treatment plans can be pre-printed in the case of a generic plan, or custom-made and presented to the client for a specific plan. A specific plan for a particular client will likely have to be presented to the client at a second or subsequent treatment; at the first treatment, explain that at the next appointment you will present her with a plan to address her complaint or condition. This helps with rebookings. Of course, if you are working in an airport or at a one-time event, treatment plans are virtually impossible. In these cases, just create a treatment to best address the immediate needs of the person you are working on at the moment. It will impress them that you customized the treatment just for them, and you may be pleasantly surprised when they stop by your business place again and again.

Putting Together a Treatment Plan

The first part of your treatment plan should be to provide the client with some immediate relief from her complaint. This involves treating the symptoms, the tender areas, and any trigger points you can find that refer into the tender areas. If your treatment reduces her complaint, she most likely will reschedule. You should also take a few minutes and try to determine a cause for the symptoms. Does she perform repetitive activity at work or at home? Are her posture and gait patterns correct? What sport or work activities does she perform? Does she work out? Do any of these things relate to her complaint?

For example, a client, Mary, comes for a seated massage. She says she just wants to relax and have a break from a stressful day, but when asked if she has any specific areas that are causing her discomfort, she admits she has a suboccipital headache and a pain between her shoulders. You ask her to stand comfortably for a minute or two. You observe that she internally rotates her shoulders and arms. You see all four knuckles of both hands facing anterior. Her ear is one inch anterior to her shoulder joint on each side. Based on this input, you might put together a treatment plan such as the one presented in Figure 5-8.

Notice that the plan in Figure 5-8 allows for Mary to progress to the next phase as rapidly as possible, based on her symptoms. A treatment plan should never be used to "string people along" just to sell treatments. It should always be for the purpose of maximizing client benefit, as rapidly as possible. Below is a summary of how you would develop this treatment plan and communicate it to the client.

Treatment Plan

Phase 1: 3-6 treatments, 20 minutes/treatment, 3 treatments/week

A General relaxation of paraspinal muscles and arms to begin treatment

B Reduce the headache and ache between the shoulders

    1 Examine rhomboid upper and mid-trapezius
    2 Examine posterior cervical muscles
    3 Examine suboccipital muscles
    4 Treat any ischemic areas and trigger points found

C Reduce postural distortion of shoulders, arms and head

    1 Stretching of pectoralis major- horizontal abduction
    2 Stretching of pectoralis minor- external rotation
    3 Stretching of subscapularis- external rotation
    4 Stretching of anterior cervical muscles- hyperextension (if appropriate) and posterior oblique

D Homework

    1 External rotation, retraction, depression exercise
    2 Pectoralis major stretch

Phase 2: To begin once headache and ache between shoulders is reduced and does not return for 2 days, or after 6 treatments. Two treatments/week should be performed for 3 weeks or until postural corrections are achieved and Mary reports no symptoms of headache or pain between shoulders between treatments.

A General relaxation of paraspinal muscles and arms

B Check any tender points and trigger points found last time. If they have reformed, treat and reduce them

C Shoulder routine, examining pectoralis major, pectoralis minor, subscapularis, anterior deltoid, and posterior deltoid

D Active isolated stretching shoulder routine, cervical hypertension (if appropriate), and posterior oblique

E Homework

    1 External rotation, retraction, depression exercise / 3-step postural correction exercise
    2 Pectoralis major stretch
    3 External rotation stretch
    4 Posterior oblique stretch
    5 Hyper-extension (if appropriate)

Phase 3: Maintenance and Wellness- to begin after achieving correction of postural distortions and elimination of symptoms (headache and pain between shoulders). Regular 15-minute massage as Mary feels necessary. Recommended minimum of 1 treatment/month.

Figure 5-8 An example of a client-specific treatment plan.

Since Mary came to you thinking she just wanted to relax, you need to quickly educate her about her posture and how it might correlate with her headache. Explain to her that her suboccipital muscles are fatigued and overloaded as they work to hold her head up. If they did not contract along with other cervical extensor muscles in the back of her neck, she would be looking down at the ground from her head-forward posture. Her shoulders have rounded forward, putting additional load on the extensor muscles of her spine as they work to keep her from falling forward and on the rhomboids, and mid-trapezius as they work to keep the shoulders from going farther anterior.

Tell Mary that you will provide her the relaxation she seeks but that you will also try to reduce her headache and see if you can find any dysfunctional tissues that contribute to her posture and headache. As you massage her, you examine the suspect muscles, and when you find tender points or trigger points you treat them, explaining to Mary what you are finding and how it relates to her pain and posture.

For the last three to five minutes, reduce your conversation to a minimum and change to very sedating techniques. When Mary gets up, hopefully feeling as relaxed as she had hoped for, and with her headache reduced, you suggest that she reschedule in two days and at that time you would like to give her a treatment plan to correct her posture and eliminate her headaches. She agrees, as she admits it would be wonderful to be free of these daily afternoon headaches. (Remember, there is no such thing as a "normal" everyday headache, and headaches are not caused by aspirin deficiency.)

CLINICAL TIP

Condition the Client's Response

It is good to explain to new clients that the relaxation effects of massage escalate over successive treatments as the nervous system becomes familiar with the experience and develops a conditioned response to the stimulus of massage. Soon they are conditioned to relax as soon as they sit in the chair and you begin your treatment, especially if you begin nearly the same way each time, thus giving their nervous system "the cue." You might try recommending a "starter pack" of either four or eight treatments in the next month (either one or two each week) and give your clients a discount for advanced purchase. Explain that this allows the nervous system to be trained to respond to massage and allows them to maximize their massage experience. Then they can spread the treatments farther apart, as they will be able to "feel" when they need their next appointment. From then on, regularity becomes more important than frequency. Even once every month will have a more powerful effect if they go through the initial "starter series." Remember Pavlov's dog!

You write up her plan that night and when she returns, you give her a copy and briefly explain it to her. Be sure to make it clear that every individual is different, and some people will respond faster than expected while some will respond more slowly. The plan is a guide and an estimate that may have to be adjusted once you begin working together. Answer her questions and ask if she would like to try your suggested plan. Do not get too long-winded with this, as she came for a massage and you have other clients after her.

The professional presentation of a treatment plan is an offer to help someone improve their health and well being. It benefits both you and the client by establishing communication, direction, and measurable goals. Try using treatment plans where appropriate.

SUMMARY

Effective communication with the client before, during, and after the treatment is of the utmost importance. Before the massage you must decide if seated massage is appropriate for the client and what techniques will be of the most benefit to him, based on the intake information he communicates to you, and instruct him on how to get on the chair. This is also an opportunity to educate the client about the services that you can offer him, from relaxation to rehabilitation, based on your level of expertise.

During the massage, you must solicit feedback on tenderness, improvement, referred pain, and pressure. Therapeutic communication can be verbal or by hand signals, such as raising a hand or a number of fingers to indicate tenderness and lowering them as it gets better. After the massage, you should advise the client on how he may feel the next day, assign and explain homework, and schedule future appointments.

Assessment is a specific type of communication in which you acquire information from the client on his complaint or condition. Assessment may be as simple as having the client point to the area of discomfort or as extensive as orthopedic testing, depending on your abilities and the extent of the client's complaint(s).

Another specific type of communication is record-keeping or documentation. Charting the client's appointments is extremely important. Charting allows you to remember the client's condition(s) from one appointment to the next. It also helps other therapists who may work on the client to know what has been done and how the client responded. Charting can be done extensively using the S.O.A.P. format or more simply using the HxTxCx method. Use the S.O.A.P. system with clients who have significant problems, who are referred from a physician or other provider, or who are in some way billing insurance for your fees. Use the HxTxCx system for all other clients. Business records of income, expenses and scheduling must also be kept.

Finally, treatment plans help you organize your techniques so as to best serve the client. They are also used to educate the client about his condition and the services you can provide for him. Treatment plans can also help to get clients involved in their own healing. They encourage compliance with homework and client commitment to a series of appointments.

Become proficient and comfortable with all these communication skills and you will likely find you practice growing and your retention rate improving.

CASE STUDY

Treatment Plan for Relaxation Routine

You have a contract to provide massage for three hours every Friday at an insurance company. During your second visit, a 35-year-old female department manager stops by and asks if massage would relax her and make her feel better. You assure her it would. She fills out a client intake form and reports nothing of note. Her posture is slightly head-forward and internally rotated at the shoulders, but she reports no back or neck pain. You perform the relaxation routine from Chapter 9 on her. When she gets off the chair she reports that she hasn't been this relaxed in years and asks whether she can get a treatment each week when you are there.

1. Is there a need to develop a treatment plan for this client? If so, what would it be?

REFERENCES

1. Thompson DL. *Hands Heal: Communication, Documentation and Insurance Billing for Manual Therapists*, 2nd ed. Baltimore: Lippincott, Williams & Wilkins, 2002.

SUGGESTED READINGS

Kendall F, McCreary E, Provance P. *Muscles—Testing and Function*, 5th Ed. Baltimore: Williams & Wilkins, 2004.

Lowe WW. *Orthopedic Assessment in Massage Therapy*. Sisters, OR: OMERI, 2005.

Notes

CHAPTER 6

Body Mechanics and Injury Prevention

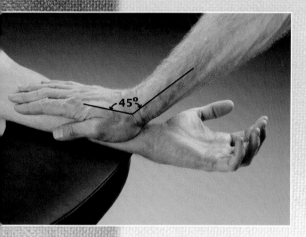

"Flexibility is experienced when the subtle energies, free to move without obstruction through the body, link the joints together like pearls on a string."

LIZ KOCH, *THE PSOAS BOOK* (1997)

Objectives

■ Use correct posture and movement while performing seated massage.

■ Demonstrate the two primary working stances for seated massage.

■ Describe proper breathing techniques to use when giving a massage.

■ Define repetitive strain injury and describe how to prevent it.

■ Explain the importance of proper physical conditioning for massage therapists and discuss the key elements of a personal fitness program.

Key Terms

Body mechanics: the proper use of posture, movement, and joint alignment to perform massage therapy efficiently and with minimum stress and trauma to the practitioner; also called *biomechanics*. The use of correct body mechanics reduces the chance of injury to the practitioner and improves the quality of touch to the recipient.

Biomechanics: the science concerned with the action of forces (internal or external) on the human body. In massage, it concerns the forces placed on muscles and joints of the therapist while performing massage.

Carpal tunnel syndrome: the most common nerve entrapment syndrome. It results from repetitive activity, causing inflammatory swelling or hypertrophy in the carpal tunnel that puts pressure on (entraps) the median nerve. Symptoms include pain, tingling, burning, prickling, and/or numbness, sometimes with sensory loss and wasting in the median distribution of the hand (part of thumb and first three fingers, along with proximal palm). Usually worse at night.

Compressive force: an action that results in the two sides of a joint being pushed together.

Extensor: a muscle or a group of muscles that causes extension of a joint or joints. Extension causes a limb or the body to assume a more straight line, or causes the distance between the parts proximal and distal to the joint to increase. An extensor is the antagonist to the flexor.

Flexor: a muscle or a group of muscles that causes flexion of a joint or joints. Flexion is the bending of a joint or the bending of the spine forward. A flexor is the antagonist to the extensor.

Hypertonic: a state of excessive muscle tonus (hypertonus) that causes discomfort, restricts range of motion, and wastes body energy.

Isometric: a muscle contraction with no movement of the involved body parts; force development at constant length.

Lateral epicondylitis: an injury to the extensor tendons of the forearm at or near their attachment on the lateral epicondyle of the humerus. Often called "tennis elbow."

Medial epicondylitis: an injury to the flexor tendons of the forearm at or near their attachment on the medial epicondyle of the humerus. Often called "golfer's elbow." In young baseball players, often called "Little League elbow."

Muscular dysfunction: an abnormal state of a muscle, most commonly resulting in local discomfort and restricted elongation, but sometimes also involving trigger points and referred pain. Hypertonicity and the resulting ischemia is the most common muscle dysfunction. Cramps, contractures, or the inability to respond are the most severe dysfunctions.

Nerve compression: pressure placed on a nerve by bone or cartilaginous structures, compromising the nerve's function and usually causing pain. Nerves may also be compressed by muscles as they pass through them, when the muscle is in spasm. Also called nerve entrapment.

Neuropathy: a disease or disorder, sometimes degenerative, that affects the nervous system.

Plantarflex: extension of the ankle, to point the foot and toes.

Repetitive strain injuries: tendon, muscle, joint, and nerve damage resulting from the body being subjected to direct pressure, vibration, or repetitive movements for prolonged periods; also called cumulative trauma disorders.

Shearing forces: a force or strain which pressures a joint to move across its axis instead of on or around it. This abnormal movement or pressure, when coupled with compressive force, is destructive to joint capsules.

Subluxation: an incomplete or partial dislocation of a joint; contact between joint surfaces remains, but not in the ideal or correct position. Correction is typically achieved through a thrusting manipulation (adjustment) by a chiropractor.

Tendonitis: an inflammation of a tendon, a tendon capsule, or a tendon sheath.

Thoracic outlet syndrome: compression of blood vessels and nerves of the brachial plexus at any point between the neck and the armpit, most commonly between the first rib and the clavicle or under the pectoralis minor, causing discomfort, compromised function, and often swelling.

Do you want to use your body to maximize efficiency when giving a massage? Do you want a long, injury-free career as a massage therapist? Do you want your massage to feel the best it possibly can to your client? If so, this chapter will benefit you greatly.

Massage is sometimes called "manual therapy" because it is done using the hands. Massage is strenuous and repetitive activity which, if done improperly, can cause the therapist great pain and significant injury. In fact, many therapists have to leave the massage profession and give up the work they love due to massage-related injuries. This is especially unfortunate because most of these injuries were avoidable. Massage-related injuries are less likely to occur if the therapist takes proper care of his body and uses it correctly.

Often these injuries occur as a result of the therapist's poor physical condition and lack of proper self care. Consider the following scenario: A therapist's practice starts out slowly, with just a few sessions per week. The therapist's body adapts to this low level of activity. As his practice grows, the number of sessions per week can rapidly increase. If he is not in proper physical condition for this level of activity, his body cannot adapt fast enough to support and withstand it and he begins to experience pain, typically in his thumb, wrist, elbow, shoulder, or back. Since he is finally busy, he does not take time off to treat the injury himself, as he would probably recommend to one of his clients with s similar problem. He keeps working, never allowing the his body time to heal and adapt. His pain becomes chronic and soon he cannot stand it. In trying to help others, he injures himself, and within one to three years he leaves the profession. This is a disappointment not only to himself but also to his clients, teachers, colleagues, and family. In most cases this does not have to happen. Please, do all you can to prevent it from happening to you.

There are a few massage therapists who are very lucky. They pay no attention to body mechanics or physical fitness and never sustain a massage-related injury. Good for them. Some of these therapists become instructors and because of their own experience, they place no emphasis on body mechanics. Unfortunately, most of us are not that gifted and if we follow their example, we will wind up in pain and possibly out of work.

This chapter teaches you to protect yourself from massage-related injuries. Topics include proper use of your body (body mechanics), including body alignment, stances, and injury prevention. Mastery of these concepts will benefit both you and your client.

EXPERIENTIAL EXERCISE

Good versus Poor Body Mechanics

With another therapist, take turns giving each other a massage. Work in good body mechanics, properly aligned and breathing correctly. Then work the same tissues in poor body mechanics and awkward alignment, with no attention to breathing. Notice how the two different styles feel to both the receiver and giver of the massage. Also note the difference in the amount of effort expended to do massage incorrectly and correctly.

BODY MECHANICS

The terms **body mechanics** and **biomechanics** are used in massage therapy to describe the efficient alignment (posture) and use of the body while performing massage. As a massage therapist you should use your body in the most efficient manner while minimizing the stress and trauma it receives. Using proper body mechanics will make a massage feel better to both the giver and the receiver.

Body mechanics are especially important in chair massage compared with table massage, due to the intensity of short treatments done over and over, sometimes with very little time in between. While the same principles apply to both, in seated massage the strokes are shorter and more repetitive because you are restricted to a smaller working space. Thus, chair massage is generally more hand-intensive than table massage. Furthermore, massage chairs do not currently have effective overall height adjustments, and the client is seated vertically in the chair. Tall therapists must "get down" to work closer to the hips, whereas short therapists must "get up" to work the neck and shoulders. Therefore, to avoid injury it is important for the chair massage therapist to use proper body mechanics. Three aspects of body mechanics are considered below: body alignment, stance, and breathing.

EXPERIENTIAL EXERCISE

Body Mechanics Self-Evaluation

Practice seated massage in front of a full-length mirror. Notice your posture as you work. Are you in good posture most of the time? If not, change your habits. Alternatively, have someone videotape you doing a seated massage. Watch yourself in the video and critique your posture, movement, flow, and communication with the person in the chair, and change your habits as necessary.

Body Alignment

Body alignment, or posture, is a critical aspect of body mechanics. For the massage therapist, a properly aligned skeleton will provide the support necessary to do massage without injury to the soft tissues. Massage should be done in a manner that minimizes the **compressive force** placed on the involved joints. Compressive force is the least harmful when it passes straight through the axis of the joint and is more harmful when it puts angular or sideways stress on the joint capsule.

While our primary focus here is doing massage efficiently, these same principles apply to all activities in life. Thus, massage therapists need to correct their own posture, not only to protect themselves from occupational injury but also to be an example to their clients. Awareness of your postural distortions is the first step toward correcting them. Have your posture assessed by a chiropractor or another therapist trained in techniques that correct postural distortions, and begin working to correct it. Postural correction takes time, as it requires old habits to be broken and new ones learned.

To perform massage, you assume an internally rotated posture, even in perfect working stances. While the spine is ideally kept straight and head-up (looking down at the client by flexing at the Occiput-C-1 joint and by looking down with your eyes), it is impossible to not have a head-forward posture occasionally as you lean forward in the lunge position. Sometimes you must bend forward or kneel down, at least for short periods of time. The same is true when driving, computing, washing dishes, and other common activities. Over time, these positions lead to the postural distortions seen in the standing posture that clients bring to you, as they become habits to the nervous system which remain even when the you stand up straight. Correct working postures minimize the effects of the internally rotated position you must assume to perform massage. Correct joint alignment minimizes the strain placed on your joints, particularly your wrists, fingers, and thumbs. In the next section we will discuss proper working stances. Later in

this chapter fitness techniques will be presented. Learn to take care of yourself so you can take care of others.

Stances

There are two stances used in table and seated massage that help us maintain good posture and thus use our bodies efficiently while doing massage. They are the lunge stance (also called the archer stance, the asymmetric stance, or the bow stance) and the straight stance (also called the warrior stance, the symmetric stance, or the horse stance). For seated massage, the lunge stance is preferable most of the time.

Lunge Stance

In the lunge stance, one foot is placed in front of the other one. Both feet point forward, with the rear foot comfortably angled outward and supporting most of your body's weight, as shown in Figure 6-1. As you move toward the client in the lunge stance, you actually lean onto the client's body, controlling the amount of weight (pressure) you place on the client with your front knee, as shown in Figure 6-2.

A common error made in this posture is angling or externally rotating the rear foot too far and thus losing the ability to **plantarflex** the ankle. See Figure 6-3.

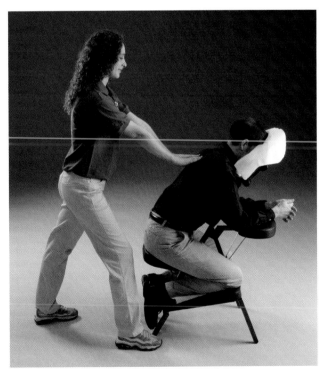

Figure 6–1 Lunge stance showing correct posture between strokes. Note that weight is mostly on rear foot.

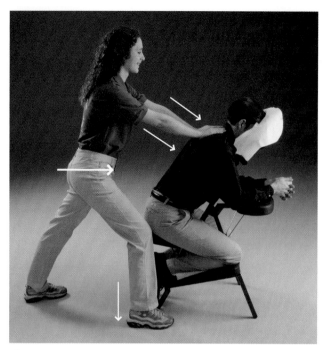

Figure 6–2 Lunge stance showing correct posture while in contact with client. Note that the therapist is leaning into the client, with weight primarily on front foot and hands.

The ability to "push off" with the back foot is a primary source of strength and power in massage. Your feet should be pointing along the line of force you are applying to the client's body. In fact, your entire body should be aligned along the line of force you are applying. Your arms should be out in front of you. Your

elbows should be straight but not locked, positioned directly over or in line with your hand and thumb.

When using your thumbs, they should be straight, their bones aligned with the radius bone of your forearm, so that your bones support the weight you are applying to the client's body, not your muscles. See Figures 6-4 and 6-5A and B.

Avoid applying pressure with a flexed thumb, as shown in Figure 6-6, as this position overstresses the joints of the thumb and places excessive strain on the adductor pollicis, flexor pollicis, flexor pollicis brevis, and opponens pollicis (1). It can also bring the thumbnail in contact with the client's body.

Some people are naturally able to hyperextend the interphalangeal joint of their thumb. Therapists who find it is easy (almost natural) to be able to hyperextend are sometimes called being "double-jointed." They tend to apply thumb pressure with the interphalangeal joint while in the hyperextended position, as shown in Figure 6-7. Working in this position creates excessive strain on the thumb joints and can cause nerve compression in the interphalangeal joint. You should apply pressure only with the tip of the thumb. Therapists who easily hyperextend should keep their thumbs in a slightly flexed position when applying pressure and either close the hand into a loose fist to support the thumb, as shown in Figure 6-8, or elevate their palms off the client's body using the four fingers for support.

If you must flex (bend forward), do so from the hips, not from the waist or mid-back. You should be

Figure 6–3 Lunge stance showing incorrect rear foot position and hyperextended wrist.

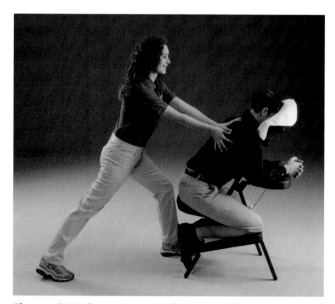

Figure 6–4 Correct upper body working posture. Elbows are straight, but not locked. Note proper wrist/thumb alignment relative to the elbow.

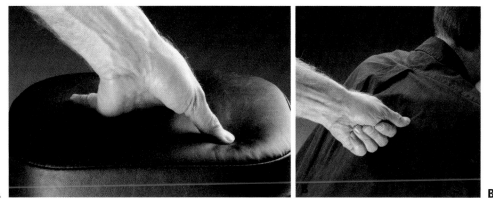

Figure 6-5 Correct thumb posture. (A) Joints are "stacked," transferring force through thumb joints and wrist to radius bone. Note the correct finger positions: hand is open with palm elevated, supported with other four fingers. **(B)** Closed hand with straight wrist.

standing "behind the stroke." Your back should be relatively straight, maintaining the lordotic (anteriorly convex) curvature of the lumbar and cervical spine. This means the head is erect and, if looking down, flexed at C-1; do *not* bend the entire neck anterior. Do not push by flexing (bending) the back, and try not to twist the back to reach the client or to change angles of pressure. Instead, reposition your entire body so you are aligned with and behind the area you wish to examine or treat.

The movement in the lunge stance comes from the knees, primarily the front knee, moving forward and back in a manner that keeps the pelvis moving along a line that is parallel to the floor. This movement is transferred through your torso to your arms and allows

pressure to be applied to the client's body without bending your back or straining your shoulders. Your power in this stance comes from your legs transferring your weight. Your weight is primarily on your back foot when you are not applying pressure to the client's body. As you bend the front knee you are not transferring your weight to your front foot. Instead, you are leaning forward into the client's body, and your weight is transferred to whatever part of your arm is touching them. This could be your elbow, hand, fingers, knuckles, or thumb. Straightening your front knee then removes your weight from the client's body and transfers it to your back foot again. The more you bend your front knee, the more of your weight leans on the client's body. To generate additional power (pressure)

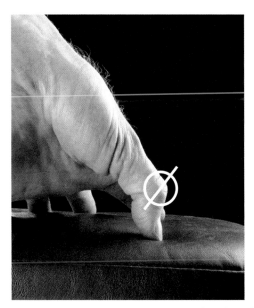

Figure 6-6 Incorrect thumb posture, showing flexed thumb. This improper posture can cause joint, muscle, and nerve injury.

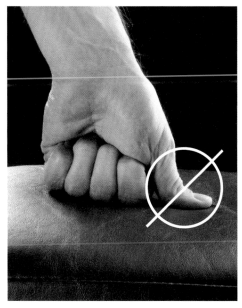

Figure 6-7 Incorrect thumb posture showing hyperextension at the interphalangeal joint of the thumb.

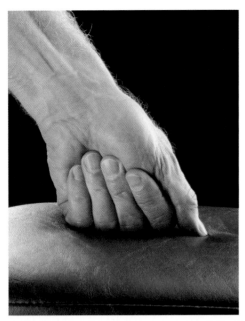

Figure 6–8   Correct thumb posture, especially for "hyperextenders." Note that the thumb is supported by keeping the interphalangeal joint slightly flexed and the hand closed.

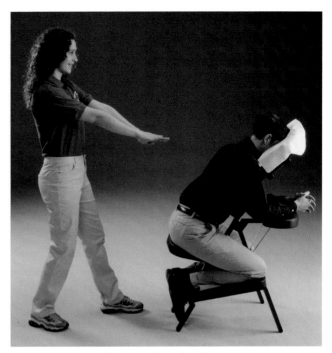

Figure 6–9   Starting position for lunge movement. Note that the back knee is bent, front knee is fairly straight, shoulders are relaxed, and elbows are straight but not locked.

you can "push off" by plantarflexing your rear foot. For some techniques, you can lean forward (transferring your weight to your front foot), grasp the client's body, and pull away by straightening your front knee. Keeping the movement primarily in the large muscles of the legs, thighs, and hips reduces strain and fatigue on your back and shoulders.

Practice the lunge position in front of a large mirror. Keep your forward/backward pelvis movement parallel to the floor, your back straight, and head up. Transfer your weight smoothly from your back foot to your front foot and to your back foot again by bending your knees, as shown in Figures 6-9 and 6-10.

Then, with a person on a chair in front of you, or using the wall, transfer your weight from your back foot through your body to your hands, onto the person or wall, and back to your rear foot smoothly in a fluid motion, moving from the knees. Exhale as you move forward and inhale as you move backward.

Once you build the required strength in your legs, this posture becomes very easy to work in and protects you from injuries. The smooth, efficient flow of energy and force through the joints when doing massage in the lunge stance makes the massage treatment feel much more pleasant to the receiver.

This is the position you should be working in most of the time when doing seated massage. This posture will be shown throughout the book as different areas and muscles are addressed.

Straight Stance

The straight stance, also called the warrior or horse stance or symmetric stance, is the other standing position used in seated massage (Fig. 6-11).

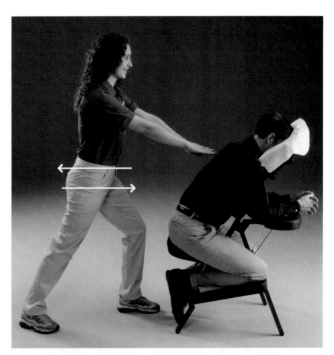

Figure 6–10   Forward position of lunge stance. Note that the front knee is bent and the back knee is fairly straight. Weight is balanced over feet, easily and smoothly controlling the amount of weight (pressure) applied to the client.

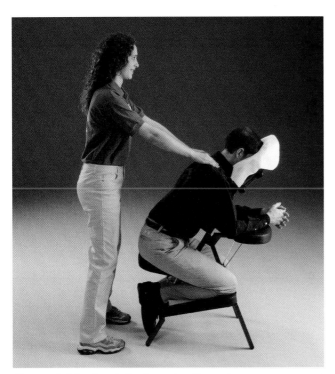

Figure 6-11 **Straight (warrior/horse) stance, correct posture.**

In this stance, your feet point forward with front tips aligned, about shoulder width or a bit farther apart, and your body faces the area you are working on. The knees are straight (in the normal knee lock position in the last 15 degrees of extension) but not hyper-extended. Your spine is erect. If you need to look down, flex your head forward at the C-1, not with the entire neck. The shoulders are relaxed, with arms out in front of you and your hands working the client's tissues. Your elbow should not be rotated outward and raised above your shoulder, as this does not deliver good leverage and flow of force from your body to the client's. The primary movement should be rotation of the pelvis, in sync with the hands for petrissage strokes. Avoid bending forward at the hips or lumbar spine and do not rotate (twist) the torso to reach; instead, move your feet. See Figure 6-12 for an example of incorrect posture in the straight stance. How many poor habits can you identify in the photo?

Do not generate pressure by pushing from your back, shoulders, or arms, as this is fatiguing to you and not as pleasant for the client. The symmetrical standing position with the weight equally distributed on both feet is fatiguing, interferes with circulation, and should be avoided or only used briefly. The straight stance can be used for applying the petrissage

stroke to the arms and shoulders and when standing close to the client to briefly perform some precise technique that does not require a significant amount of strength. Whenever it is practical, it is best to use the lunge stance. Become comfortable in these two stances, primarily the lunge stance.

Working in proper posture is a habit. Be conscious of your working posture until you develop this habit, keeping in mind that it takes about a month to form a new habit. If you experience pain or discomfort while doing massage, especially in the hand or thumb, check your posture; you are probably out of the stance. Get back into alignment, breathe, move with your legs and pelvis, and you will probably feel better. Your massage will feel better to the person receiving it, as well.

Wrist Posture in Both Stances

Wrist posture is important in both the lunge and straight stances. Most therapists must be very careful not to overextend their wrists, as doing so often leads to injury. However, therapists who have strong, flexible wrists are less likely to experience this discomfort. Try to minimize the angle of extension in your wrists when doing massage. It is best to keep them at 45 degrees or less above the line of the forearm, as shown in Figure 6-13.

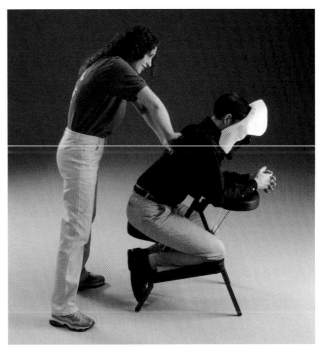

Figure 6-12 **Straight stance, incorrect posture.** Note that the knees are locked, the spine is bent forward and twisted, the head/neck is flexed, the elbows are bent, the thumbs are hyperextended; each of these can lead to injury.

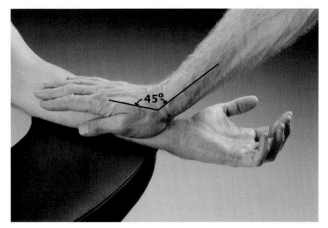

Figure 6–13 Correct wrist alignment. Forty-five degrees of extension or less is ideal.

Occasionally you must increase this angle, but do not stay in this position for long or use it often. If you experience discomfort while working with extended wrists, switch to a loosely clinched fist, which gives good, straight wrist alignment, as shown in Figure 6-14. Be careful not to flex or extend wrists in the loose fist position. If slightly flexed, the wrist can buckle due to the **shearing forces** across it, injuring muscles, ligaments, tendons, fascia, and even the joint itself.

Shearing forces across the wrist joint are damaging over time. The line of force should flow from you to the client, parallel to your radius and ulna bones, then through the wrist joint and into the hands parallel to the metacarpal bones, as shown in Figure 6-15.

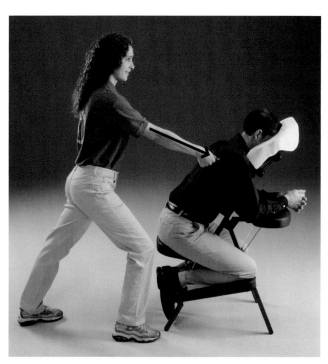

Figure 6–15 Correct line of force through the arms, wrists, hands, and thumbs.

Do not rotate the forearm internally, and radially deviate the wrist so that pressure flows across the wrist, as shown in Figure 6-16. This puts significant strain on the ulnar side (little finger side) of the wrist capsule that over time may lead to hyper-mobility

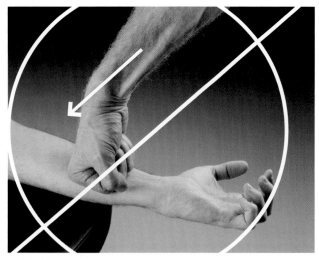

Figure 6–14 Incorrect wrist posture when using loosely clinched fist. Flexed wrist can buckle, causing injury. Lack of support can also cause ligament injury.

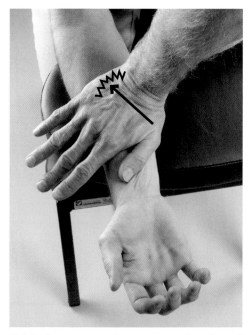

Figure 6–16 Incorrect wrist posture showing shearing forces across the wrist.

and injury, including possible nerve compression in the wrist. This improper wrist alignment also compromises the alignment of the elbow and shoulder, which can lead to pain in these joints as well.

Keep your hands and wrists relaxed as you do massage. Allow your hands to conform to the tissues they are touching. Do not stiffen or tense the part of your hand or fingers that is not applying pressure to the tissues, as the resulting rigidity and tension in the tendons of the extensor muscles reduces the quality of touch to the client and increases your chances of fatigue and injury.

Developing and maintaining strength and flexibility in your wrists is well worth the time and effort, as it helps ensure a longer and less painful career. Utilize the forearm, wrist, and hand stretches along with the exercises in this book or other methods of your choosing.

Breathing

Most people take breathing for granted. It happens automatically, right? Fortunately, it does occur in some form automatically, controlled by the autonomic division of the nervous system. However, we do have the ability to consciously control our breath and, to some degree, this ability can be of great benefit to our practice of massage and our own well-being. Below are some tips on how to breathe most effectively during a massage.

Maintain a full, deep breathing pattern, through the nose. Not an exaggerated one, but a full one. Breathe from the diaphragm, the muscle of inhalation that is deep in the abdomen. Your breath should go into your abdomen first. Then, as your lungs fill, allow them to lift and open the chest. This does not mean you are huffing and puffing over your client. Just learn to take full and smooth breaths. Of course, this deep breathing will be interrupted when you talk, but when you are finished talking revert to full, smooth, nostril breathing. It is best to make the transitions from inhalation to exhalation as smooth as possible. You do not want your breath to stop or pause between inhalations and exhalations. This is true whether you are doing massage or not. Neither you nor the client should hold their breath (stop breathing) anytime during the massage. If the client is holding their breath during the massage, it probably means you are working too hard or they are uncomfortable for some other reason. Gently remind them to breathe and ask about your pressure and their comfort.

Furthermore, you should breathe through your nose as much as possible. The nose cleans, warms, and adds moisture to the incoming air. Full breaths through the nostrils allow for better oxygenation of the blood and, therefore, better physical performance. Mouth breathing dries the vocal folds and can contribute to bad breath (2,3).

When performing massage, breathing is most effective while in the lunge stance. As you move forward toward the client, exhale. As you move backwards or pull away from the client, inhale. When doing shorter or more detailed strokes that have little full body movement, this technique will not work; however, you can keep breathing regularly and smoothly, which will help maintain your posture and energy. Use your breath to maintain an erect, "open heart" posture of the torso. If you take full breaths from the abdomen and fill the lungs, it will naturally lift the chest and open the shoulders. Allow these things to occur and utilize the power and strength the full breath gives you.

Yoga science teaches us a great deal about breathing and Hatha Yoga includes breathing exercises called pranayama (4), which teach how to control the breath. Learning to control your breathing can help you improve your mental focus and concentration. Our emotions affect our breathing. For example, if startled, we tend to gasp and hold our breath. If we can learn to control our breath we can learn to better control our emotions. Emotions can be dangerous things, especially when out of control. Breath is the link between the body and the mind. You cannot underestimate the importance of proper breathing and control of the breath. Yoga and pranayama are subjects well worth studying by the massage therapist.

Besides helping the therapist provide a more effective massage, proper breathing techniques can benefit the clients, as well. Teaching your clients proper breathing techniques from the abdomen (diaphragm) can help them improve health, gain focus, and feel better. People in shock, fear, and pain tend to breathe shallowly, using just the upper portion of their lungs. They breathe mostly with the accessory breathing muscles instead of the diaphragm. People with fibromyalgia, in particular, usually have shallow breathing patterns with internally rotated (rounded or slumped) shoulders. These improper breathing patterns are habits and must be broken and consciously replaced with corrected habits. This takes about 30 days of conscious effort, but is well worth the time and energy required.

Proper Breathing

Have another student or person sit up straight or stand and place, one hand on the upper chest (above the breasts) and the other hand on the abdomen. Have her inhale normally, and notice which of her hands moves first and most. It should be the lower hand. If it is the upper hand, she needs to correct her breathing. The breath should fill the abdomen, then fill the mid-chest, and finally lift the clavicles. On exhalation the reverse should occur: the clavicles should lower, the chest contract, and finally, the abdomen draw in. On inhalation, have her imagine her lungs are balloons and that she is inhaling helium. Allow her lungs to fill from the bottom up, lifting the chest and clavicles.

INJURY PREVENTION

Use of proper body mechanics, of course, is a type of injury prevention in and of itself. This section covers one of the most common types of injury sustained by massage therapists, repetitive strain injuries, as well as how to prevent injury through conditioning, flexibility, and strength training.

Repetitive Strain Injuries

Because **repetitive strain injuries** (RSI) are so common among massage therapists, it is critical that you learn what causes them, how to prevent them, and how to treat them. Basic background information on RSI is provided below, followed by specific considerations for massage therapists.

Background

RSI, also known as repetitive motion injuries and cumulative trauma disorders, are injuries resulting from performing the same movement over and over again. Some of the most common RSI include **carpal tunnel syndrome, medial epicondylitis** (golfer's elbow), **lateral epicondylitis** (tennis elbow), some rotator cuff problems, and **thoracic outlet syndrome.** Such injuries are generally related to inefficient biomechanics, poor posture, repetitive movements in sports and work, and poor work habits. In particular, repetitive motions preformed

while the body is under compressive forces or joint hyperextension, or both, tend to cause soft tissue injury. The risk factors associated with RSI include exertion, frequency, duration, force, posture, low temperatures, and vibration (5). These conditions build up over time, and the cumulative result is **muscular dysfunction, tendonitis**, and in the case of carpal tunnel syndrome, **nerve compression** (6).

Taking Deeper Breaths

Lie supine and place a weight of several pounds on your abdomen (a velcro-on ankle weight band works well for this). Inhale to lift the weight, counting until you begin to exhale. Then, count to the same number as you exhale. See how high you can count (how long an inhalation you can take) while still maintaining a smooth transition between inhalation and exhalation with no jerk or pause. Perform 12 breaths per session. Gradually increase the amount of weight on your abdomen until you are using 10 to 12 pounds. Eventually, try to have your exhalation time double your inhalation; for example, inhaling to a count of 6 and exhaling to a count of 12. Work to lengthen both inhalation and exhalation times a second or two each week until you can do 12 smooth breaths with 16 seconds of inhalation and 32 seconds of exhalation with 10 to 12 pounds of weight.

An alternate version of this is to lie face down with your forearms crossed and on top of one another. Pull your crossed arms inferior until you can comfortably rest your forehead on your folded forearms. Now inhale, counting like above. Notice the expansion of your abdomen at the sides of your waist line. As above, work to lengthen your breaths and smooth the transitions between inhalation and exhalation. In Hatha Yoga this is called crocodile pose (Makarasana). This relaxation pose is an excellent position to gain breath awareness and learn diaphragmatic breathing. This pose also releases tension in the lower back and mid-torso.

The activity causing RSI is usually not a maximal contraction or a ballistic activity, but rather a seemingly easy or normal movement such as using a computer mouse or doing massage. Therefore, tissue tearing (strains and sprains) is not the cause of these injuries. It is the repetitive activity or constant **isometric** activity of the muscle(s) creating sub-maximal mechanical overload of constant tensile stress placed on the tendon(s), causing a breakdown in the collagen fibers (7).

While some RSIs have evidence of mild inflammation, many do not and there is now evidence that the classic inflammatory treatments are of little value if inflammation is not clearly present (8). This is good news for massage! Massage is contraindicated where there is clearly inflammation, but where there is little or no inflammation massage is very effective.

The pain associated with RSI, usually experienced in the course of performing the repetitive activity, is minor at first but gradually gets worse as the activity is repeated over time. The injury typically progresses from ache or soreness to increased tonus (tightness), to the formation of trigger points, and possibly to nerve compression. As the condition becomes chronic, it can lead to **neuropathy, subluxation,** deterioration of the involved joint(s), bursitis, arthritis, and even stress fractures of the involved bones (9). Recovery from RSI requires cessation of the repetitive motion that caused it, therapy, and rest. If an RSI is ignored and the repetitive motion continues, the injury will become more severe, require longer recovery, and be less likely to heal completely. Therapy for RSI includes use of an ice pack, stretching, strengthening, postural correction, and activity modification (changing the motions that caused the injury).

RSI and the Massage Therapist

As noted before, massage involves much repetitive motion, especially in the hands and wrists. This repetitive activity, along with the compressive forces involved in applying pressure to the client's body, can rapidly cause RSI to develop in your body. This is especially true if you do not practice proper body mechanics.

EXPERIENTIAL EXERCISE

Breathing and Visualization

In some of the energetic models of the body, the hands are considered to be the extension of the heart and are energized by the heart energy center. The heart energy system is believed to bring vitality to the heart, lungs, circulatory system, and upper back and to vitalize the sense of touch. Visualize your breath bringing life force energy into your heart as you inhale, and see some of that energy flowing down your arms, through your hands, and to the client as you exhale. Thinking of the heart center as the seat of love, and love as the most powerful force in the universe, become a channel for love to flow through from the universe to the person in the chair. Attach no intentions except the highest good and have no attachment to a desired outcome. Let love do the work. However, you must keep your breath full and regular.

I learned another effective visualization for this concept from by one of my early massage instructors. He taught that you should visualize a gold goblet in the center of your heart. As you inhale, you fill your goblet to full and overflowing. Keep your cup full so you have all the energy you need and let your cup "runneth over" through your arms to the person in the chair. Share only the abundance, which is limitless. If you empty your cup on them, you may find yourself empty and drained energetically.

The best way for you to prevent RSI is to work in the proper biomechanical postures for massage which were covered earlier. Furthermore, keeping your body, especially your shoulders, elbows, wrists and hands, physically fit and strong by doing regular weight and flexibility training will also help prevent these injuries. You need to develop a "reserve capacity" of physical endurance to manage the stress of massage. This topic is covered in detail later in the chapter.

The use of massage tools can also help prevent RSI. These are small, hand-held tools designed specifically to be used by the therapist during massage to prevent excessive strain and overuse injury in the wrists, thumbs, and fingers. Figures 6-17 and 6-18 show an assortment of massage tools.

Although you lose some touch sensitivity when using tools, the protection they provide against the debilitating effects of RSI makes them well worth it. If you do decide to use a tool, it is important that you find one that properly fits your hand; an ill-fitting tool can cause more stress to your joints and muscles than going without one.

Other preventative measures include using a variety of strokes, resting your hands by scheduling extra

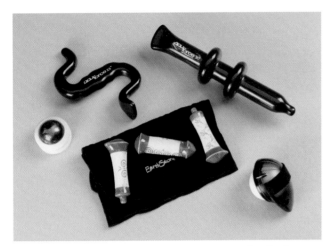

Figure 6–17 Assorted large massage tools. Tools courtesy of Scrip Massage Supply, Peoria, IL, www.scrip-inc.com.

time between your appointments, taking regular breaks, stretching between sessions, and receiving regular massage. Remember that to successfully take care of your clients, you must first take care of yourself.

Should you sustain an RSI, do not go into denial; immediately begin an aggressive treatment program. Ask another therapist (or an instructor) who understands body mechanics for massage to evaluate your working posture and style. If you are not already receiving regular massage (which is recommended), begin a regular massage program and start stretching and strengthening your muscles. Massage must be frequent at first, and specific. General relaxation massage will be of little value as far as resolving the injury but can be somewhat beneficial because of its parasympathetic effect if done throughout the kinetic

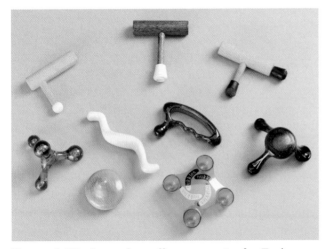

Figure 6–18 Several small massage tools. Tools courtesy of Scrip Massage Supply, Peoria, IL, www.scrip-inc.com.

chain of the injury. The kinetic chain of most RSI caused by performing massage would be upper extremity, shoulder, neck, and upper thoracic areas. All of these areas are appropriate for seated massage. If you do not take immediate steps to correct an RSI, it may jeopardize your career. What you do as a massage therapist is important and needed; do not let RSI end your career and deprive your clients of the help you provide them. Specific therapeutic massage techniques for addressing RSI in the forearm, wrist, and hand are given in Chapter 12.

EXPERIENTIAL EXERCISE

Improving Balance

The following is a simple exercise to improve balance. Stand with your feet hip-width apart. Raise one knee straight up toward your chest (hip flexion with knee flexion), lifting your foot off the floor as high as you can. Hold for 5 seconds and return to standing on both feet. Repeat with the other side. You should be able to do this easily, smoothly, and without loss of balance. However, you initially may need to do this near a wall or chair and use one arm for balance. Do 6 to 10 lifts of each foot twice a day until you can do them smoothly and without the need for a balance support.

Conditioning, Flexibility, and Strength Training

Massage therapy is a physically challenging occupation. Massage is repetitive and uses the entire body. You are on your feet most of the time you are doing massage. You will be carrying a massage chair around, along with the gear you chose to have with you (briefcase, appointment book, computer, face cradle covers, water, lunch, etc.). Because the work is strenuous and repetitive, it is essential that you invest the time necessary to develop and maintain your flexibility, strength, stamina, and balance. Failing to do this greatly increases your odds of injury. Developing these attributes will make you healthier as well as a better massage therapist.

To accomplish this, it is essential that you invest time in a personal fitness program, preferably before you sustain an injury. You need to develop full-body strength and stamina. Specifically, you must develop

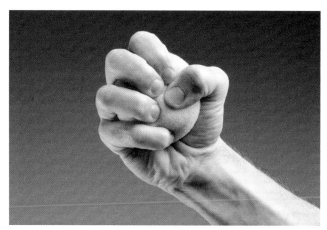

Figure 6–19   Entire hand squeezing a small rubber ball to develop finger flexor strength.

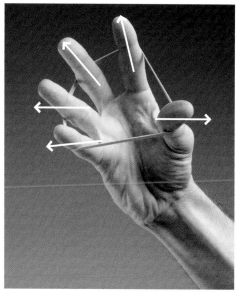

Figure 6–21   Rubber band providing resistance for thumb and finger extension exercises.

strength in your legs, back and abdominal wall, shoulders, arms, and hands. A balanced weight routine for the entire body is advisable. If you do not like using weights, there are several excellent resistance band systems available. These systems use elastic bands to create resistance to movement. There are very good full-body workouts using these elastic systems, which come complete with diagrammed routines. Additionally, inexpensive items such as rubber bands and small rubber balls can be used to develop hand strength. The rubber band may be wrapped around the fingers and thumb to provide resistance to finger extension, and the rubber ball held in the hand and squeezed repetitively. See Figures 6-19 and 6-20 for exercises with a rubber ball.

Special attention needs to be given to conditioning wrist and finger extensor muscles. Massage therapists tend to become strong and **hypertonic** in their fore-

arm **flexor** muscles and relatively weak in their forearm **extensor** muscles. This imbalance can lead to wrist and elbow problems. To build finger extensor strength, use rubber bands, as shown in Figure 6-21.

To build wrist extensor strength, it is best to use resistance bands. Using a dumbbell (weights) requires the use of the flexors to hold onto it, minimizing the effect on the extensors. On the other hand, resistance tubing or bands, such as a TheraBand® (Fig. 6-22) allows contraction of the extensor muscles without engaging the flexors. This actually allows you to stretch the flexors as you strengthen the extensors, if you go through the full range of extension motion.

Of course, general conditioning and exercise can be accomplished with minimal resources. Pushups

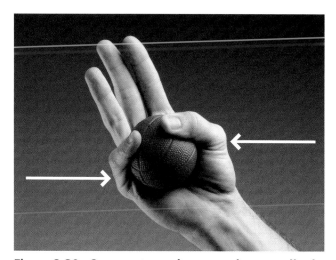

Figure 6–20   Opponent muscles squeezing a small rubber ball to develop thumb strength.

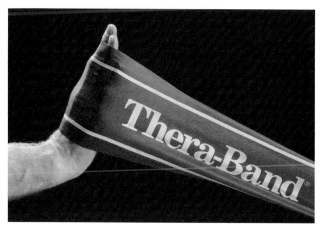

Figure 6–22   Wrist extension using TheraBand® for resistance to strengthen hand extensor muscles.

and situps require no investment in equipment. Walking 20 to 30 minutes a day only requires a decent pair of walking shoes. The important thing is to find a system and routine that works for you and use it regularly.

In addition to conditioning, stretching is a vital part of any fitness program. The repetitive contraction of strength training and work activity needs to be counter-balanced with a stretching routine to prevent loss of range of motion and possible repetitive strain injuries.

The best stretching system for massage therapists is the Active Isolated Stretching—Mattes Method (AIS). Routines from this system are presented in Chapter 8 of this book. It is highly recommended that you do these routines at least once a day (it only takes 10–15 minutes). It is best to do the forearm/wrist stretches before and after each day's work. Many of the stretches can be done while walking to the bathroom, walking across the parking lot, going to or from lunch, and sitting in traffic at stop lights or traffic jams, so there is no valid excuse for not stretching every day. The AIS system also includes lower body stretches, which are available in books, videos, and wall charts.

Yoga is another excellent system for improving flexibility. Yoga teaches strengthening, balance, relaxation, and meditation techniques. It is a centuries-old, full-body wellness system, probably the first holistic body-mind-spirit system. Therefore, yoga is very compatible with massage, for both therapists and massage clients. For a brief description of yoga, see Box 6-1.

Stamina and endurance are also necessary for seated massage. You should have enough endurance to not be exhausted at the end of the day. To be a

---

Box 6-1

What is Yoga: A Brief Overview

Yoga means "union between the individual self and universal consciousness." The goal of yoga is gaining control over the modifications of the mind and finally gaining direct experience of one's inner self, or self-realization. There are many different types and systems of yoga taught by various organizations, ranging from purely physical to completely metaphysical. As with most things, somewhere between the extremes lies the best path for most people. One of the most common systems, due to the fact that it has the most universal appeal, is Hatha Yoga. Initially, Hatha Yoga involves mostly physical teachings and uses static stretching and breathing to increase flexibility, strength, stability, and body awareness. There are several areas of study in Hatha Yoga, the most common being the postures called asanas. Each asana is a position or pose that stretches particular muscles and joints while strengthening the opposite muscles. Done in routines, a yoga class typically lasts 60 to 90 minutes and gives a complete full-body workout. Some personal yoga routines can be as short as 15 to 20 minutes. Beginning yoga classes are quite gentle. Advanced classes can be very strenuous. When done regularly, the postures create the flexibility, strength, and stability to allow you to sit calmly in one of several meditative poses, keeping the head, trunk, and spine aligned vertically for significant periods of time without distraction from an uncomfortable or fatigued body. Of course, this also creates general flexibility and good-quality movement patterns which are beneficial during all activities. Learning and using the many asanas is an interesting course in self-awareness, as you will learn your limitations and restrictions as well as your abilities and capabilities.

In addition to the postures, Hatha Yoga also teaches controlled breathing (pranayama). The controlled breathing patterns not only help to gain conscious control over the mind, but also the emotions. Some of the breathing exercises provide health benefits such as improved digestion, relaxation, and increased circulation and lung capacity.

Properly taught, yoga classes include relaxation techniques as part of their routines, usually at the end of the class. Yoga relaxation exercises help expand body awareness, reduce stress, improve sleep, and facilitate healing through visualization and the parasympathetic response. When you learn them well, you can share them with clients when appropriate.

Meditation is another yoga technique. Meditation helps focus and control the mind, turning its focus inward, away from the sensory bombardment of the external world toward the calm, peaceful awareness within. Meditation helps reduce stress, lower blood pressure, and has many other positive physical benefits as well as potential spiritual benefits. If you are interested in yoga and how it can benefit you, find a good yoga instructor or center in your area that is certified or affiliated with Yoga Alliance or the Himalayan Institute Teachers Association (HITA).

Box 6-2

Personal Fitness Program

Don't procrastinate! Begin a personal fitness program today. Although it is beyond the scope of this book to give detailed exercise programs, below is a basic plan to get you started. Of course, check with your physician before beginning any exercise program.

A. Gain Flexibility

1. Active Isolated Stretching—Mattes Method: see Chapter 8 for application of this method to the upper body. Lower body stretches and strengthening methods are available in books and videos by Aaron Mattes and by this author. Forearm, wrist, and hand stretches should be done every day, before and after doing massage.

2. Yoga: a great system for massage therapists, which combines static stretching, breathing, and relaxation techniques. Yoga classes are also a great place to meet new clients.

B. Build Strength

1. Weight training
2. Elastic band and tubing systems: light, simple, inexpensive, and easy to use; they usually include good, full-body strengthening workout instructions for no extra charge.
3. Exercise balls: can provide good workouts that emphasize core strength (low back and abdomen).

C. Build Stamina

1. Brisk walking: 20 minutes or more each day
2. Aerobic sports: bicycling, swimming, running, racquet sports, etc.
3. Aerobic classes

4. Aerobic gym equipment: treadmills, bicycles, etc.
5. Rebounding

D. Build Balance

1. Yoga
2. Pilates
3. Tai Chi
4. Balance boards
5. Posture Correction: most people are internally rotated at the shoulders, with head bent forward and lower chest collapsed ("slouched") into the abdomen. Neuromuscular therapy, Rolfing, and other posture and movement corrective systems can help improve posture. Lengthen shortened muscles using Active Isolated Stretching—Mattes Method and strengthen long and/or weak muscles using weights or resistance.
6. Foot strengthening and stabilization: you need stable feet and ankles when practicing. This protects your knees, hips, and even your low back. Get orthotics if you overpronate or oversupinate until you can strengthen your feet with exercises. If you have lax or weak ligaments in your feet or ankles you may need orthotics permanently.
7. Proper shoe selection: wear supportive, shock-absorbing shoes when doing massage. High-quality walking shoes are recommended.
8. Treatment of structural misalignments: chiropractic or manipulative osteopathy can be helpful in restoring joint alignment and movement.

---

bit tired is normal, but physical fatigue is a sign of lack of endurance. Begin a walking program, take aerobic classes, ride a bicycle (stationary or on the road), run, or engage in other aerobic activities that will help build up your endurance to support your level of work comfortably. Box 6-2 provides some suggestions for putting together a personal fitness plan.

Again, seated massage is repetitive, strenuous work. Think of yourself as a "massage athlete" and realize that you must train (work out) regularly to develop and maintain the strength, flexibility, and endurance required to perform massage all day, day after day, without injury.

CASE STUDY

Effects of Poor Body Mechanics

A massage therapist comes to you for a massage at your kiosk at the shopping mall. She has been practicing table massage for about a year, initially doing about 10 hours of massage a week. She attended a continuing education program two months ago on how to treat the cervical region. Since then, her practice has grown dramatically and she is now doing 20 hours of massage a week. However, in the last two weeks she has started to have thumb pain, wrist pain, and upper thoracic pain.

1. What might be a significant contributing factor to her pain complaints?
2. Besides recommending that she see you for massage and stretching on a regular basis, what else can you do to help her?
3. What things should you look for while observing another therapist perform massage to determine whether they are using proper body mechanics?
4. Practice tactfully making suggestions to a colleague regarding their body mechanics, or lack of them.

chronic and possibly career-ending. Massage, stretching, ice, rest, and behavior modification are all important treatments for RSI.

Because massage is strenuous, repetitive activity, you should engage in a regular stretching and strengthening program. You need enough strength and stamina to easily handle your daily work load and to have some reserve capacity. You should stretch your hands, arms, and shoulders before and after you work each day, whereas strength and endurance training should be done several times each week.

Your ability to sustain a long career in massage therapy is dependent on your willingness to develop proper working habits and maintain your body's fitness to perform massage. You must take care of yourself so you can take care of others.

SUMMARY

Chair massage is a very repetitive activity that puts significant stress on the entire body. Body mechanics allows you to use your body in the most efficient way possible, minimize your chance of massage-related injury, and improve the feel of the massage to the client.

Proper posture is when the body is aligned on the mid-sagittal and coronal planes with the hands at the side of the thighs, thumb side of the hand facing forward. Poor posture contributes to pain and injury. Work to correct or maintain your own proper posture and also educate clients about theirs. The primary working postures for seated massage are the lunge stance and the straight stance. The lunge stance should be used most of the time when performing seated massage.

Repetitive Strain Injuries (RSI) occur from submaximal, repeated motions. These injuries are painful and, if not treated at onset, can become

REFERENCES

1. Mochizuki S. *Hand Maintenance Guide for Massage Therapists.* Boulder, CO: Kotobuki Publications, 1999.
2. Sivasankar M, Fisher KV. Oral breathing increases breath and vocal effort by superficial drying of vocal fold mucosa. *J Voice* 2002;16(2):172–181.
3. Kanehira T, Takehara J, Takahashi D, et al. Prevalence of oral malorder and the relationship with habitual mouth breathing in children. *J Clin Pediatr Dent* 2004;28(4):285–288.
4. Swami R, Ballantine R, Hymes A. *Science of Breath.* Honesdale, PA: Himalayan International Institute of Yoga Science and Philosophy of the U.S.A., 1988.
5. http://www.aaos.org/wordhtml/research/comittee/research/rsrch_5c.htm. Accessed April 13, 2005. http://orthoinfo.aaos.org/main.cfm
6. Lowe WW. *Orthopedic & Sports Massage Reviews*, issue no. 12. Corvallis, OR: Pacific Orthopedic Massage, 1996:35.
7. Kahn KM, Cook JL, Bonar F, et al. Histopathology of common tendinopathies—Update and implications for clinical management. *Sport Med* 1999;27(6):393–408.
8. Almekinders LC. Anti-inflammatory treatment of muscular injuries in sport—An update of recent studies. *Sport Med* 1999; 28(6):383–388.
9. Lowe WW. *Orthopedic & Sports Massage Reviews*, issue no. 38. Corvallis, OR: Pacific Orthopedic Massage, Jan/Feb, 2001.

Notes

CHAPTER 7

Strokes

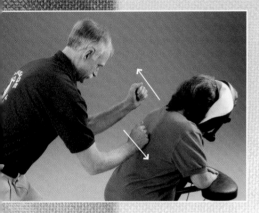

"If you're going to be a healer, it's not enough to read books and learn allegorical stories. You need to get your feet wet, get some clinical experience under your belt."

DIANE FROLOV AND ANDREW SCHNEIDER,
***NORTHERN EXPOSURE, HEAL THYSELF* (1993)**

Objectives

▪ Explain the two primary stimuli that massage can provide to the nervous system.

▪ List the eight strokes used in seated massage.

▪ Associate each stroke with the stimulus it has on the nervous system.

▪ Select the stroke(s) appropriate for a selected client's needs and state the therapist's reason for choosing the stroke(s).

▪ Assemble a sequence of massage strokes to effectively sedate or invigorate a selected client.

Key Terms

Acetylcholine: a chemical normally present in many parts of the body, playing a role in vasodilation and in nerve impulse transmission from one nerve to another across the synaptic junction.

Bracing massage: a refreshing or invigorating massage, typically faster-paced.

Histamine: a powerful dilator of the capillaries.

Hyperemia: an excess of blood or increased circulation in tissue, increasing oxygen and nutrient delivery and improving waste removal.

Stimulus: any agent, act, or influence that produces a functional or tropic reaction in a receptor or a tissue.

Vasodilation: the widening or opening of a blood vessel.

As with table massage, seated massage involves the use of a few basic techniques or strokes. Although these strokes are known by different names and have been classified in different ways, the actual techniques themselves are practiced fairly consistently throughout the field of massage and bodywork. In this book, the strokes are identified by their traditional western names and grouped in eight categories: compression, effleurage, friction, nerve strokes, petrissage, sustained pressure, tapotement, and vibration. Given that you should already have a basic understanding of the massage strokes, the purpose of this chapter is to review the strokes and their physiological effects and to present specific applications of each to seated massage. Before turning to the strokes themselves, however, we shall consider the stimulating effect of massage strokes on the nervous system.

STIMULATING THE NERVOUS SYSTEM

Massage is a powerful **stimulus** to the nervous system. Since, in part, the nervous system is a stimulus-response mechanism, we can expect the stimulus of massage to a elicit a significant response. It is important to know what response you are trying to elicit in your clients and apply the appropriate stimulus.

Each stroke of massage provides a different stimulus to the nervous system and elicits a different response. The speed of a stroke can change the amount of effect it has, as can the pressure. To obtain a desired response, you must apply the correct stimulus, at the correct rate and level of pressure. Therefore, as the strokes are discussed, their effects on the nervous system are also explained. This is important in all forms of massage, but in seated massage it becomes extremely important because of the short session time. Seated massage therapists must be efficient and maximize their therapeutic impact by selecting and using appropriate techniques.

In this textbook, the term "stimulate" is used to indicate the application of any technique to a client. There are two primary types of stimulus in massage: invigorating and sedating. "Invigorating" describes a massage technique that intensifies nervous system activity and brings alertness. The definition of invigorate is: "To fill something with energy or life." A sedating stimulus is one that brings about a state of restfulness, calm, or drowsiness, so a relaxation massage is one that is sedating, quieting, and soothing.

All massage strokes are divided into these two primary categories.

Relaxation, the most common response desired from massage, requires a stimulus that is sedating to the nervous system. However, in many cases, it is appropriate to invigorate the client by giving him a more **bracing massage**. This would be appropriate in pre-event sports massage and for someone who is returning to an intense job or activity immediately following the massage.

Combining both invigorating and sedating strokes in a massage routine can create an effect somewhere between the two extremes. A great state to leave a client in after a seated massage is a state of relaxed alertness. Research by Dr. Tiffany Field and the Touch Research Institute, University of Miami, has proven that this is possible to accomplish (1).

By studying each stroke and understanding what response it will elicit, you can create a massage that best fits the needs of the specific individual you are working on. This makes you a more effective therapist with a higher likelihood of becoming successful.

COMPRESSION

Compression is a rhythmic, pumping technique that is applied to a muscle belly or tendon by the palm of the hand, heel of the hand, or loosely clenched fist. See Figure 7-1A–D for examples of compression.

This stroke causes a sustained increase in blood flow at the capillary level for several hours by causing the release of **histamines** and **acetylcholine**, both of which cause **vasodilation**, which is the widening of the blood vessels. For the massage therapist, creating a general state of increased blood flow (called **hyperemia**) in the muscles makes it easier to treat localized areas of tenderness and trigger points.

The client's nervous system perceives compression as an invigorating stimulus. Compression is warming due to the increased blood movement it causes. In terms of technique, the pumping action is always directed toward an underlying bone. This spreads the muscle fibers and squeezes blood out of them as they are compressed between the bones of the therapist's hand and the bones of the client, similar to water being squeezed from a sponge. As the compression is released, fresh, oxygenated blood rushes back in and displaces and dilutes pain-inducing substances which may be present (2,3).

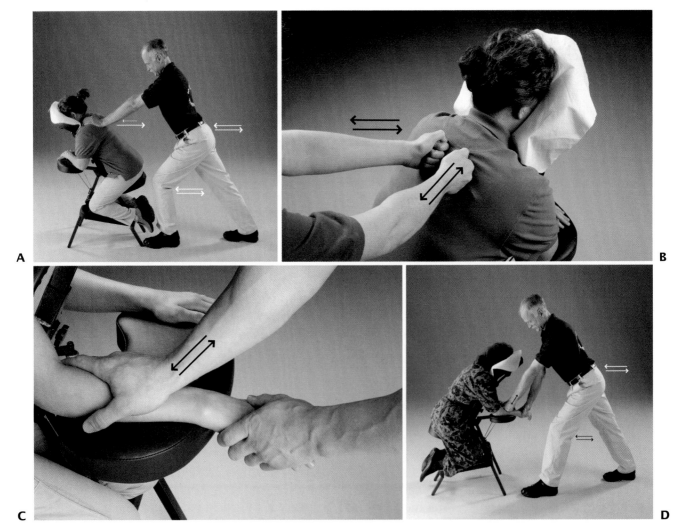

Figure 7–1 Compression. (A) Palms of hands on paraspinal muscles. **(B)** Loosely clinched fists on paraspinal muscles. **(C)** Heel of hand on forearm. **(D)** Loosely clinched fists on forearm.

Compression Stroke

Stand in the lunge position (sometimes called the bow or archer stance) alongside a massage table or padded piece of furniture that is not quite waist-high. With the arm closest to the table held straight but not quite locked at the elbow, and with the wrist bent at about 45 degrees if using the palm or straight if using a loosely clinched fist, press into the padded material. Your movement should be coming from your legs. As you compress, bend your front knee, and as you release, straighten your front knee. Your back should be straight, with virtually no flexion-extension movement occurring. Your shoulders should not be moving much, either. Keep your head up and level, looking down only with your eyes.

As your hand sinks in, feel the ever-increasing resistance until you just barely "hit bottom." As soon as you hit bottom, reverse and pull back out. Do not stop and hold at the bottom. The "end feel," where the hard structure stops your penetration, is similar to the end feel where the client's bone stops your penetration into the muscle tissue. You must reach this end feel for the stroke to be effective. You must spread or squeeze the fibers of her muscles between the bone of your hand and the bone under the muscle. "Take it to the bone" describes this technique very well.

Practice a rhythmic pumping on the table for a few dozen pumps. Get the feel for hitting bottom and bouncing off at various tempos. The stroke should be smooth, not jarring to the client. Compression should be firm, but not so hard as to be painful to the client.

To be thorough, compress each "handful" of tissue three times. This can be done by pumping three times in one spot and then moving, or by pumping one time in each spot until you have covered the entire area, and then repeating the whole sequence two times. To be effective, compress into the tissues until you just feel the "hard bottom" of the muscle tissue against the bone. Keep in mind that the faster the rhythmic pumping, the more invigorating the stroke becomes.

In seated massage settings in which a less invigorating effect is desired, compression is applied slowly, in the rhythm of the breath, or about one pump per second. This approach may be used on the paraspinal (erector spinae) muscles to begin a seated massage. This initiates touch with the client while warming and relaxing the large muscles along the spine. Compression is also used extensively in chair treatments as the warmup stroke on the flexor and extensor muscles of the forearms and the posterior and lateral shoulder muscles. This warms and prepares the tissues for strokes such as deep friction.

In pre- and post-event sports massage treatments, compression is used extensively to generate a sustained hyperemia. For pre-event sports massage or for a more bracing massage, do the compressions at the tempo of 2 to 3 pumps per second, to invigorate and "pump up" the athlete. The hyperemia helps provide nourishment to the muscle cells well into the event. Compression is done slower in post-event treatments to be more relaxing and soothing to the athlete while creating a sustained hyperemia to assist in the removal of muscle waste products.

CONTRAINDICATION

COMPRESSION

Compression is contraindicated over the following:
- Bony prominences
- Joints
- Abdominal wall muscles
- Quadratus lumborum
- External oblique
- Internal oblique
- Rectus abdominis

These are very logical contraindications if you think about them. Bony prominences, like the acromion process, the posterior superior iliac spine (PSIS), spinous processes of the vertebrae, the epicondyles of the elbow, etc., have no muscle tissue directly over them to compress. It is very uncomfortable for the client if you compress on the bony spots. In fact, it could cause a significantly painful injury by bruising the superficial tissue and possibly subluxating or dislocating a bone. In the case of joints, compression right over the joint will create a strong shearing force on the joint capsule which could injure ligaments or cartilage. In the abdominal wall, beneath the muscles mentioned above, the only bone is the spinal column. Between the spine and the muscles mentioned are the abdominal organs (viscera). Thus, it could cause a life-threatening injury to apply the compression stroke to the abdominal tissues and organs. Furthermore, compression on the quadratus lumborum can cause injury to the small twelfth rib, possibly breaking it, and can bruise the muscle attachments on the rather sharp transverse processes.

Use the compression stroke only where it is appropriate—over muscle belly and tendon tissues only. Never use it directly over bony prominences, joints, or the unsupported tissues of the abdominal wall.

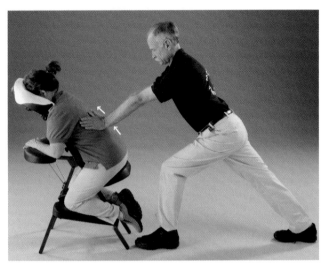

Figure 7–2 Effleurage. Using both hands, moving up the back.

EFFLEURAGE

Effleurage is a smooth, even, sliding/gliding stroke performed through the client's clothes or directly on the skin using the fingertips, thumb, or the entire hand. Pressure is usually constant throughout the entire length of the stroke, but may be increased or decreased on successive strokes. The most sedating stroke in all of massage, it is usually done parallel to the superficial muscle fibers and/or toward the heart (proximally/medially/centripetally). The direction of movement is especially important in the extremities because of the somewhat fragile venous valves, which resist distal blood flow. In seated massage, the direction of the effleurage stroke on the back is not significant.

In general massage applications, effleurage can be used to induce relaxation or to smooth a tender area before, but most often after, deep work. Effleurage is also effective in reducing fluid congestion. Moderate pressure strokes tend to move venous fluids, whereas light strokes tend to move lymphatic fluids. Deep strokes are used for affecting muscle tissue.

Effleurage, particularly the deep strokes, is not used extensively in seated massage because it is not as effective without lubrication or over clothing as it is directly on the skin. Traditionally, lubrication is not used in seated massage, even on areas of exposed skin such as the arms, neck, and face. Of course exceptions can be made, but you must be careful not to get any lubricant on the client's clothing, the chair surfaces, or the floor, or to alter the client's makeup without permission.

When effleurage is used in seated massage, it is mostly used as a soothing, finishing stroke to conclude working on a particular area or as part of the conclusion of the entire treatment (Fig. 7-2). Sometimes, it can be beneficial to glide over an area to help move edema. Edema and lymph fluids move with just ounces of pressure, so effleurage can be effective through clothes or on the skin without lubrication. Effleurage is an appropriate stroke to use when the client is too sensitive to receive strokes that penetrate deeper, such as compression and friction. Because of the light pressure and generally non-specific way effleurage is used in seated massage, at least in this text, there are no specific contraindications for this stroke other than to avoid moving distally on the forearms. Of course, the standard contraindications for massage in general always apply.

EXPERIENTIAL EXERCISE

Effleurage Stroke

To experience effleurage yourself, try this exercise. Sit down and place an exposed forearm across your legs, palm down. Grasp the "top" side of the forearm just above the wrist with your other hand and glide from wrist to elbow. Vary the degree of grasping pressure and downward pressure. If both your hand and forearm are dry, you should be able to slide quite comfortably. If either are slightly sweaty, there will be quite a bit of drag (especially if hair is present), and this would be quite uncomfortable. Either dry your hand and forearm or add some lubrication for this exercise.

Also try effleurage with your fingertips and then with one thumb. Now perform the same exercise on the other forearm with the arm covered with your shirt sleeve. Notice the difference in feeling and effect between the covered and uncovered arm. The stroke can still be quite effective through the clothes; however, you are limited to the amount of pressure you can apply without bunching up or damaging the clothing. Always be respectful of this limit.

In seated massage, effleurage is usually done through the clothes, but can be performed on exposed areas such as the arm, hand, neck, or face. If working on the face, be careful not to smear the client's makeup.

FRICTION

Friction comes from the Latin *frictio*, meaning "to rub." Used to warm the tissues for palpation and examination and for treatment, friction techniques are powerful tools for affecting the body. These strokes are used extensively in seated massage. There are two primary types of friction strokes: superficial and deep. Superficial friction and deep friction do not refer to the amount of pressure used, but to the layers of tissue affected by the stroke. Superficial friction primarily affects the skin and superficial fascia, whereas deep friction primarily affects the muscle layers.

Superficial Friction

Superficial friction, also called "general friction" or "palmar friction," is an invigorating stroke to the nervous system. Its primary effect is to produce heat in the skin and superficial layers of fascia and muscle. This improves cutaneous circulation and makes the fascia more pliable. This stroke is done by sliding the hands back and forth rapidly, usually in an alternating pattern, until heat is felt in the tissues. It may be performed using the palmar side of the hand flat on the tissues, as shown in Figure 7-3, or by using the ulnar side (knife edge) of the hand, as shown in Figure 7-4. The ulnar edges of the hand are particularly effective in applying superficial friction to the trapezius

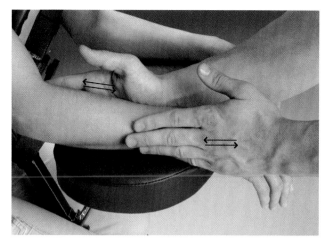

Figure 7-3 Superficial friction. Using the palms of the hands to warm the tissues of the forearm, with rapid strokes sliding from wrist to elbow and back with moderate to light pressure.

muscles and the upper paraspinals. The palms are used to treat the arms, shoulders, and back.

While not as effective through the clothes as it is directly on the skin, this technique is still useful in seated massage. It is used in pre-event sports massage as part of a more bracing (invigorating) treatment, or whenever heat is desired in the superficial tissues. Unless you are working in a very cold environment, if a client reports he is cold during a massage, superficial friction and compression will quickly warm him up.

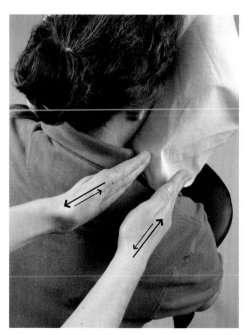

Figure 7-4 Superficial friction. Using ulnar edges of hands on upper trapezius muscles in an alternating, "sawing" motion.

Superficial Friction

Sit in a chair with one forearm across your lap, palm down, as in the effleurage exercise. Using the palm of your other hand, slide rapidly from wrist to elbow and back repeatedly, using a light to moderate pressure. Notice the heat that is generated in the skin.

Using the ulnar (little finger) side of one hand, rapidly rub your opposite upper trapezius muscle (top of your shoulder) in an anterior to posterior direction (forward-backward sliding over your skin or clothes). Again, feel the heat being generated by the friction between your hand and the clothes and skin over the shoulder.

Superficial friction is a great way to warm up the superficial tissues quickly. It is also an invigorating stimulus to the nervous system.

Deep Friction

Deep friction does not mean hard, intense pressure; actually, it can be done very lightly. Deep friction is a sedating stimulus that treats the deeper, myofascial and periostial layers of tissue as opposed to the superficial fascia and skin. It can be performed with the entire hand, the palm, a loose fist, fingertips, the thumb, forearm, or elbow.

When using this stroke, apply enough pressure to engage the clothes and skin, and then add movement to shift the skin back and forth over the deeper muscle layers. This can be done with ounces of pressure, just enough to engage and shift the skin, or with several pounds of pressure, to get to the deepest layers. Never go beyond the client's ability to tolerate pressure without tensing up. The tempo is usually moderate. Slow tempos are more sedating, whereas fast tempos are less sedating.

Generating Heat

Deep friction at fast tempos using light to moderate pressure can be used to generate significant heat in the deeper myofascial layers and around joints. This is done extensively in pre-event sports massage applications.

Deep friction is used first as an examination tool to palpate the tissues in search of tender points (TePs), trigger points (TrPs), tight bands of tissue, and bony landmarks, and to assess the client's sensitivity. This examination phase is done using a light to moderate pressure, shifting the skin over the muscles while gradually working deeper into the tissues. This warms the tissues as you examine them. You have found abnormal tissue when the client reports sensitivity (tenderness) at normal massage pressure. Healthy, normal tissue is not tender to the touch at moderate to firm pressure. Abnormal tissue is usually contracted and feels tighter, denser, harder, or thicker. Sometimes it feels like a tight band running through the tissues. This often indicates a trigger point that sometimes exists as small, taut, palatable band. Scar tissue, which forms to heal injuries and surgeries, is often adhered to surrounding tissues and restricts the mobility of the tissues so they feel stiff or have less mobility than surrounding tissues. The deep friction stroke helps new scar tissue form in a more organized manner, with fewer unwanted adhesions to surrounding tissues and structures. Deep friction can also mobilize old scar tissues and break unwanted adhesions. Tender tissues are ischemic. This ischemia needs to be reduced by relaxing the muscle and restoring blood flow. Deep friction can be used as a palpatory technique to find abnormal, ischemic tissues.

When abnormal tissues are found, deep friction can be used as a treatment technique. Start lightly, or at the examination pressure where the client reported the tenderness. Gradually work deeper into the tissue by applying more pressure as the tissue warms up and relaxes from the movement. Since it is often difficult to feel this warming through the clothes, a good guideline is to perform five to seven strokes, then increase your pressure. Do another five to seven strokes and increase pressure again. Another method is to perform the deep friction stroke until the client tells you the spot feels better, then increase pressure, melting your way into the tissue. The client's feedback, not the amount of pressure you apply, is the relevant indicator. If the client reports significant sensitivity, 5 to 7 on a 10-point scale or 3 to 4 on a 5-point scale, but is below the threshold at which the client begins to tense up, and the tissue is relaxing as you treat it (becoming less tender), your pressure is appropriate. If the client reports pain, is tensing up, or the tissue is not relaxing, you are working too hard; lighten up! Do not work any point for more than 25 seconds at once or the client will likely be quite sore the next day. If the tissue has not relaxed within 25 seconds, release your pressure and move on to the next area, letting the tissue "rebound." Return to the stubborn area again after a minute or so and repeat the procedure for another 25 seconds. Return again for a third time if necessary. If after a third application of friction the tissue has not changed for the better (become less tender), do not treat it further with friction. Use another stroke, try stretching, or move on, treating surrounding tissues and tissues on the other side of the joint (antagonists). Deep friction is often alternated with sustained pressure to treat TePs and TrPs. (See the section on "Sustained Pressure" below.)

CLINICAL TIP

Combining Strokes

Sustained pressure is usually alternated with deep friction to treat TePs and TrPs. You find abnormal tissue with deep friction and treat it with sustained pressure.

There are three main types of deep friction strokes: deep longitudinal, deep circular, and deep cross-fiber friction.

Deep Longitudinal Friction

Deep longitudinal friction moves the superficial layers of tissue over the deep layers in directions that are parallel to the deep fiber (Fig. 7-5). On the

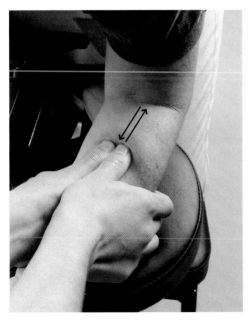

Figure 7–5 Longitudinal deep friction. Using both thumbs to apply longitudinal friction to the forearm.

paraspinal muscles, this would be superior to inferior direction. Because the stroke moves parallel to the muscle(s) being treated, longitudinal is the least invasive form of deep friction and can be used when other forms are too painful. Longitudinal deep friction lets you penetrate the muscle more easily because of its movement is parallel to the muscle fibers. Done at equal pressure over the same tender tissue, longitudinal friction is the least painful of the three types of friction. It is best used when circular and cross-fiber cause too much discomfort. Longitudinal friction can be used over recent injuries, as sensitivity of the client allows, before the other versions of deep friction can be tolerated by the client.

Deep Circular Friction

Deep circular friction engages the tissues and moves them in a circular motion, either clockwise or counterclockwise (Fig. 7-6A). Overlapping circular deep friction around a trigger point is very effective at reducing the TrP. Visualize that you are pulling the taut fibers apart a layer at a time as you work all around the TrP (Fig. 7-6B). Circular friction can also be used on tender points in the same manner. Another application of deep circular friction is to create heat deep in the tissues. An example of this is to place one of your hands on the front of the client's shoulder joint and the other hand on the posterior side. Using a moderate pressure and speed, press toward the joint with both hands and shift the tissue in circles until the client reports that he feels warmth in the joint. This is an excellent warmup procedure for pre-event sports massage as well as a great way to warm a joint before examination and treatment. It can also be used as a finishing stroke to leave the joint warm after treatment.

CLINICAL TIP

Clockwise or Counterclockwise Circles?

Some Asian bodywork philosophers believe that a counterclockwise circular movement loosens, de-tonifies, and sedates the tissue while a clockwise circular motion tightens, tonifies, and strengthens tissues. Be observant and notice what results you get from each direction.

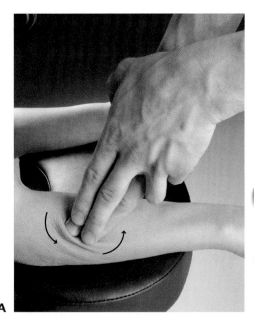

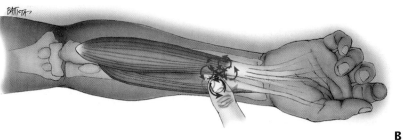

Figure 7–6 Deep circular friction. (A) Using braced fingertips on forearm. **(B)** Treating a trigger point with overlapping applications of deep circular friction.

A

B

Deep circular friction over tender tissue will cause more discomfort to the client than longitudinal friction, but less than cross-fiber at comparable pressure. It is a more powerful stroke, causing more movement in the deeper layers of tissues, and should only be used when the client's sensitivity in the area allows it to be done within his pain tolerance.

Deep Cross-fiber Friction

Deep cross-fiber friction, also called "deep transverse friction," engages the tissues and moves them back and forth across, or perpendicular to, the deeper fibers. On the paraspinal muscles this would be a medial to lateral movement. This is the most powerful form of deep friction. However, at the same pressure on the same tissue, it will be the most uncomfortable for the client. It is very effective in treating scar tissue from old or recent injuries.

There are two ways to perform deep cross-fiber friction. One way is to stroke back and forth over the tissues with equal pressure in each direction, like a windshield wiper (Fig. 7-7A). The other is to stroke

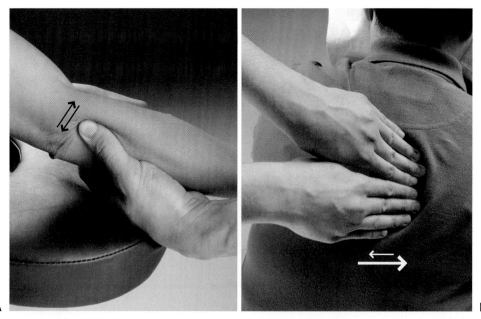

A

B

Figure 7–7 Deep cross-fiber friction. (A) Using the thumb to treat tendons just distal to the lateral epicondyle of the humerus, moving back and forth like a windshield wiper. **(B)** Using fingertips to stroke in one direction, ("strumming") laterally, on the paraspinal muscles.

across the tissue in one direction, such as medial to lateral, then reset and again stroke lateral, strumming or plucking the tissues. This is sometimes called "flat palpation" and is very effective in finding trigger points (Fig. 7-7B).

Both techniques are effective and provide similar results. Some clients respond better to the windshield wiper-like motion, whereas others prefer the strumming motion. Whatever technique is the most effective for the therapist and the client is the one that should be used.

Deep cross-fiber friction can be done with a light to moderate pressure as a palpatory stroke to examine tissues. When using this stroke for examinations, start lightly and work your way into the tissue as it warms up and relaxes. The stroke can also be performed at moderate to firm pressures, within the client's pain tolerance, for therapeutic work.

CONTRAINDICATION

FRICTION

Friction is contraindicated for the following:

- Superficial friction has no stroke-specific contraindications in seated massage; however, the general contraindications for massage apply.
- Clients with multiple sclerosis, due to the nerve damage caused by the disease, do not respond well to superficial applications of heat. Therefore, superficial friction should not be used on these clients.
- Deep friction should never be done over blood vessels that are large enough that a pulse can be felt when they are palpated.
- Deep friction is also contraindicated near significant-sized nerves. You will know you are on such a nerve when the client reports an electric, tingling sensation usually radiating inferior or distal from where you are working. The sensation is quite intense for the client and she will usually jump or recoil.
- Deep friction should be avoided or at least done lightly and sparingly on clients taking blood thinners, anticoagulants, and pain medications, as bruising can result.
- It is also contraindicated near acute inflammation or within 72 hours of a significant injury.

EXPERIENTIAL EXERCISE

Deep Friction

Exercise 1: The Effectiveness of Deep Friction

To experience the effectiveness of deep friction, try the following exercise. Using the fingertips of one hand, palpate the brachioradialis muscle of your other forearm. Starting about 4 to 5 inches distal to (below) your elbow, press into the tissues with a few ounces of pressure and move the skin distal to proximal (elbow to wrist) parallel to the fibers of the muscle. This is longitudinal deep friction. Move as far as the skin will let you go without your fingers sliding over the skin. Notice how this feels.

Now move one inch closer to the elbow. Engage the skin, using the same pressure as before, but this time slide the skin around in a circular motion. You are now doing circular deep friction. Make as big of a circle as the skin will let you without sliding over the skin. Notice how this feels. Most people report that this feels like they are working deeper with the same amount of pressure. This is a more powerful way to perform deep friction, but it is more invasive, as it feels deeper with the same pressure.

Move another inch closer to your elbow. Engage the skin, again being careful to use the same pressure as before. This time shift the skin back and forth across the muscle, moving lateral to medial or perpendicular to the fibers. Move back and forth across the muscle with equal pressure in each direction, like a windshield wiper. Notice how this feels. You are now performing cross-fiber deep friction (or deep cross-fiber friction). Most people report that this feels even more powerful than circular deep friction. Typically it feels more invasive, or as if you are working deeper at the same pressure.

A variation of cross-fiber deep friction is to stroke in only one direction. Engage the tissue and slide it from medial to lateral across the brachioradialis. Then, lightening up on your pressure until you are just barely touching the skin, move back to the starting point, engage again, and repeat the slide. You are strumming the muscle in one direction only. Notice how this feels compared with the "windshield wiper" method.

Now switch arms and, in the upper part of the brachioradialis, repeat the four techniques right in a row on the same spot, using the same amount of pressure. Do four or five strokes of longitudinal, then four or five circles of circular, then four or five strokes of cross-fiber in both directions, and, finally, cross-fiber in only one direction.

Exercise 2: Creating Heat in Joints with Deep Friction

To experience the heat generation potential of deep friction, place the palm of one hand on the front of the opposite shoulder. Apply a light to moderate pressure, enough so your hand does not slide on the clothing or skin. Now move the tissues lateral and medial very rapidly, 5 to 6 cycles per second. Notice the warmth created deep in the shoulder tissues. This is usually a very pleasant experience and is beneficial to the joint tissues. Now try a similar technique on your own knee. Put one hand on each side of one of your knees. Press hard enough to prevent sliding on your skin or clothes. Move your hands distal to proximal or in circles very rapidly. Feel the heat building up in the knee joint. This warms all the way to the ligaments and periosteum. In seated massage, this two-handed technique works great on the shoulder joint and elbow joint.

Exercise 3: Deep Friction as a Palpatory Technique

To gain an appreciation for the power of deep friction as a palpatory technique, try the following exercise. Roll up the shirt sleeve of your non-dominant forearm and slide the fingertips of your dominant hand back and forth across the skin of the forearm in a lateral to medial direction. Try to feel the deeper layers of tissues as you slide across the skin. Now engage the skin using a light to moderate pressure and shift it back and forth across the deeper layers. First you were sliding over the skin (effleurage), and now you are sliding the skin itself over the deeper layers (deep friction). Notice what you can feel using this technique. Most people report dramatically increased perception of the layers, bands of muscles, and textures of the tissues when using deep friction. This is the most powerful palpatory stroke we have with which to examine tissue; it can be used to identify abnormal (ischemic) areas. Thus this stroke, used as an examination technique, is an important tool in therapeutic massage.

SUSTAINED PRESSURE

Sustained pressure is also called ischemic compression, direct pressure, digital pressure, static pressure, acupressure, inhibition, and trigger point pressure release. This technique involves pressing on a specific spot on the body and holding the pressure for a period of time, usually for 8 to 12 seconds. Typically this is done with a thumb or finger (hence the term "digital pressure"). However, it can be done with the elbow, forearm, heel of hand, loosely clenched fist, or a massage tool (Fig. 7-8).

The pressure is directed toward an underlying bone and applied and released slowly, so the client is not jarred, poked, or startled. This action squeezes fluids out of the immediate area, causing a temporary ischemia (hence the term "ischemic compression"), and spreads fibers. The body reacts to this stroke by sending more blood to the area, causing a reactive

Figure 7–8   Sustained pressure. (A) Using thumb to apply sustained pressure to the quadratus lumborum muscle in the low back. Note proper alignment of thumb and wrist joints. **(B)** Using braced fingertips to apply sustained pressure to the lateral erector spinae in the low back. Note correct posture using "stacked" (aligned) joints of fingers and wrists. **(C)** Using elbow to apply sustained pressure to the left rhomboid. "Guide" elbow with other hand. **(D)** Using forearm to apply sustained pressure on "top" of shoulder, treating upper trapezius. Note good therapist posture. Generate pressure by flexing front knee. **(E)** Using heel of hand to apply sustained pressure to flexor muscles of forearm. Note incorrect posture: wrist is more than 45 degrees extended while focusing pressure through heel of hand. Also note incorrect tense hand: fingers are flexing and not conforming to tissues of forearm. This is a common mistake that is less comfortable for the client and stressful on the therapist's wrist. **(F)** Applying sustained pressure to flexors of forearm using loosely clinched fist. Note correct wrist posture. **(G)** Using a massage tool to apply sustained pressure to the left rhomboid. (AcuForce 2.5® tool courtesy of Scrip Massage Supply, Peoria, IL. www.scrip-inc.com)

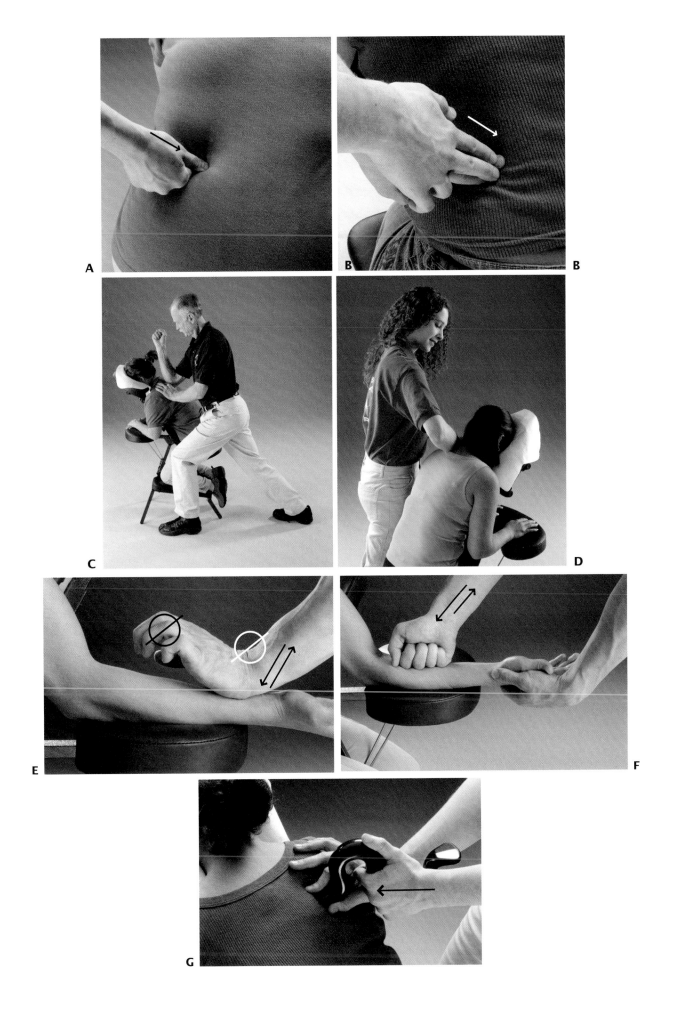

A

B

B

C

D

E

F

G

hyperemia as pressure is released. This brings oxygen and nutrients to the compressed area and flushes out metabolic waste products. The slight stretching of the muscle or tendon that occurs as pressure is applied elicits an inhibition response from the golgi tendon organ, facilitating relaxation of the treated area (4).

Sustained pressure is used to treat tender points and trigger points. Sustained pressure can also be used to hold a point while shortening or lengthening a muscle, either passively or actively. Effective pressure is usually firm, but should never cause the client to tense up or pull away.

CONTRAINDICATION

SUSTAINED PRESSURE

Sustained pressure is contraindicated for the following:

- To a pulse or to a significant nerve.
- For clients on blood thinners or anticoagulants or who have a history of bruising easily.
- Over acutely inflamed areas or on injuries sustained in the last 72 hours.

Duration of Sustained Pressure

Practitioners of different modalities of massage and bodywork disagree about how long to maintain sustained pressure in one spot. Some recommend a time period as short as three seconds, whereas others recommend as long as two minutes. Various times have probably developed from different philosophies and goals. For example, to affect energy flow in a meridian by pressing on an acupressure point will not require the same time it takes to elicit a relaxation response in a muscle. This text focuses on affecting the nervous system and the myofascial tissues, specifically. You will learn how to examine tissues, attempting to locate abnormal areas of tissue (tender points and trigger points) that cause pain and dysfunction and restrict movement. You will also learn to eliminate (or at least reduce) these areas, thus providing the client more normal movement. And relief from her pain.

With these goals in mind, it has been found by this author and others that a time of 8 to 12 seconds is the most effective stimulus. Compressing tissues for longer periods of time than this with heavy pressure

can cause a temporary reduction of pain. It creates a local anesthetic effect in the tissues, likely from endorphin release and fatigue of nerve receptors. This reduction of pain will last for about one hour, but usually results in subsequent increases in pain and irritation. According to Paul St. John (5), clients often report increased pain and decreased mobility the day following a treatment with heavy sustained pressure held for long periods of time (over 15 seconds). This result is obviously undesirable. To maximize effectiveness and minimize client discomfort, maintain sustained pressure on tender points and trigger points for 8 to 12 seconds. This is typically long enough to cause a therapeutic stimulus from which the body should respond and relax the tissues. To the client, the relaxation response will feel as though you are letting up on your pressure, even though you are not. If a reduction in sensation does not occur in 8 to 12 seconds, you are working too hard, overstimulating the client, and causing her to tense up, not relax. Release your pressure, move on in your routine, and come back to the spot in 30 to 60 seconds with less pressure. If the relaxation occurs in less than 8 seconds, you could apply more pressure, accessing deeper layers of tissue, until the time for the relaxation is in the 8 to 12 second range. This approach will allow you to treat clients effectively and they will experience minimal post-treatment soreness.

A modification of this technique can be done by compressing the tissue between your thumb and fingers in a pincer-like grip. This is still applying a sustained pressure and is very effective on the upper trapezius muscle and the axillary areas of pectoralis major, latissimus dorsi, teres major, and teres minor. This will be shown in the routine chapters.

Trigger Points

Trigger points are most commonly treated using pure sustained pressure, called ischemic compression in trigger point literature. However, in recent years authors have been introducing modified versions of sustained pressure, often combining pressure with subtle movement or varying pressure. These techniques are used specifically for treating trigger points and include variable ischemic compression and trigger point pressure release.

Variable Ischemic Compression

Sometimes trigger points do not respond to pure sustained pressure. Chiatow and Delany-Walker (4) present this technique, which involves cycles of alternating pressure in which sustained pressure hard enough to elicit pain but not so hard as to cause the client to tense up is held for 5 seconds, with the pressure then being eased for 2 to 3 seconds. This cycle is continued until the local or the referred pain diminishes or until 2 minutes have elapsed. If after 2 minutes of this cycle there is no change, move on. Examine surrounding tissues and apply a sedating stroke over the area, such as a few passes of light effleurage, slow vibration, or some gentle deep circular friction with your entire hand or fist. Allow the tissue to "rebound" and treat again, with less pressure.

CLINICAL TIP

Start Out Simple

Variable ischemic compression and trigger point pressure release are techniques that require strong palpatory skills. This is particularly true in seated massage, when the therapist is working through clothes. Until you have practiced extensively and developed a high degree of sensitivity, it is recommended that you use the 8 to 12 second method described initially. This will help minimize post-treatment soreness in your clients. As your skills evolve, begin integrating these additional techniques into your treatments.

Trigger Point Pressure Release

Travell and Simons, in their later writings, introduced a technique known as trigger point pressure release for the treatment of trigger points (6). To use this technique, begin by slowly applying pressure to a trigger point while sensing for resistance in the tissue. You should feel this resistance before pain is elicited. Once you do feel this barrier of resistance, hold steady pressure until you sense it releasing (softening), usually after a few seconds, then increase pressure until a new barrier is felt and then repeat this process until the trigger point tension and tenderness is eliminated.

Experiment and see which technique works best for you. Keep in mind that some clients may not respond to your favorite, so it is useful to learn more than one way to treat trigger points.

EXPERIENTIAL EXERCISE

Sustained Pressure

To experience sustained pressure and the relaxation response it evokes, try the following exercise. Find an area of tender tissue on your body that is fairly accessible. The brachioradialis muscle is a good one to try, if it is not already overtreated from previous experiential exercises. Find a tender point (TeP). As you exhale, take your thumb or finger(s) and press into the tender area. Press straight into the tissue, perpendicular (90 degrees) to the skin. Apply pressure until you experience a mild discomfort but not a level that is painful. Now, continue breathing and hold the point for 12 seconds. You should have the sensation that you are letting up on the pressure even though you are not. The discomfort should lessen. If the sensation of discomfort did not lessen, you are pressing too hard. Release the pressure, shake out your forearm (or whatever area you are using), wait a minute or two, and press on the same place again, this time using less pressure. You should perceive the relaxation response this time. If not, repeat again with even less pressure until you do experience some tenderness and then, in 8 to 12 seconds, a lessening of the tender sensation.

If the TeP responded and relaxed very rapidly (in under 8 seconds), it means that you could have been pressing harder, accessing deeper layers of the tissue. Of course, you do not have to press harder on a TeP that released rapidly, but you do have this option.

Another way to apply sustained pressure is by compressing the tissue between your thumb and fingers in a pincer-like grip. This method works very effectively on the upper trapezius muscle and in other areas where you can grasp the muscle effectively.

PETRISSAGE

Petrissage is grasping, kneading, and rolling tissues between the thumb and fingers, using one hand, both hands together, or with alternating hands. This technique lifts the tissues away from the bone or off the deeper tissues separating layers of tissues, thus enhancing tissue movement and blood flow. It is a mildly invigorating stroke to the nervous system; the faster you work, the more invigorating it becomes. Petrissage is also a warming stroke, generating heat in the tissues similar to the way deep friction does, but to a lesser degree. It is usually done across the fibers to improve fluid exchange in the treated tissues. In seated massage, petrissage is used on the upper and middle trapezius, anterior and posterior axillary areas, and the upper extremity (Fig. 7-9).

Petrissage can be used as a palpatory stroke for examination of the tissues and as a treatment technique for abnormal tissues. Sometimes this examination technique is called "pincer palpation." To apply this technique, grasp the tissues between the thumb and fingers of one or both of your hands and move your fingers and thumb side to side, feeling the layers of tissue between them. Start gently and work deeper and deeper into the tissues until you reach a normal massage pressure or until the client reports tenderness. If tenderness is reported, you can either stop and hold the pincer grip for 8 to 12 seconds ("pincer compression") or continue to knead the tissues at an acceptable level of discomfort until the sensitivity lessens or the density of the tissue is changed.

Another application of the stroke is to hold the thumb relatively still and flex the fingers, as if you were grasping a roll of nickels. Use this cross-fiber movement in the same way as described above for the side-to-side movement.

Petrissage is also a form of passive exercise that may be used for rehabilitation. To perform this application, lightly and gradually apply more pressure, working deeper into the tissue. After warming and examining the tissues with petrissage, if tenderness persists in the tissues, switch to sustained pressure. The traditional method of alternating hands in petrissage can be effectively used in seated massage on the upper extremity as well as the upper trapezius and deltoid muscles.

CONTRAINDICATION

PETRISSAGE

Petrissage is contraindicated for the following:
- Near a significant blood vessel. As you grasp the tissue and apply pressure, be sure to feel for any pulsing. If you feel a pulse in your grasp, release immediately and re-position. Never compress or massage tissue where you feel a pulse.
- Nerves

EXPERIENTIAL EXERCISE

Petrissage

To practice petrissage on yourself, sit erect and place your non-dominate hand on your ilium at the waistline. Reach across your chest with your dominate hand and grasp the pectoralis major muscle between your thumb and fingers. The pectoralis major is the muscle that makes up the anterior web of the armpit, and it is this web of tissue that is available to treat in seated massage. Compress the tissues gently between your thumb and fingers and begin moving the thumb and fingers back and forth, in and out, kneading the tissues. Gradually apply more pressure until you feel you are working at a sufficient pressure to

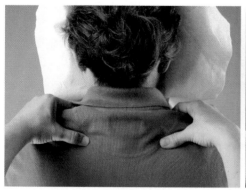
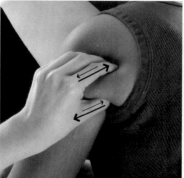
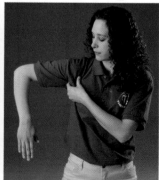

A,B **C**

Figure 7–9 **Petrissage. (A)** Kneading and rolling the upper trapezius fibers with petrissage, working both sides at once. **(B)** Using one hand to apply petrissage to latissimus dorsi, teres major, and teres minor with a pincer-like grip, kneading the tissues between the thumb and fingers. **(C)** Using petrissage on yourself to examine for trigger points and tender points in pectoralis major.

thoroughly examine the handful of tissue you are holding or until you elicit tenderness. If tenderness is found, stop the kneading movement and hold for 8 to 12 seconds. During this time, take a deep breath or two. You should experience a lessening of the tender sensation.

If no tenderness was found, or after it has been reduced, move your hand a few inches and examine another section of the muscle. Examine lateral to the humerus and medial to the chest. If you are female, do NOT compress and knead breast tissue, as you can damage it. It is common to find TrPs in the pectoralis major. They typically refer into the breast area and down the arm. If you notice referred sensations, stop and treat them just as you would a tender point, by holding a sustained pressure for 8 to 12 seconds. In seated massage, petrissage is usually applied to the pectoralis major, latissimus dorsi, teres major and minor, upper and mid-trapezius, biceps, and triceps.

TAPOTEMENT

Tapotement involves sharply striking the body in a rhythmic, typically rapid pattern with loose wrists and fingers. Sometimes categorized as a percussion technique, tapotement can be done with both hands at the same time or alternating hands in a one-two pattern (Fig. 7-10).

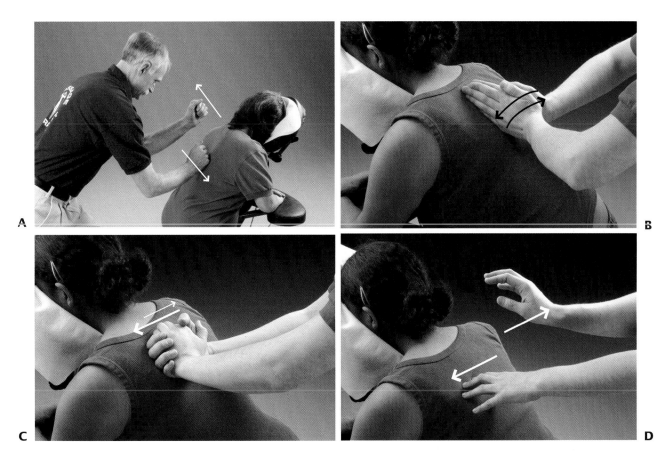

Figure 7–10 Tapotement. (A) Beating tapotement done with alternating hands to the upper back. Caution: do not strike on the spinous processes of the spine. **(B)** Hacking to upper back using both hands together. **(C)** Beating to upper back using clasped hands. **(D)** Tapping on the shoulders, using alternating hands. This is an excellent technique to use on the head, just be careful not to mess up the client's hair.

Tapotement is very stimulating to the nervous system. As you strike the muscle, a slight but very rapid stretch occurs. This rapid stretch causes the muscle spindle cells to fire, causing a momentary contraction of the muscle cells as a protective response to the rapid stretch. This warms the tissues by causing them to contract (work) slightly. In seated massage, tapotement is usually done with the fingertips (tapping), loosely clenched fists or clasped hands (beating), or the ulnar edge of a loosely held hand (hacking) (Fig. 7-10A–D).

Although tapotement can be done with the palms cupped (cupping) or flat (slapping), these techniques are generally not appropriate for seated massage. Cupping is a respiratory therapy technique that is very effectively used over the lungs; however, it has no significant effect on muscles. Therefore, only use it if your client has a respiratory condition. Likewise, slapping is generally not used in seated massage because it is not effective when done through the clothes.

Tapotement is typically used in seated massage as a finishing stroke to invigorate the client at the end of the treatment, or as part of a more bracing, energetic treatment when finishing each area and then again at the end. In sports applications, tapotement is used extensively for pre-event treatments. Tapotement should never be done in post-event sports massage treatments. The muscle spindle cell response described above can set off cramps in exhausted muscles. Also, due to the sensitivity from lactic acid buildup in the athlete's muscles during prolonged, strenuous activity, tapotement will be very uncomfortable, possibly quite painful. In post-event sports massage, it is generally best to use sedating strokes and tempos to spread fibers, move fluids, and relax and soothe the exhausted athlete.

CONTRAINDICATION

TAPOTEMENT

Tapotement is contraindicated for the following:

- Post-event sports massage.
- Over the lumbar region. This can be very painful for the client if they have exhausted adrenals, kidney problems, low back muscle spasms, or unstable lumbar discs.
- Over an area you have just treated for trigger points; tapotement can reactivate the trigger points. In this case, just use it on other muscles that did not have TrPs.
- For deep relaxation treatments, because it is too invigorating.
- On the spinous processes of the spine, or other bony prominences.

EXPERIENTIAL EXERCISE

Tapotement

Sit down and practice the different types of tapotement on your own anterior thigh. Notice the difference in penetration achieved with the different types: slapping and cupping, hacking, beating, and tapping. The objective is to impact the muscle enough to cause a slight reaction of the muscle spindle cell that causes a momentary contraction of the muscle fibers. Notice that cupping and slapping do not penetrate enough to accomplish this. Experience using both hands impacting at the same time. This slower version of tapotement, usually done as tapping or beating, can be slowed down to one strike per second.

VIBRATION

Vibration involves the use of shaking, jostling, trembling, oscillating, or rocking movements. This stroke can be done rapidly and vigorously or slowly and gently. Vibratory massage movements can be done fine and isolated, as with one finger on a spot trembling back and forth or moving straight in and out like a piston, or coarse and general, as in shaking a whole arm (Figs. 7-11 and 7-12).

Vibration is invigorating to the nervous system when done rapidly. It increases circulation in the affected area and relieves tension in joints. As the vibratory movements become slower, the invigorating effect is lost and the movement becomes sedating.

One vibratory method, "shaking," involves grasping a muscle such as the biceps with one hand and

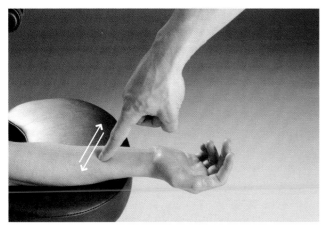

Figure 7-11 Fine vibration. Using one finger to apply fine vibration, "pointing" to the extensor muscles of forearm. Stroke is fairly light, straight in and out, as fast as possible.

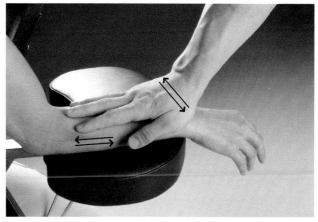

Figure 7-13 Shaking vibration. Applied to forearm extensor muscles by grasping muscle with entire hand and moving back and forth while moving proximal and distal.

shaking part or all of it. The hand can stay in one spot while shaking back and forth or move along the muscle (Fig. 7-13).

Rocking, a vibratory technique that is typically done slowly, causes a body part or area to gently rock back and forth, loosening the tissues and joints involved.

Rolling is a vibratory technique that is sometimes classified as a form of petrissage. The therapist's

hands grasp opposite sides of the muscle and move back and forth, rolling the muscle tissues around the underlying bone. Rolling is relaxing if done slowly, but becomes invigorating when done rapidly. In seated massage, rolling is used on the arm, from wrist to shoulder, as an opening or finishing technique, or for both (Fig. 7-14).

Jostling is an even more invigorating form of vibration than rapid rolling and shaking. This technique is done rapidly and vigorously, throwing

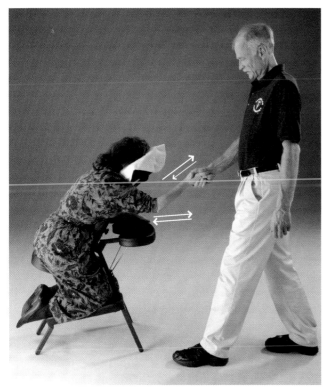

Figure 7-12 Shaking vibration. Shaking entire arm, with movement in all directions.

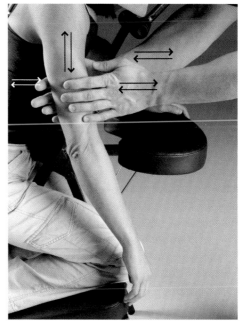

Figure 7-14 Vibration. Rolling vibration applied to arm, with hands moving back and forth, opposite each other, rolling the muscles around the bone.

the body part back and forth between your hands. Jostling is primarily utilized on the extremities. In seated massage, vibration is used primarily on the arms, but can also be used on other areas as appropriate for a particular client. Slower, gentle vibration is used in seated massage to relax tissues and joints. More vigorous forms of vibration are used to provide a more bracing treatment to leave the client in a more alert state when returning to work. Very rapid vibration is used extensively in pre-event sports massage treatments to prepare the athlete for competition.

Another interesting use of vibration is to combine a slow to moderate fine vibration (a trembling-type movement) with sustained pressure when treating tender points and trigger points. The vibration provides additional stimulation, which activates mechanoreceptors in the fascia; they respond to the vibration by increasing local proprioceptive attention. This seems to facilitate the nervous system's recognition of the pressure and results in quicker relaxation of the point (7).

CONTRAINDICATION

VIBRATION

Vibration is contraindicated for the following:

- Near or on an injured or degenerated joint.
- Vigorous vibration on clients with a history of strokes and blood clots. However, gentle, slow vibratory movements are acceptable for this category of clients.

EXPERIENTIAL EXERCISE

Vibration

Experience vibration on your body by sitting erect in a chair and applying the various types of vibratory movements to your thigh. First, using just one finger, press on a spot in the quadriceps muscle. Move back and forth very rapidly without leaving the spot, as if you were "buzzing" on the spot. Now change the movement to straight in and out of the tissue as rapidly as you can without ever completely breaking contact with the tissue. This fine, piston-like movement is called pointing.

Now, place you hand flat on your quadriceps. Lightly grasp the tissues and move your hand back and forth, staying in one spot. Increase the tempo to a rapid movement. Notice how this feels. Then slow the tempo down. How does this feel? Now, continue the shaking movement but lighten your grip and move your hand along the length of the thigh, working the entire muscle. Experiment with the pressure and tempo and notice how different it can feel. This technique is called shaking.

To experience rocking vibration, remain seated but slide up to the front of your chair and straighten one leg, placing the heel on the floor. Place one hand on each side of the thigh and rotate (twist) it internally and externally. Keep the heel on the floor. Notice that there is a speed (tempo) at which the legs moves the most freely. This is the ideal speed for rocking your leg. Your arm will have a different ideal speed. Each client will have a slightly different speed at which his body rocks the easiest. This tempo is the most relaxing for him to be rocked at and, therefore, has the most powerful sedating effect. Try using this technique at a slower and then a faster pace on yourself. You will notice that as you rock slower the range of movement increases and the feeling becomes monotonous. Notice that as you increase the rocking speed, the range of hip joint movement decreases and the sensation becomes more enlivening.

Jostling takes this movement to the extreme. Go faster and faster, with more energy, until you are throwing the thigh back and forth between your hands. This is very invigorating!

NERVE STROKES

Nerve strokes can be considered a form of effleurage. However, since effleurage is generally considered to be a stroke used to move fluids, nerve strokes (being too light to accomplish even lymph movement) are given their own category in this text. They are very light, sliding strokes, usually done with the fingertips over the clothes or skin at slow to moderate speeds. Nerve strokes are so light they do not require lubrication on exposed skin, so they work very well over clothing. These strokes are very soothing and calming, so they are used to sedate the nervous system. They are usually used as finishing strokes for relaxation treatments, a nice "icing on the cake" method to end contact with the client. When performing this technique to relax your client at the end of a massage, make your strokes lighter and lighter until your fingertips are off the body.

However, nerve strokes can also be done quickly with slightly more pressure to provide an invigorating stimulus. This is usually done in conjunction with tapotement to leave the client in a more alert state, or invigorated, as in pre-event sports massage or when the client needs to return to an activity that requires alertness (Fig. 7-15).

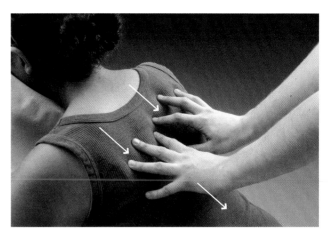

Figure 7–15 Nerve strokes. Nerve strokes being done lightly and slowly with fingertips. Moving from superior to inferior, both hands at the same time, one on each side of the spine.

CLINICAL TIP

Nerve Stroke Application

Rapid nerve strokes would be appropriate in pre-event sports applications or in other similar situations in which the goal is to leave the client in a more alert state at the end of a massage.

CASE STUDY

Strokes for Clients with Anxiety Disorder

You are working on-site at a factory. A woman comes to you and confides that she has an anxiety disorder and is particularly worried about a meeting she will be attending later that day. She wonders if a massage might relax her and "settle her nerves down."

1. What strokes should you select to have the greatest therapeutic impact on this woman?
2. What speed (tempo) would be best to accomplish the goals of this treatment?

SUMMARY

Massage is a form of manual medicine that provides stimulus to the nervous system to bring about profound responses. Massage techniques are called strokes. The different types of strokes used in seated massage are compression, effleurage, friction, nerve strokes, petrissage, sustained pressure, tapotement, and vibration. Each stroke has specific effects on the nervous system. The two main effects are sedating and invigorating (Fig. 7-16). Typically, increasing the tempo or pressure causes a stroke to become more invigorating, whereas slowing the tempo or reducing pressure causes a stroke to be more sedating. Strokes are selected and combined to create a treatment appropriate for the needs of each client.

CASE STUDY

Strokes for Pre-Event Sports Massage

It is 5:00 p.m. and a middle-aged, athletic man stops by the salon you are working in, seeking a chair massage. He is from out of town and says he has had a massage before. He says he is out of energy but wants to play racquetball at 6:00 p.m. with his host, an important customer of his business. He wonders if you could pump him up and loosen his shoulders before he goes to the Racquet Club.

1. What should you select as your primary strokes to help this man get ready to play racquetball?
2. What tempo would be the most appropriate for the majority of the massage?

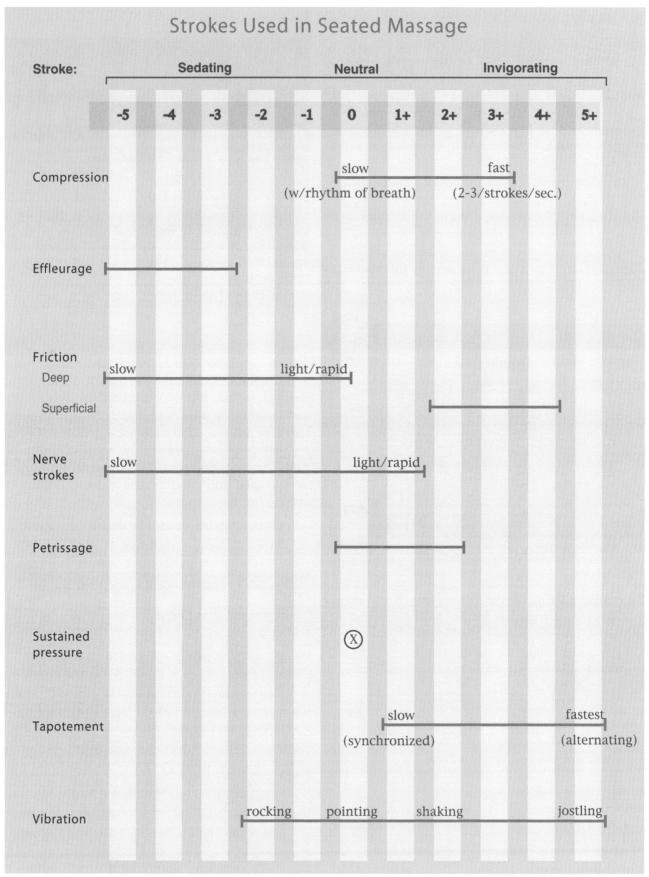

Figure 7–16 Strokes used in seated massage. Listed is each stroke used in seated massage, as discussed above, showing the relative stimulus each stroke applies to the nervous system of the client.

REFERENCES

1. Field T, Ironson G, Scafidi F, et al. Massage therapy reduces anxiety and enhances EEG patterns of alertness and math computations. *Int J Neurosci* 1996;86:197–205.
2. Hovind H. Effects of massage on blood flow in skeletal muscle. *Scand J Rehabil Med* 1974;6:74–77.
3. Xujain S. Effects of massage and temperature on permeability of initial lymphatics. *Lymphology* 1990;23:48–50.
4. Chaitow L, Delany-Walker J. *Clinical Applications of Neuro-muscular Techniques*. Volume 1—The Upper Body. Edinburgh, UK: Harcourt Publishers, Ltd., 2000.
5. St. John P. NMT 1 Cervical injuries, postural analysis and pelvic stabilization. Largo, FL. St. John Neuromuscular Therapy Seminars: 1999.
6. Travell J, Simons D, Simons L. *Myofascial Pain and Dysfunction: The Trigger Point Manual*, vol. 1, 2nd ed. Baltimore: Williams & Wilkins, 1999.
7. Schlep R. Fascial Plasticitya new neurobiological explanation, Part 2. *JBMT* 2003;7(2):104–116.

CHAPTER 8

Stretching Techniques

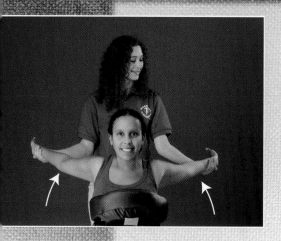

"The manual stretch of muscles and fascia creates mechanical, bioelectrical and biochemical responses that promote improved vascular and lymphatic circulation, increased oxygenation, removal of body toxins, and a more efficient nervous system."

AARON L. MATTES (1,2)

Objectives

- Explain the role of fascia and muscles in flexibility.

- Explain and demonstrate each of the four types of stretching techniques presented.

- Select the appropriate stretches to be used for each client.

- Explain the importance of drinking enough pure water.

- Perform complete Active Isolated Stretching—Mattes Method stretching routines for the neck, shoulder, forearm, wrist, and hand.

Key Terms

Areolar tissue: loose, irregularly arranged connective tissue that consists of collagenous and elastic fibers, a protein polysaccharide ground substance, and connective tissue cells including fibroblasts, macrophages, mast cells, and sometimes fat cells, plasma cells, leukocytes, and pigment cells.

ATP (adenosine 5′-triphosphate): a body chemical that is the primary source of energy (fuel) for the cell.

Joint: the point of union, more or less movable, between two or more bones. There are three types of joints, each with several divisions. See an anatomy text for details.

Inhibition: a signal from the nervous system telling a muscle to relax.

Innervation: a signal from the nervous system telling a muscle to contract.

Ligament: a specialized form of fascia that connects two or more bones, thus holding a joint together. An injury to a ligament is called a "sprain."

Normal range of motion: the amount of movement, usually measured in degrees, that a healthy joint should be able to perform without pain or injury.

Reciprocal: something that is mutual or done in return; in this application, the neurological communication mechanism between opposing pairs of muscles signaling contraction (innervation) in the agonist while signaling relaxation (inhibition) in the antagonist.

Tendon: a specialized form of fascia that connects the contractile part of a muscle to its attachment site, usually a bone. An injury to a tendon (or a muscle) is called a "strain."

Life is movement. A sign of death is the lack of movement. In one sense, massage is a very static or low-movement experience for the client. If an entire massage treatment consists of only massage strokes, nothing in the client's body moves more than a few inches, except maybe lymph and venous fluids. To put more life into a massage, add movement by including stretching techniques as part of your massage routine. Stretching techniques provide movement in joints and elongation of muscle and fascial tissues, greatly enhancing the therapeutic impact of the massage. This is true for both relaxation and therapeutic massage on either a chair or a table.

When stretching is included in a massage, positive results are achieved faster and last longer. Frequently, stretching brings the desired results when massage strokes do not.

Furthermore, stretching is one of the best methods for maintaining the therapist's own body. In addition to the use of proper body mechanics, stretching can help you prevent repetitive strain injuries, which often result from the practice of massage. Make stretching a part of your daily life, both personally and professionally.

Several systems of stretching are available for use in conjunction with seated massage. The most popular are Active Isolated Stretching—Mattes Method (AIS), proprioceptive neuromuscular facilitation (PNF), static stretching, and passive stretching. Also available to a limited degree in seated massage is myofascial stretching, which could be considered "micro-stretching." Unfortunately, myofascial stretching is only minimally effective when done through the clothes; therefore, in seated massage, its use is limited to areas where skin is exposed, such as the neck, forearm, wrist, and hand.

In this chapter you will learn a systematic stretching routine using AIS, as well as other types of stretching techniques. You will learn the physiology behind restricted range of motion and the nervous system's response to the stimulation stretching provides, both of which are imperative to understand when stretching a muscle.

"Stretching is beneficial only if it is done correctly."

AARON L. MATTES

UNDERSTANDING FLEXIBILITY

The human body is designed to be remarkably flexible (Fig. 8-1).

Each **joint** allows a certain amount of movement in various directions. "**Normal range of motion**" is

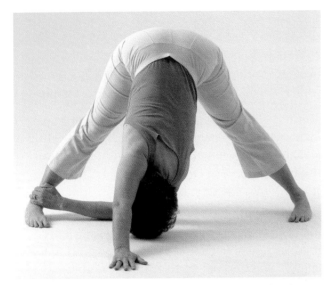

Figure 8-1 The human body has the potential to be remarkably flexible. (Photo courtesy of Yoga International Magazine.)

Factors Affecting Flexibility

What causes a person to lose their ideal flexibility and range of motion?

- Flexibility is related to body type, sex, age, bone and joint structure, and medical history.
- Females, on the average, are more flexible than males of the same age.
- Work or exercise that produces repeated overuse of the same muscles day after day confines joints within a restricted range of motion and tends to reduce flexibility (2).
- Trauma, overuse, and the effects of age are the most common causes of muscle tightness, resulting in protective flexor postures. Our upright, biped stance and constricted gait pattern further contribute to functional muscle weakness and contractures.
- Sedentary living habits and the repeated (habitual) use of flexor muscles are often major reasons for lack of complete range of motion (2).
- Abnormal chronic posturing such as a head-forward, round-shoulder posture, which will restrict normal raising of the arms (forward elevation).
- Muscle imbalances on opposite sides of a joint, such as overly strong shoulder internal rotators (pectoralis major, subscapularis) with weak external rotators (infraspinatus, teres minor), will restrict external rotation.
- Chronic sitting at work, when traveling, or resting creates an overflexed posture which resists extension and external rotation movements.

In other words, lack of movement may cause loss of ability to move.

what we will call the full amount of movement each joint is designed to allow. Unfortunately, a relatively small percentage of people can perform the normal range of motion of every joint in their bodies.

The goal of stretching techniques is to gain or maintain range of motion. Massage and stretching techniques are the most effective methods of restoring normal range of motion. To fully understand flexibility, we must first consider what does and does not restrict normal range of motion. Joints are designed to allow normal range of motion, not restrict it. **Ligaments** hold a joint in proper position. They allow normal range of motion and only restrict abnormal or excessive movement. When ligaments are stretched by excessive force, they allow abnormal (excessive) movement and unstable joints. Only if restricted by excessive scar tissue adhesions resulting from injuries do ligaments restrict normal range of motion. **Tendons** are the connective fibers between muscles and bones. They do not restrict normal movement unless scar tissue adhesions bind them to surrounding tissues. Skin is quite pliable, an unlikely restrictor of movement. Therefore, the primary obstacle to normal flexibility is tightness of the fascia and muscles surrounding a joint.

Fascia's Role in Flexibility

Fascia plays a vital role in the flexibility and homeostasis of the body, and conditions affecting the fascia can lead to a loss of flexibility. Specifically, the

integrity and proper tensile tone of the fascia directly affects the body's muscular performance and ability to move. Below, we will consider the basic properties of fascia, what conditions in the fascia can affect flexibility, and what treatments are useful in addressing these conditions.

Description of Fascia

Sometimes called dense irregular connective tissue, fascia is often referred to as our organ of form (3,4). There are two basic types of fascia, subserous and subcutaneous. Subserous fascia is loose **areolar tissue** that covers the visceral organs and lines body cavities. Its small circulatory channels carry fluid that lubricates the surfaces of the internal viscera (5). Subserous fascia is not directly addressed by typical massage techniques.

The subcutaneous fascia is a continuous sheet from region to region, which surrounds and connects all other elements of the body, including skin, muscles, bones, and joints, giving our body structural integrity and strength. Although it is continuous, it has specialized elements such as ligaments and tendons. These elements have unique characteristics but share the general makeup of fascia, that being collagen fibers, elastic fibers, cellular elements, and ground substance. Fascia is highly innervated and the ground substance contains many substances that contribute to the immune mechanisms of the body.

Subcutaneous fascia is interconnected to the subserous fascia, so, ultimately, fascia creates a connective matrix that ties the entire body onto one continuum from the skin to the deepest viscera. Fascia provides support for vessels and nerves and enables adjacent tissues to move upon each other while providing stability and contour. This fascia also encompasses the sensory organs of the nervous system, blood vessels, and lymph channels and serves as an extensive water storage system. Oxygenation of the cells and tissues is regulated by fascia. Furthermore, this fascial network facilitates the removal of our body's metabolic wastes.

Fascia consists of a three-dimensional fibrous matrix that provides interconnections throughout all cells in the body. It is densely innervated by mechanoreceptors, which are responsive to manual pressure. Fascia is also populated with smooth muscle cells embedded within the collagen fibers. Furthermore, there is a rich intra-fascial supply of capillaries, autonomic nerves, and sensory nerve endings. It seems likely that these fascial smooth muscle cells enable the autonomic nervous system to regulate a fascial "pre-tension" that is independent of muscular tonus. Fascia is an actively adapting organ that responds to pressure, vibration, and stretch (6). We must affect the fascia in order to effectively address the muscles.

The subcutaneous fascia is divided into two layers: superficial and deep. Superficial fascia is very elastic due to the crisscrossing pattern network of fibers. It is attached to the underside of the skin and is loosely knit, fibroelastic, areolar tissue. Within the superficial fascia are found fat, capillaries, lymphatic channels and other vascular structures, and nerves, particularly pacinian corpuscles (skin receptors). Within this layer is potential space for the accumulation of fluid and metabolites. Many palpable tissue texture abnormalities are the result of changes within the superficial fascia. It is effectively the membrane or bag that holds the body together. The myofascial release techniques primarily affect the superficial fascia.

Deep fascia is tough, tight, and compact. Denser than superficial fascia, the subcutaneous deep fascia layer protects vital internal organs from trauma and envelopes and separates the muscles (with the exception of the superficial muscles of the neck, head, and palmar brevis), nerves, blood vessels, lymph vessels, nodes, and glands. It is able to store water and, when well hydrated, creates a smooth coating allowing fascial structures to glide over each other without friction (7).

The deep fascial system is continuous with the subcutaneous fascial system, connecting the superficial layer to the interior, integrating within the deeper body cavities, spinal canal, dura, and meninges. Thus, a woman who experiences pain of menses through uterine congestion creates fascial tension that disrupts the normal tensile forces and refers pain to as far away as the top of her head (2).

Conditions Affecting the Fascia

Certain conditions in the fascia can adversely affect flexibility. Specifically, if the fascial matrix is distorted by trauma, aging, poor posture, hormonal or metabolic imbalances, injuries, and dehydration in localized areas of the fascia, it can disrupt the homeostasis of the entire body. If these localized conditions are left untreated, they may in turn decrease flexibility by compromising fascial integrity and tone. Then, as in a "daisy-chain effect," they can possibly lead to more generalized (systemic) dysfunctional conditions of severe postural distortions, inflammation, detrimental contractures, lymphatic congestion, peripheral vascular obstruction, hypertension, and a host of other disease states (2).

Trauma creates micro-bleeding that heals into aberrant scar tissue, which changes the tensile tension of the musculoskeletal system. Additionally, this scar tissue interferes with bioelectric communication channels, which flow along the fascial lines in patterns that seem to correlate with the meridian system of Eastern medicine (8).

Dehydration, inflammatory processes, and trauma deplete the smooth, hydrated matrix and cause adherence between tissues, as if they were partially glued together. This adherence creates tension and fatigue and leads to ischemia and a build up of metabolic toxins (2). These disruptions in the fascial web create tensile forces where tender points or trigger points become manifest in myofascial tissue. If the disruption manifests within the internal organs, disruption of physiological function may result in a disease state.

Treating Fascia

Fortunately, these conditions affecting the fascia are treatable. The superficial fascia responds well to therapeutic modalities such as heat, ultrasound, and massage, which promote restoration of energy fields allowing for facilitation of flexibility and movement. The deeper layers of fascia do not, however, respond to these superficial modalities. This is where stretching comes in. The therapist must stimulate the deep fibrous fascial matrix through precise application of active stretching techniques, such as Active Isolated Stretching—Mattes Method, done in the proper order (2). In seated massage, modalities such as heat and ultrasound are seldom available. However, massage and stretching techniques combine to make a very powerful, positive agent of change for the improvement of fascia health.

Muscle's Role in Flexibility

In addition to fascia, muscles also play a critical role in flexibility. Muscles cause movement and restrict movement and hold the body in whatever position it is in. Thus, it is necessary for a muscle to maintain its flexibility in order to move the body into its many different postures.

First, consider how muscles work. Muscles contract (shorten) actively and elongate (lengthen) passively in response to stimulation from the nervous system. When a muscle fibril is stimulated by a nerve,

---

Box 8-2

Fascial Perforations and Acupuncture

German researchers, using electron photomicroscopy, found that the superficial fascia has numerous perforations where a triad of a nerve, an artery, and a vein pass through on the way to the skin. The majority (82%) of these perforations are topographically identical with the 361 classical acupuncture points in traditional Chinese acupuncture (2,6).

Box 8-3

Importance of Water

Lack of sufficient water intake has many negative effects on the body. Loss of flexibility is one result. You will have better results with clients who are properly hydrated. Encourage your clients to consume water, especially before and after massage appointments. Six to eight glasses of water per day is ideal for the normal individual.

Among its many essential functions, water acts as a lubricant in between the layers of tissue and as a solvent to help with waste removal. Water serves as a solvent when waste products bind to the two parts of hydrogen in H_2O and are filtered out of the body by the urinary system. This means water can help reduce post-exercise and post-massage soreness. The purer the water, the fewer chemicals are bound to the hydrogen atoms, making for a more powerful solvent. Municipal tap water is the least pure, safe drinking water. Distillation with carbon filtration and reverse osmosis with carbon filtration makes the purest and safest drinking water.

As a therapist, it is important that you remain hydrated yourself. Massage is hard work, often in warm environments, causing more perspiration loss than if you were sedentary. Breathing naturally depletes water from the body. Breathing through the mouth depletes water faster than breathing through the nose and is particularly drying to throat and vocal membranes. You will find you energy levels and your ability to concentrate will be better maintained throughout the day if you are well hydrated.

---

it contracts to its fully shortened position. It holds that contraction as long as it continues to receive stimulation from the nervous system, and **ATP** (fuel) is available. When stimulation stops, the fibril relaxes and waits to be passively lengthened by its antagonistic muscle or gravity.

Spasms

One factor that can affect muscle flexibility is spasms. When a mild spasm is present in a muscle, it means some of its fibers are still being stimulated by the nervous system and are contracted (shortened). A spasm can be any involuntary contraction, from just a few fibrils in one area of a muscle to a full contraction (often called a cramp) by most of the fibrils. A cramp-type spasm usually causes involuntary movement and pain as it shortens and will not allow elongation.

Partial spasms, which are much more common, can become ischemic and are tender to palpation and possibly movement.

Often, a spasm will begin in a small area of the muscle. However, over time, and if left untreated, more fibrils will join the spasm, thus increasing the resistance to elongate and leaving the muscle continuously "locked on" and very fatigued. The fibrils in these isolated spasms, when suddenly called upon to elongate rapidly in athletics, at the work place, during a fall, etc., will instead rupture, causing soft tissue injury. To relieve the pain and restore flexibility and normal range of motion, the massage therapist must be able to use stretching techniques that relax and "turn off" these muscle spasms.

Scar Tissue

Scar tissue is another factor that can reduce muscle flexibility. Muscles can be lengthened up to 1.6 times their resting length. If forced beyond that amount, muscles may tear or rupture, resulting in bleeding at the injury site. The body will heal by forming scar tissue. It does not build new muscle fibril cells. Once injured, the muscle fibers are lost forever and are replaced with scar tissue, which is a type of fascia. Scar tissue is less flexible than uninjured muscle tissue and cannot actively contract or elongate. In the process of creating scar tissue to heal the injury, adhesions to surrounding tissue usually occur, especially if the area is immobilized. These adhesions restrict flexibility. Wherever flexibility is compromised, muscle weakness and contractures develop (2).

CLINICAL TIP

Correcting "Slumped Posture"

Where muscle weakness and contractures develop, postural distortion is soon evident. In conditions of postural distortion, there is always one muscle concentrically contracted (shortened) while its antagonist (opposite) muscle is eccentrically contracted (lengthened). During the brief moments when no movement is occurring, both are in isometric contractions (unless the person is lying supine, very relaxed). The most common postural distortion pattern is the head-forward, internally rotated shoulders—the "slumped posture." Figure 8-2 shows an extreme version of this posture. Most clients' patterns are more subtle than those shown.

The client with this pattern (which will be the majority of people you will see) usually complains of discomfort or pain in the eccentrically contracted muscles, which are fatigued and most likely ischemic from holding the load. The eccentric muscle is more likely to develop trigger points due to its chronic overload. Typically, the eccentric muscles will be in the posterior neck, shoulders, and back. However, the client will often gain the most relief from lengthening of the concentrically contracted muscles by massage and stretching techniques, thus correcting posture and reducing the load on the lengthened (eccentric) muscles. Since the

Box 8-4

Controlling Muscle Force

The more strength someone desires to apply to a particular movement, the more fibrils her body calls into contraction in a muscle or muscle group. To pick up a feather, the nervous system will only contract part of the available fibrils. To pick up a heavy weight, most of the fibrils will be stimulated to contract. To try to pick up an immovable object, possibly all available fibrils will be recruited. The nervous system initially calls on the fibrils in the center of the belly of the muscle. As more and more strength is needed, fibrils farther and farther from the center of the mus-

cle are recruited. Finally, for the maximum effort, the most distant fibrils in the musculotendinous junction are called into play. Unfortunately, these fibrils, which are used the least, are called upon to do the most. This is one reason why so many injuries occur in the musculotendinous junction area. These areas need to be warmed up before heavy exertion. They should be examined for ischemia and trigger points during massage sessions. Precise stretching movements, such as those in AIS, also help to keep the musculotendinous junction healthy.

Box 8-5

Types of Muscle Contraction

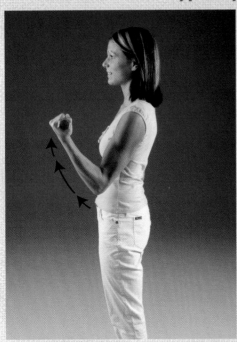

(A) Concentric contraction of the elbow flexor muscles causing shortening of the muscles and flexion of the joint.

Concentric Contraction: A shortening contraction in which a muscle's attachments are drawn toward one another as the muscle contracts and overcomes an external resistance (10). An example is lifting a weight by flexing a joint, as the muscle insertion is brought closer to the muscle origin, as shown in Figure *(A)*.

Eccentric Contraction: A lengthening contraction in which a muscle's attachments are drawn away from one another by an external resis- tance, even though the muscle is activated (10). An example is slowly lowering a weight by ex- tending a joint, causing the muscle insertion to move away from the muscle origin in a controlled manner, as shown in Figure *(B)*.

Isometric Contraction: Force development at constant length (10). This is a contraction against resistance where no movement occurs.

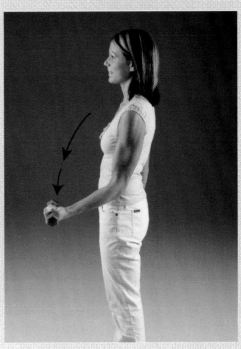

(B) Eccentric contraction of the elbow flexor muscles allow- ing controlled elongation of the muscles and extension of the joint.

anterior muscles are less available for massage in the seated position than when on a massage table, stretching is the ideal method to lengthen them with.

To maintain the correction, the client must strengthen the long, eccentric muscles and regu- larly stretch the shortened ones in between mas- sage sessions. In the upper body this usually means stretching the anterior muscles and strengthening the posterior muscles. Therapists are tempted to only work the posterior (eccentric) muscles in response to the client's complaint of pain in the back of their neck or between their scapulas. Doing so will bring the client temporary relief. However, by only relaxing the eccentric muscles, the concentric muscles on the anterior side will usually pull the person further anterior into their distortion pattern, taking up the newly created slack, ultimately making the distorted posture worse over time. Do not do this to your clients. Cer- tainly examine and treat the eccentric muscles, but spend more time lengthening the concentric muscles. Teach the client the stretches and give them one or two as "homework." They must maintain what we gain.

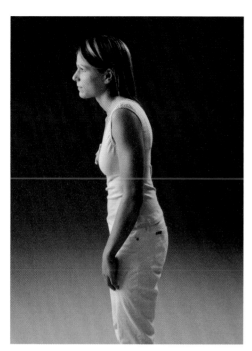

Figure 8-2 Demonstration of the head-forward, internally rotated posture. Note the forward lean of the torso, the ear forward relative to the shoulder, the bent elbow, the internally rotated hand and arm resting on the anterior thigh. This is an exhausting and uncomfortable position, which places damaging stress on joints and soft tissues.

Treatment of Muscles

The nervous system controls muscle tonus and the number of fibrils that are contracted in a muscle at any given moment. This is done automatically, not consciously, by the autonomic nervous system. With few exceptions, it cannot be controlled voluntarily. Have you ever tried to consciously think away a muscle cramp? If you try to stretch a group of contracted fibrils, you will find they will not elongate. If enough force is applied it will cause ruptures (injury) to the fibers, but not elongation. The more you try to stretch a cramp the more it tenses. The cramp will remain unless you can convince the nervous system to turn it off.

So how do you treat a muscle cramp or spasm? The nervous system is a stimulus response mechanism. To get it to turn off a muscle you must provide it with a relaxing (sedating) stimulus. Correctly applied stretching and massage techniques can be that stimulus. The massage technique of sustained pressure, usually performed with a loosely clinched fist or heel of the hand at the site of the cramp, is effective in cramp management. The PNF stretching technique of reciprocal inhibition is the stretching technique of

choice for cramps. For a description of how to use reciprocal-inhibition to treat an active muscle cramp, see Box 8-7.

For low-grade spasms, the increased tension or hyper-tonus type, all sedating massage strokes and correctly applied stretching techniques are effective. Note that incorrectly applied stretching techniques will not relax the muscle(s), but will instead result in increased muscle contraction; at worst causing injury, at best providing no gain in movement. While muscles have an elastic component to them, in that they can shorten and elongate mechanically, they cannot be stretched like a rubber band or even like fascia, which will deform (elongate) to some degree in response to pressure. Therefore, in stretching, just as in massage, our access to the body is through the nervous system, not through brute force.

Scar tissue adds the additional problem of undesirable adhesions, which restrict movement. Desirable adhesions are the ones that bridge (repair) the rupture (tear) of muscle fibers or fascial components such as ligaments and tendons. Undesirable ones bridge to adjacent, uninjured tissue or structures, binding them together so they can no longer move independently. Over time these can be reduced by repeated stretching. Early mobilization (movement) of injuries, through stretching, exercise or deep friction massage techniques, helps prevent unwanted adhesions from forming. Adhesions also form between layers when there is a lack of movement or no movement, even if no injury occurs. The layers seem to stick together. This type of adhesion can be broken by stretching or possibly assisted by massage.

WHEN TO USE STRETCHING IN SEATED MASSAGE

Just as with massage strokes, stretching techniques can be used for both general relaxation and for specific therapeutic treatments. The use of stretching for each of these goals is discussed below.

Relaxation Treatments

When the goals for the massage are relaxation and stress reduction, stretches are most effective when performed toward the end of the treatment. Static, PNF, or AIS methods may be used. Muscles most commonly stretched for relaxation are the anterior cervical and shoulder muscles and the internal rotators of the shoulder.

Suggested stretches for relaxation are as follows:

- Passive stretches: shown in Figures 8-3 and 8-4
- PNF stretches: shown in Figures 8-5A–C and 8-6A,B
- AIS stretches: shown in Figures 8-9A,B, 8-23A, 8-25A,B, 8-26A–D, 8-27A–C, and 8-31A,B.

Of course, you may perform any stretch you feel appropriate for the client. Do not feel limited to this list. Also understand that you do not have to do to all the stretches listed. You may choose to do only one stretch. However, it is recommended that you do at least two stretches to address the anterior of the neck and chest.

Therapeutic Treatments

When doing therapeutic treatments, stretches are valuable tools. If performed at the beginning of a treatment, they serve as a quick assessment technique showing you which muscles are tight, which movements are restricted, and where in a given movement pain occurs. Of course, never stretch the person into the pain; stop at the edge of pain.

If stretches are performed toward the end of a therapeutic treatment, they serve to elongate the tissues you have specifically massaged. This helps reduce the likelihood of a spasm or a trigger point returning. Stretches can also be done in the middle of the session. It is common to stretch the specific muscle you have just massaged, then move to the next muscle in your massage routine. To sum it up, use stretches whenever you believe they will do the most good for the client you are working with.

TYPES OF STRETCHING

There are many types of stretching, most of which can be adapted to seated massage. All the various systems of stretching can be categorized into four major types: static, passive, proprioceptive neuromuscular facilitation (PNF), and Active Isolated Stretching (AIS). Static and passive stretches are recommended only for relaxation routines where no injury, postural distortion, or muscle spasms are evident. PNF and AIS can be used in either relaxation or therapeutic routines. AIS is recommended by this author because of its ease of use, versatility, effectiveness, and the fact that the client can do AIS unassisted or self-assisted for "homework." PNF requires assistance from another person. We will now study each of the four types, see several applications of each in seated massage, and then study comprehensive Active Isolated Stretching routines for the forearm, wrist and hand, neck, and shoulder.

Static Stretching

Static stretching is probably the most commonly done form of stretching. There are many systems of flexibility that use static stretching, among them yoga. Static stretching is best described as a low-force, long-duration stretch in which the stretcher is actively performing the stretch.

The common mistakes made when doing static stretching are not going far enough into the stretch or lengthening the muscle too far. If the stretcher does not go far enough, no lengthening will occur. If the stretcher goes too far (stretching too hard), the spindle cells will fire, causing the muscle to contract to protect itself from injury. The protective contraction prevents any elongation and may create more tension and less range of motion than existed prior to stretching. If the stretcher pushes past this protective resistance, injury in the form of muscle strain may result, leaving the body with tissue memory that will resist elongation in the future. Stretching too far (too hard) is the most common mistake.

To perform a static stretch, move into the stretching position just far enough to feel a gentle (moderate) stretch and breathe while holding the position. In 10–15 seconds, you should feel the lessening of the stretch sensation. This lessening of sensation is believed to be the muscle relaxing from the inverse stretch reflex of the golgi tendon organ. Now move further into the stretch, breathe, and wait for another inverse (relaxation) response. Two or three responses are sufficient. Once achieved, slowly return to the starting position. If no relaxation occurs, you have moved into the position too far and have set off the spindle cell response. Return to the starting position and begin again, this time not going as far into the stretch. In a seated massage session, you (the therapist) may assist the client in performing stretches by providing guidance to the movement for accuracy. However, the stretch must be done actively by the client to have the proper effect on the client's nervous system. Clients can be taught this method and given a particular stretch or two after each session to do as homework between appointments.

Box 8-6

The Myotatic Stretch Reflex

To further complicate our efforts to elongate muscles, they have built-in sensors that protect them from elongating too far or too fast. These sensors are to prevent injury. However, they will also prevent elongation of the muscle during stretching exercises if they are activated by movements done too fast or too forcefully.

The two sensors involved in stretching are the muscle spindle cells in the muscle belly and the golgi tendon organs or golgi bodies, which are arranged in series with the fascial fibers in the myotendinous junctions, in attachment transitions of aponeuroses, in capsules and ligaments of peripheral joints, and in tendons (9). Together, these two sensors make up the myotatic stretch reflex.

The muscle spindles monitor how fast and far muscle fibrils are elongating. When a muscle is elongating too far, too fast, or both, the spindles inform the cord through the gamma fibers. The cord then reflexively sends back stimuli to the muscle, causing it to contract to resist lengthening, thus protecting both the muscle and the associated joint. This is called the stretch reflex. If stretching movements are done too fast or too hard, spindle cells will fire, the muscle will contract and no "stretch" will occur. Unfortunately, this is the way stretching is most commonly done: too fast and too forcefully. It should be easy to understand why most people are not rewarded with success from their stretching program.

The golgi tendon organ (GTO) provides the inverse stretch reflex (also called autogenic inhibition). It measures the strain being applied to the tendon. When a strain (stretch) is applied, the GTO measures this strain and reports it to the cord. Golgi organs respond to slow, active stretch at physiologically safe levels of strain by influencing the alpha motor neurons via the spinal cord to lower their firing rate. If the strain is deemed safe, the cord inhibits the contraction of the muscle (relaxes it), allowing it to elongate.

The dialogue between the cord and these two sensors is continuous, going on to some degree with every movement we make. In order to successfully stretch muscle tissue, we must understand and respect the myotatic stretch reflex and stimulate it in a way that causes it to allow elongation of tissue to occur. Muscle spindles cause a muscle to contract. Golgi tendon organs cause a muscle to relax. For stretching to be successful, we want to activate the golgi without firing the spindles protective reflex (2,9).

Please realize that the above is a very simplistic explanation of the mechanism. The central nervous system does not operate one muscle at a time. The mind sees the muscular system as one huge muscle, capable of being activated in an infinite number of ways using learned functional units or groups of contractile fibers. The motor system of our nervous system has as its functional units not individual muscles, but motor units comprised of the many muscles throughout the body required to perform a specific movement. To raise our arm from our side to our ear requires more than just a few shoulder muscles. Abdominal muscles must contract to balance us and, if we are standing, muscles all the way to the feet will be used to prevent us from falling over. We have millions of these motor units.

Movement is a learned skill. We learn which muscles to contract to close our hand, to bend over and touch our toes, or to do any particular movement. The nervous system calls into play all the muscles it has learned are necessary to make a desired movement and does so at a level unconscious to us. Stretching positions attempt to isolate a certain muscle, but cannot help but involve sensors in other surrounding tissues (ligaments and joints) as well as the entire motor unit required to balance and stabilize as the stretch is performed. Therefore, it is important to always keep in mind the importance of providing the nervous system with the proper and sufficient stimulus to achieve a desired response, usually relaxation and elongation, without causing overstimulation or injury.

Passive Stretching

In passive stretching, the subject is passive (relaxed) while the stretch is performed on them by another person, usually a therapist or a workout partner. The same principles that apply to static stretching apply to passive stretching. The danger is that the person doing the stretch has no direct feel of the intensity of the stretch. Therefore, it is very important that the person doing the stretch ask for feedback from the person being stretched and be careful not to overstretch (injure) the tissues.

For example, if you perform passive stretching on your client, you should ask, "Tell me when you feel a comfortable level of stretch." Then hold the stretch and ask, "Tell me when you feel the stretch sensation going away." When the client reports the lessening of the stretch sensation, return her to the starting position. If a relaxation response doesn't occur in 15 seconds, she is being stretched too far (too hard); return to the starting position and begin again, this time with less force.

This form of passive–static stretching may be used effectively in seated massage on the neck and shoulder areas. However, due to the lack of active nervous system involvement, passive stretching is seldom as effective as other types of stretching.

The limitations of passive stretching are:

1. The dependence on a therapist/partner to perform the stretch.
2. There is no motor learning and no improvement in the motion capacity of the tight muscle or its opponent.
3. Golgi organs do not respond to passive movement.

Two passive stretches commonly used in seated massage relaxation treatments are shown below in Figures 8-3 and 8-4.

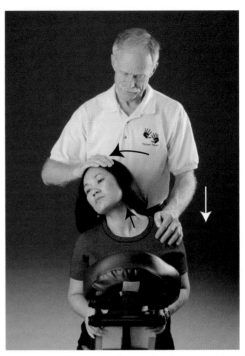

Figure 8-4 Passive stretch–cervical posterior oblique performed by therapist to stretch scalene and sternocleidomastoid muscles. Therapist rotates client's head 45 degrees to the right and then slowly pulls client's head posterior and lateral at a 45-degree angle to the right, moving client's ear toward the lateral border of their scapula. Stop when client reports a comfortable stretch. Hold for five seconds. Note therapist's hand stabilizing client's shoulder. Return client to upright, forward facing position. Repeat stretch on other side.

Proprioceptive Neuromuscular Facilitation (PNF)

PNF was developed in the 1950s by Dr. Henry Kabat, MD, PhD, a neurophysiologist, and by two therapists, Margaret "Maggie" Knott and Dorothy Voss. PNF is a complete system of stretching and was originally developed to help rehabilitate polio patients suffering from paralysis (9). Its objective is to stimulate the neural mechanisms of contraction and relaxation. The developers of PNF noticed that most of the natural movements in life are done through three planes: front–back, down–up, and right–left. They developed precise protocols to isolate muscles and at the same time duplicate the spiral diagonal movement patterns of the body. PNF uses two primary neurological phenomena: tense and relax, and reciprocal inhibition. Several combinations of tensing, relaxing, and movement have been developed based on these two principles. Additional range of motion can usually be quickly gained using PNF methods.

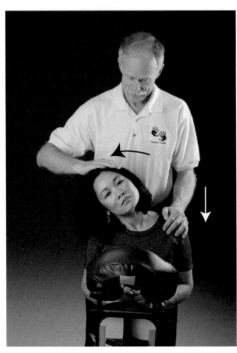

Figure 8-3 Passive stretch–lateral cervical flexion performed by the therapist with the client passive. Ask the client to indicate verbally when a comfortable stretch has been achieved. Therapist slowly moves client's head toward client's shoulder until client reports a comfortable stretch. Hold for five seconds. Note therapist's hand stabilizing client's shoulder. Return client's head to upright and stretch client to the other side.

Tense and Relax (Contract and Relax)

It was discovered that if a muscle was tensed without movement (an isometric contraction), it would then relax and elongate further than if it were not tensed prior to elongation (stretching). To utilize this mechanism, the client moves into the stretching position as far as he comfortably can. Then the therapist (or a partner) holds him in such a manner that he cannot move back toward the neutral (starting) position. The client then tries to move back to the neutral position, with no movement allowed. This is tensing the muscle to be stretched. After 8–10 seconds, the client relaxes but the therapist continues to support the client, preventing any movement. Still relaxed, the client inhales and then, as he exhales, he moves further into the stretch and the therapist assists this movement to the next "barrier." This cycle is repeated two to four times. For an example of a tense and relax PNF stretch, see Box 8-7.

Box 8-7

Application of PNF Stretches

Description of a Tense and Relax PNF Stretch. For example, a client with restricted range of motion in cervical rotation cannot comfortably look over her right shoulder to back her car out of a parking stall.

- With the client sitting up straight, have her turn her head toward her right side as far as she comfortably can.

- Then hold her head with one of your hands on her left temple and the other on her right occiput.

- Now ask her to turn back to the left (to center). Do not allow her to move. This is tensing the muscles that are restricting her movement to the right. She only needs to use 10% of her strength. It is a mechanism that is being activated, not a strength contest between the client and therapist. She will not improve the results by pushing harder. If she is pushing too hard and you are struggling to resist her, tell her not to push so hard. If she is barely pushing at all, ask her to push harder.

- After 8–10 seconds (it is helpful to count the seconds out loud for her), ask her to slowly relax and inhale. There should be no movement during this relaxation as she breathes.

- Then tell her to exhale and try to turn further to the right as you assist her with a light to moderate pressure. This stretches the muscles that were just contracted. Help her move until resistance is felt (the next "barrier").

- Have her repeat the contraction by turning back toward center again as you hold her, preventing movement.

- Repeat the process 2–3 times.

 You can easily remember tense and relax as a zig-zag or back and forth active movement: tense one way, then move the other. In this case, tense left, then relax and move right, or left, right, left. Tense and relax helps build strength, but does so equally on both sides of the joint or movement as both muscles groups are contracted, one and then the other.

Description of a Reciprocal–Inhibition PNF Stretch. Using the example above again, reciprocal inhibition could be applied as follows:

- Ask the client to sit up straight and turn her head as far to the right as she comfortably can.

- Hold her head so that she cannot move any further to the right by putting one hand on her right temple and the other on her opposite occiput. (Note: this is the opposite of tense and relax!)

- Ask the client to try to look further to the right with 10% of her strength as you prevent any movement from occurring. This is tensing the muscles that are trying to turn the head to the right, sending an inhibition signal to the opposite (antagonist/reciprocal) muscles that are restricting the movement, turning them "off."

- As before, hold the contraction for 8–10 seconds, counting the seconds for the client.

- At the end of your count, tell the client to slowly relax and inhale.

- Do not allow any movement during this relaxation and inhalation.

- Ask the client to exhale and try to turn her head further to the right, assisting her as she moves, stopping at the next barrier. This active movement again sends an inhibition signal to the opposite muscles, allowing them to elongate further.

- Repeat 2–3 times.

Cramp Control using Reciprocal–Inhibition PNF.

- Determine which muscle or muscle group is in spasm; for example, let's say the forearm flexors.

(continues)

Box 8–7

Application of PNF Stretches (Continued)

- Grasp the client's hand so that it cannot move and ask her to contract her forearm extensor muscles. Since she probably does not know what extensor means, ask her to push the back of her hand against yours with 10% of her strength. She is contracting the opposite (antagonist) muscles to the ones in spasm, so an inhibition signal is sent to the spasming flexor muscles, telling them to relax. This usually "turns off" the cramp.

- Resist her attempted movement for 8–10 seconds, counting the seconds.

- Ask her to slowly relax and inhale.

- Ask her to exhale and relax, and as she does, passively stretch her into extension, 10–15 degrees, hold her again, and immediately have her contract her extensors again.

- Repeat this cycle several times until she is at the neutral anatomical position; in this case, the hand

should be straight, not flexed or extended at the wrist or fingers. If the cramping still persists in this position, hold her as before and have her contract the antagonist to the muscle in spasm, then relax and breathe. Perform some very light effleurage on the cramping muscle. If the cramp is persistent, have her activate the entire arm and shoulder in some movement to re-establish firing of a myotactic unit. Possibly have her walk around. Have her focus on breathing in to a count of 4 and out to a count of 8 (preferably through the nose if she can). This combination of techniques will alleviate most cramps. In stubborn athletic situations, it may be necessary to apply ice to the cramping muscles to slow their neurological processes.

- Notice that in cramp control, the elongation movement is passive: you perform the movement for the client. In the previous example, it was active: the client performs the movement and you assist her.

Reciprocal Inhibition (Reciprocal Innervation)

It was also found that when a muscle is contracted, an inhibition signal is sent by the nervous system to its antagonist (opposite muscle) telling the antagonist to relax. An inhibition signal "inhibits" muscle contraction. This principle can be utilized to gain range of motion. For example, when the biceps contracts, the triceps is reciprocally inhibited. In other words, if the biceps contracts (shortens), the antagonist muscle (the triceps) is told by the nervous system to relax (turn off) and lengthen in order for the movement to occur. A PNF stretch utilizing this reciprocal–inhibition principle has the client move as far into a stretch position as he comfortably can. The therapist then holds the client in a manner that prevents further movement into the stretch. The client then tries to move further into the stretch for 8–10 seconds, but is restrained as he pushes against the therapist's resistance. During this contraction, the inhibition signal is sent to the antagonist muscle. The client then relaxes, takes in a breath, and during exhalation, moves further into the stretch, assisted by the therapist to the next barrier.

You can easily remember reciprocal–inhibition PNF as always trying to move the same way. Each contraction is in the same direction, with or without resistance. This not only increases range of motion

but also builds strength on one side of the joint, helping to correct muscle strength imbalances. Reciprocal–inhibition PNF "turns off" the strong, tight muscles that are restricting movement, while strengthening the muscles creating the movement.

Reciprocal inhibition, if used properly, is a very effective method of using the nervous system to relax (turn off) a muscle cramp and is used extensively in event sports massage for this purpose. It can be used any time a client has a cramp. In seated massage, cramps are unlikely unless you are working at an endurance-type athletic event. If you intend to work such events, you should get specific event sports massage training.

These PNF protocols require considerable training to learn to do correctly. PNF also requires a therapist (or a partner) to assist with the protocol. The therapist must have a good understanding of the system and a high degree of sensitivity to fully achieve the desired effect and to avoid injuring the client. For an example of a reciprocal–inhibition PNF stretch, see Box 8-7.

Contract–Relax, Agonist–Contract (CRAC) Method

One of the simplest, safest methods of PNF, based on these principles, is contract–relax, antagonist–contract (CRAC) (9). In this method, the therapist only provides resistance to a 10% contraction of the muscle about to be stretched. The client then slowly relaxes the contraction, inhales, and moves into the stretch while exhaling. The therapist does not assist the client during the stretching phase. In this way, there is virtually no chance of overstretch injury, since the client will not overstretch himself. Because of its relative safety, the CRAC method is the most appropriate PNF technique for you to use, unless you have studied PNF techniques extensively.

The protocol for CRAC-type PNF stretching is as follows:

1. The client moves as far into the stretch as she comfortably can, as shown in Figure 8-5A.
2. The therapist then restrains the client from moving back toward the starting position.
3. The client tries to move back toward the staring position with 10% of her strength as the therapist resists the attempt for 8–10 seconds, as shown in Figure 8-5B.

4. The client then slowly relaxes and takes a deep breath. No movement occurs during this relaxation period, just a deep breath (inhalation). Therapist provides support and stabilization during the relaxation phase.
5. The client then exhales as she attempts to move further into the stretch as shown in Figure 8-5C.
6. The procedure is repeated one to two more times.
7. The client slowly returns to the starting position after performing repetitions of the CRAC procedure.

Figure 8-6A and B shows another CRAC stretch for the shoulders, specifically the pectoral muscles. These stretches are intended to be an introduction to PNF. Using this procedure, you can stretch any muscle. If the client has a range of motion restriction, have her move into the restriction as far as she can without pain and then use this CRAC procedure to increase her range of motion. Should you desire to use PNF methods extensively, it is highly recommended that

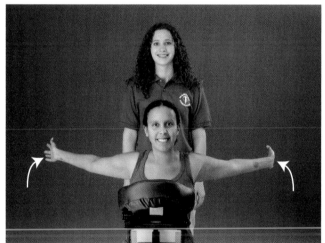

A

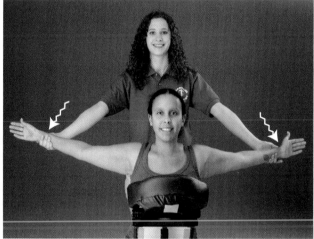

B

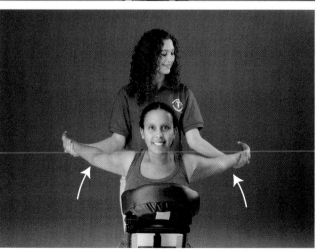

C

Figure 8-5 Contract–relax, agonist–contract (CRAC) PNF stretch for pectoralis major. (A) Step 1: Client moves as far into the stretch as she can. (B) Step 2: Therapist provides support and resistance as client contracts the muscle(s) being stretched for 8–10 seconds, then slowly relaxes. No movement is allowed. (C) Step 3: Client then actively contracts the agonist muscle, moving further in to the stretch. Therapist does not assist or pull the client in to the stretch; she only provides support and guidance.

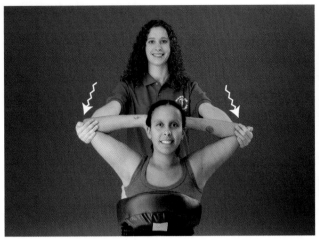
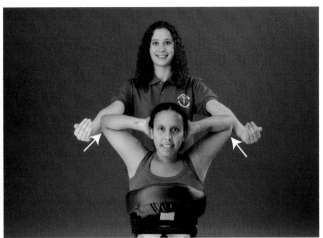

A

B

Figure 8-6   CRAC–PNF stretch for pectoralis minor and lower pectoralis major fibers. (A) Step 1: Contraction–relax with therapist support and resistance. (B) Step 2: Agonist–contract. Note the increased range of movement achieved. The therapist's hands did not move as the client contracted further into the stretch.

you invest in a complete training program on the techniques.

Active Isolated Stretching—Mattes Method

(Note: The information and the stretches below are adapted from *Active Isolated Stretching: The Mattes Method*, by Aaron Mattes and are used with permission.)

Active Isolated Stretching—Mattes Method (AIS) was developed by Aaron Mattes, a registered kinesiotherapist and licensed massage therapist, and adapts very well to seated massage. The AIS routines presented in this text provide very complete assessment, movement, and elongation techniques for the seated therapist, as well as homework stretches for the client. As mentioned above, this author believes the AIS system is the best system to use in seated massage. Therefore, this chapter will present more information and stretches from the AIS system than any other types of stretching techniques. However, to fully utilize AIS, it is recommended that you take specific training from an AIS—Mattes Method instructor.

AIS uses the principles of reciprocal inhibition, reciprocal innervation, and repetitive movement, combining them in a way that makes AIS stretches more powerful and more effective than any of the other systems alone. Done regularly, AIS not only increases flexibility, it increases strength.

AIS positions are chosen to best isolate the muscle(s) to be stretched. AIS uses reciprocal innervation of the agonist muscles to cause contraction, which will also simultaneously reciprocally inhibit contraction by the opposite side muscles, allowing them to relax and lengthen (stretch). Reciprocal innervation causes contraction, whereas reciprocal inhibition causes relaxation. Done repetitively, this increases range of motion (ROM) (2).

Local blood flow and nutrition is increased by AIS stretching. Repetitive isotonic muscle contractions increase the flow of blood, lymph, oxygen, and nutrition to specific regions more than static or isometric contractions do (2).

Muscles shorten, stiffen, or become tense from daily exposure to imbalanced posture, repetitive motion of work and sports, or stress. AIS can help restore normal joint movement, decrease tissue soreness, increase tissue pliability, and improve posture (2).

Unless the limit of existing range of motion is reached daily, range of motion will seldom be maintained. ROM can only be improved if the existing limit is exceeded repetitively. Improved flexibility can be acquired by properly performing movement techniques, such as AIS, which exceed the existing range of motion without causing injury. This is the purpose of assisting to the second barrier but only holding there for 2 seconds. Flexibility is reversible. It is lost gradually and is regained gradually (2).

Active Isolated Stretching is done in a very specific routine, no matter what muscle is being addressed. That routine is described below and summarized in a following list. A wrist-forearm stretch is then presented so you can practice on yourself and get the feel of this system of stretching. Finally, the effects of each step of the AIS routine are explained. Once you understand the AIS routine you can apply it anywhere on the body.

For chair massage, the areas most commonly addressed are the forearm, wrist and hand, neck, and shoulders. Routines for each of these areas will be given following the technique explanation section.

AIS Technique

To perform an AIS stretch, have the client comfortably inhale and begin to exhale. The client moves into the stretch as far as she can go with her own strength, contracting the opposite muscle to the one being stretched. For example, to stretch the forearm flexors, the client contracts the forearm extensors, causing the wrist to move into extension until it stops. We will call this end-of-movement point "the first barrier," as shown in Figure 8-7A.

The therapist then assists the client in the stretch with 1–2 pounds of pressure, taking the muscle to a second point of resistance or stopping point, which we will call "the second barrier." The client continues to contract (pull) into the stretch as the therapist assists the movement. Figure 8-7B shows a therapist assisting a client to the second barrier.

The stretch is held at the second barrier for two seconds, no longer. After two seconds, the client relaxes, the therapist withdraws his assistance, and the client inhales while returning to the starting position. Figure 8-7C shows the starting position or "neutral position." The sequence is repeated 6–10 times. Or, stated more concisely:

1. Client inhales.
2. Client exhales as she contracts into the stretch.
3. Therapist assists.
4. Client holds for two seconds.
5. Client inhales as she returns to the starting position.
6. Repeat.

One of the advantages of AIS is that you can perform the stretches on yourself (providing your own assistance), or, as a therapist, you can perform the stretches on your client (providing the assistance for her). Begin by assisting the client, then teach her to assist herself. In this way, she learns the stretch correctly and can then do it as "homework" between appointments with you.

The best place to learn Active Isolated Stretching is on your own wrist and forearm. You can easily assist yourself with your other hand and the sensitivity of your two hands working together will help you rapidly get the correct feel of the two barriers and the correct amount of assistance pressure.

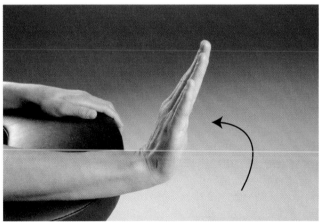

A

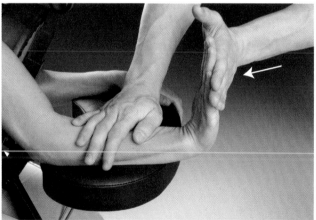

B

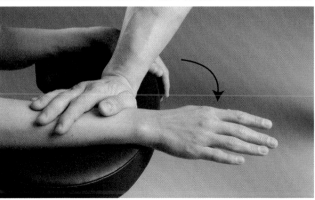

C

Figure 8-7 Active wrist extension. (A) Client's "first barrier." Exhale during this movement. (B) Therapist assisting wrist extension to the "second barrier." Hold at this position for two seconds. (C) Therapist releases assisting pressure. Client inhales as she actively moves back to the neutral (starting) position of the stretch.

Below is a sample forearm stretch.

1. Start with your non-dominate arm, elbow straight (locked), wrist and fingers neutral (straight), and palm down (pronated).
2. Inhale.
3. As you slowly exhale, extend your wrist as far as you comfortably can, this stopping point is the "first movement barrier."
4. Using your dominant hand, press on the palmar side of the fingers of the extended hand and press the fingers and hand further into extension. Do this slowly and gently. Feel for a point of resistance, the "second movement barrier."
5. Hold the assisting pressure at the second barrier for two seconds.
6. Release the assisting pressure and return the wrist to neutral as you inhale.
7. Repeat.

Repeat this sequence several times, usually 6–10 times. It is very important that you get the feeling of the first and second barriers. The first barrier is as far as the muscle(s) will move the joint by themselves. The second is the stopping point or point of resistance you encounter with 1–2 pounds of assistance. This should feel like a good stretch but should not be painful. The first three to four repetitions warm the tissues. Successive repetitions will usually gain a few degrees of increased movement with each repetition in the typical client. However, some clients are very tight, and many require more repetitions before their range of motion improves. In these cases, do 10 repetitions, then massage the muscles being stretched or do several other stretches, and then go back and do another set of stretches. Do not do more than 10 repetitions of a stretch in one set. Come back and do another set of 10 if necessary. This has been found to be more effective than 20 repetitions in a row.

Here is what you have done by performing the AIS routine:

1. Inhaling: brings in oxygen to the lungs for distribution to the body's cells.
2. Exhaling: a parasympathetic, relaxing response in the nervous system.
3. Contracting (innervating) the opposite muscle(s) of the one(s) being stretched: this, of course, causes the movement, but it also sends the reciprocal inhibition (relax) signal to the muscle being stretched, which helps it to turn off and relax, allowing it to be elongated to its point of resistance (first barrier).
4. Assisting: this intensifies the stretch, lengthening the fascia and resetting the nervous system

to accept moving past its first barrier to the second.

5. Holding for two seconds: allows the connective tissue to stretch, blood to flow out of the stretched tissue, and the nervous system to register the event.
6. Inhaling while returning to the neutral (starting) position: this again brings oxygen into the lungs, allows blood to flow back into the stretched tissue, and contracts (innervates) the muscle to be stretched to some degree, setting up a tense–relax event in the nervous system, all of which will allow further and further elongation with each repetition.

AIS Routines for Therapeutic Chair Massage

Below are some AIS routines appropriate for seated massage. They cover the forearm, wrist and hand, thumb, neck, and shoulder. The same protocol just described is used for each stretching position shown below. The first AIS routine is for the forearm, wrist, and hand. This entire forearm-wrist sequence is excellent for massage therapists to do on themselves before and after work to maintain the tissues of their arms and hands. It is also excellent to do on clients with carpal tunnel syndrome, hand, wrist, and elbow injuries. Practice this routine assisting yourself several times to get a confident feel of the protocol. Then perform it several times on another person, guiding and assisting him.

The client should exhale as he is doing the stretch and inhale as he is returning to the starting position. As this is true for every stretch, breathing instructions are not included in the descriptions for the individual stretches. Likewise, all stretches are held for two seconds, with the client then returning to neutral; this direction is also omitted from each description. Remember, when not talking, it is best for you to breathe in sync with your client, exhaling as you assist, inhaling as the client returns to starting position.

FOREARM, WRIST, AND HAND

1. **Elbow Flexor Stretch** (6–8 reps)
   (Stretches biceps brachii, brachialis, brachioradialis)
   - Have the client lift his arm off the arm rest and flex his elbow 45 degrees. Rotate his hand so that the palm is facing the body midline (medial), as in Figure 8-8A.
   - Have the client extend his elbow to its first barrier, then ulnar flex his wrist (moving little

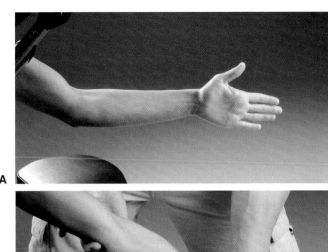
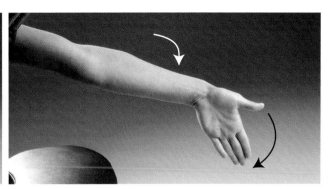

A

B

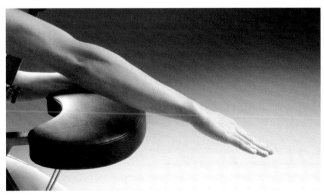

C

Figure 8-8 **Elbow flexor stretch.** (A) Starting position. Client's arm is off the arm rest, with her palm facing medial, thumb up, and elbow flexed. (B) Client at first barrier. Elbow is now extended (straight) and wrist is ulnar flexed as far as the client can move with her own strength. (C) Client assisted to the second barrier by the therapist.

finger toward the same side of the wrist) to stretch the brachioradialis, as in Figure 8-8B.
- Provide gentle assistance by supporting the client's elbow with one hand and applying pressure to the client's hand, taking both the elbow and the wrist further into the stretch (to the second barrier), as in Figure 8-8C.
2. **Wrist Extension, Prone** (6–10 reps)
   (Stretches wrist and finger flexors with emphasis at distal end attachments, including flexor

digitoriums, flexor carpi radialis, and flexor carpi ulnaris)
- Have the client lift his arm off the arm rest, elbow straight, wrist straight, and palm down, as in Figure 8-9A.
- Have the client extend his wrist and fingers as far as he can.
- Assist by supporting client at the elbow, while applying 1–2 pounds of pressure to the client's palmar surface and entire length of

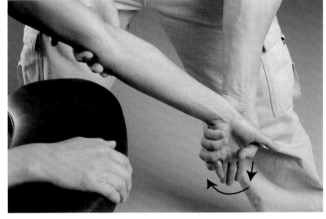
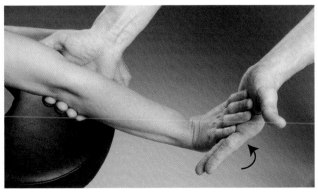

A

B

Figure 8-9 **Wrist extension prone.** (A) Starting position. Elbow is locked, wrist and fingers are straight, palm is facing downward. (B) Client assisted to the second barrier. Therapist is providing support at the client's elbow to keep it locked straight while assisting the movement by pressing against client's four fingers and hand.

fingers, as shown in Figure 8-9B. Make sure distal ends of the client's fingers do not bend.

3. **Wrist Extension, Supine** (6–10 reps)
(Stretches wrist and finger flexors as in previous stretch but with emphasis on proximal end attachments.)
   - Begin with the client's arm and wrist straight, with forearm supported by the armrest of the chair, palm up, as in Figure 8-10A.
   - Have the client extend her wrist and fingers backwards through the full range of motion.
   - Assist by stabilizing the forearm at the armrest, while applying 1–2 pounds of pressure to the client's palmar surface and entire length of fingers, as shown in Figure 8-10B.
   - Be sure that the distal ends of the client's fingers do not bend, or the effectiveness of the stretch will be lost.
   - (Note: The supine position intensifies the stretch. Perform the prone position first to warm up tissues, then progress to the supine position.)

4. **Wrist Flexion** (6–8 reps)
(Stretches wrist and forearm extensor muscles including the extensor carpi radialis longus, extensor carpi radialis brevis, and extensor carpi ulnaris.)
   - Begin with the client's arm and wrist straight, with the forearm supported by the armrest of the chair, palm down, as in Figure 8-11A.
   - Have the client flex her wrist downward, keeping her fingers straight.
   - Assist by stabilizing the forearm at the armrest, while applying 1–2 pounds of pressure to the client's dorsal hand surface and entire length of her fingers, as shown in Figure 8-11B.

5. **Finger Extensors** (6–10 reps)
(Stretches extensor carpi radialis longus, extensor carpi radialis brevis, extensor carpi ulnaris, extensor digitorum, extensor indicis, and extensor digiti minimi.)
   - Begin with the client's arm, wrist, and fingers straight, palm down, as in Figure 8-11A. (Same starting position as the previous stretch.)
   - Have the client make a fist and then flex her wrist downward as far as possible.
   - Assist by pressing your hand against the dorsal surface of the client's hand that is being stretched, as shown in Figure 8-12.

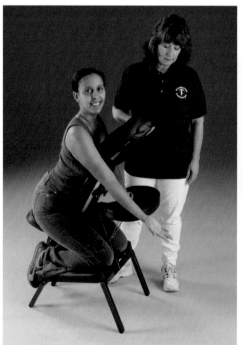 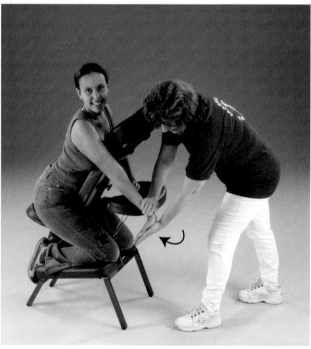

A　　　　　　　　　　　　　　　　　　　　　　　　　　　**B**

Figure 8-10 Wrist extension supine. (A) Starting position. Client's elbow is locked, wrist and hand are straight, with palm facing up. Note client's forearm is resting on the arm rest of the chair. (B) Assisted to second barrier. Therapist is providing stabilization just proximal to client's wrist while assisting movement.

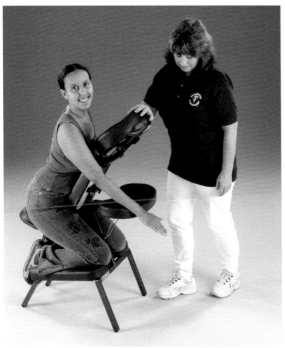 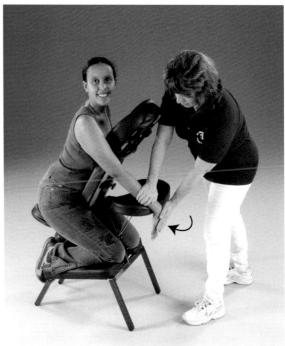

A   B

Figure 8-11 **Wrist flexion.** (A) Starting position. Client's arm is straight, elbow locked, palm down, resting on arm rest of chair. (B) Assisted to second barrier. Therapist stabilizes client's forearm while applying pressure on dorsal side (back side) of client's hand. Note client's fingers remain straight during the wrist movement.

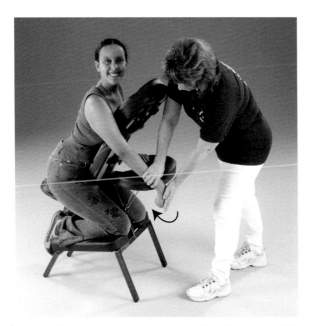

Figure 8-12 **Finger extensor stretch.** This is a modification of the stretch shown in Figure 8-11B to create a better stretch for the finger extensor muscles. With palm facing downward, client makes a loosely clinched fist, then flexes wrist. Therapist provides assistance to the second barrier by pressing on the dorsal side (back side) of client's hand.

6. **Ulnar Deviation** (also called wrist ulnar flexion or adduction; 6–10 reps)
   (Stretches flexor carpi radialis and extensor carpi radialis longus.)
   - Begin with the client's forearm resting on the armrest of the chair with the wrist and fingers straight and the palm facing the mid-line (medial), thumb up in the handshake position. (Note: stretch may also be done with the palm facing down, or prone.)
   - Have the client bend his wrist straight toward his little finger side (lateral), keeping his fingers straight.
   - Assist by grasping the client's hand and fingers (but not thumb) and applying gentle pressure in the direction of the movement (lateral and posterior), as shown in Figure 8-13.
7. **Radial Deviation** (also called wrist radial flexion or abduction; 6–10 reps)
   (Stretches extensor carpi ulnaris and flexor carpi ulnaris.)
   - Begin with the client's forearm resting on the armrest of the chair with the wrist and fingers straight and the palm facing down (prone). (Note: stretch may also be done with the palm facing medial in the handshake position.)

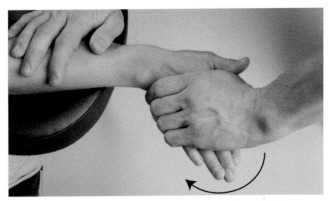

Figure 8-13 **Ulnar deviation in the "handshake position" with therapist assisting client to the second barrier.**

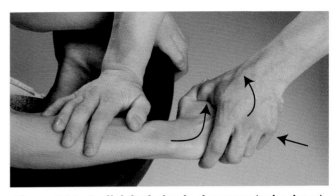

Figure 8-14 **Radial deviation in the prone (palm down) position with therapist providing stabilization and assistance.** Note therapist grasps hand and all four fingers, but not the thumb.

- Assist by grasping the client's hand and fingers (but not thumb) and applying gentle pressure in the direction of the movement (lateral and posterior), as shown in Figure 8-14.
8. **Radial-Ulnar Supination and Pronation** (6–8 reps in each direction)
(Supination stretches pronator quadratus and pronator teres; pronation stretches biceps brachii and supinator muscles.)
   - Begin with the client's forearm resting on the armrest of the chair, palm downward for both stretches.
   - Supination: have the client rotate his forearm and wrist to the palm up position and continue the rotation as far as he can go. His thumb should now be pointing lateral.
   - Assist by grasping the dorsal side of the client's hand with two of your fingers on each side of the client's thumb and gently apply pressure in the direction of the stretch, as shown in Figure 8-15A.

- Pronation: have the client rotate his forearm and wrist so that his thumb points downward and his palm points lateral.
- Assist by grasping the lateral (little finger) side of the client's hand and applying gentle rotational pressure in the direction of the rotation, as shown in Figure 8-15B. (Note: it may be necessary for you to use your other hand to stabilize the client's forearm against the armrest so that it does not move up and away from the client's body during the stretch movement.)
9. **Finger Flexors** (6–10 reps for each finger)
(Stretches flexor digitorum superficialis, flexor digitorum profundus, and flexor digiti minimi muscles.)
   - Begin with the client's hand supported on the armrest pad of the chair, palm down, wrist and fingers straight.
   - Have the client extend an individual finger as far as he can.

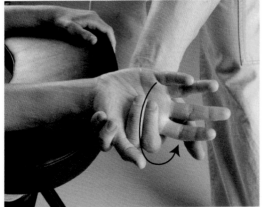
A

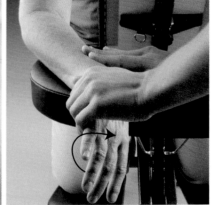
B

Figure 8-15 **Radial–ulnar supination showing therapist assisting.** (A) Note therapist's grip on client's hand—two fingers on each side of client's thumb. (B) Radial-ulnar pronation shown with therapist assisting to second barrier. Note stabilization on forearm.

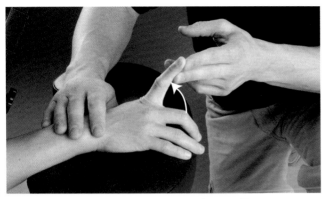 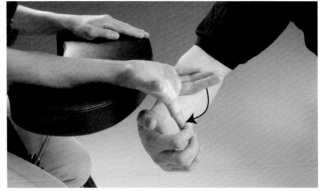

A   B

Figure 8-16 **Stretching individual finger flexors.** (A) Hand prone (down) position. Client extends one finger as far as she can, then therapist uses a few ounces of pressure to assist client to second barrier. There is usually a significant movement from the first barrier to the second. Stabilize client's hand and restrain her other fingers as necessary. (B) Supine (palm up) position. Client moves fingers off the edge of arm rest but keeps hand and wrist supported. Stretch each finger as is done in prone position (part A).

- Assist by using two fingers or your palm to move the client's finger further into the stretch. Be gentle! This stretch only requires ounces of pressure to reach the second barrier. See Figure 8-16A.
- Repeat for each finger.
- For a greater stretch, extend the client's wrist, then do each individual finger.
- For maximal stretch, rotate the client's hand to the palm up position (supination) and slide the client's arm forward so that his hand is off the front of the chair armrest, but so that the client's wrist remains supported. Repeat the stretches for each finger as shown in Figure 8-16B.
- This position will significantly intensify the stretch; therefore, it is important that six repetitions be done in the palm down position first to reduce chance of injury.
- Note the following: (1) This is an extremely beneficial stretch for clients with carpal tunnel syndrome. They should perform the wrist extension and flexion stretches first, then do this individual finger extension stretch twice or more each day. They assist themselves with their other hand. (2) Individual fingers may be stretched into flexion to stretch finger extensors. With wrist and fingers straight, flex one finger. Assist by applying gentle pressure to the dorsal side of the proximal phalange. (3) Only one pound of pressure or less is required to assist individual finger stretches.

THUMB

Note: Only one pound of pressure or less is required to assist thumb stretches.

1. **Thumb Opposition Stretch** (5–8 reps)
   (Stretches opponens pollicis, flexor pollicis brevis, and adductor pollicis)
   - Place the client's arm on the arm rest of the chair with her palm up.
   - Have the client move her thumb tip toward the base of her little finger. This is the starting (neutral) position.
   - Have the client move the thumb straight back away from the base of the little finger (horizontal abduction) as far as she can.
   - Assist by gently pressing on the tip of the client's thumb in the direction of the movement using one or two fingers. Ounces of pressure are sufficient to reach the second barrier of this movement. See Figure 8-17.
   - Note the following: (1) The therapist may stabilize the client's wrist (and heel of hand) as necessary. (2) Slightly vary the angle to achieve the best stretch.
2. **Thumb Adductor (web) Stretch** (5–8 reps)
   (Stretches web of thumb including adductor pollicis longus and adductor pollicis brevis.)
   - Begin with the client's hand palm down, fingers straight, resting on the armrest of the chair with the thumb next to the index finger.
   - Stabilize the client's hand by grasping the client's four fingers.
   - Have the client abduct her thumb horizontally (move thumb away from the index

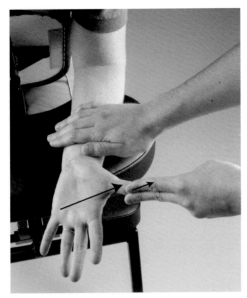

Figure 8-17 Thumb opposition stretch with therapist assistance. Tip of thumb moves away from base of little finger (horizontal abduction). A few ounces of pressure in the direction of the stretching movement is usually sufficient for thumb stretches.

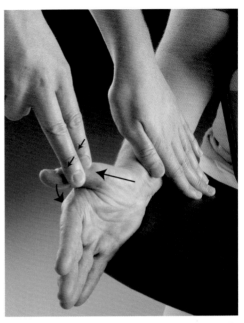

Figure 8-19 Thumb adductor stretch assisted to second barrier. Therapist stabilizes wrist as client tries to touch her first knuckle with her thumb. Therapist assists with just ounces of pressure.

finger in a plane parallel to the armrest) as far as she can.
- Assist by grasping client's thumb and applying gentle pressure in the direction of the movement, stretching the thumb and connecting web tissue as shown in Figure 8-18.

3. **Thumb Abductor Stretch** (5–8 reps)
(Stretches abductor pollicis longus and abductor pollicis brevis.)
- Begin with the client's wrist and hand supported on the armrest of the chair with the client's palm facing the midline (medially), thumb up. You may use one of your hands to stabilize client's wrist or forearm.

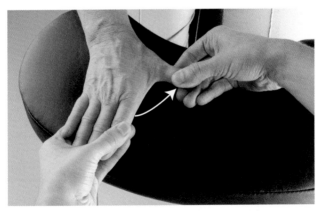

Figure 8-18 Thumb adductor (web) stretch assisted by therapist. Note stabilization of fingers by therapist during assistance of thumb movement.

- Have the client move her thumb over the first finger to the back (dorsal) side of her index finger, trying to touch her first knuckle.
- Assist with one or two fingers in the direction of the stretch, as shown in Figure 8-19.

4. **Thumb Extensor Stretch** (5–8 reps)
(Stretches extensor pollicis longus and extensor pollicis brevis.)
- Begin with the client's wrist and forearm supported on the armrest of the chair with the palm of the hand toward the midline (medial) and the thumb up.
- Stabilize the client's hand by grasping the first metacarpal bone, just proximal to the metacarpal-phalangeal joint.
- Have the client flex her thumb toward the base of her little finger as far as she can go.
- Assist by gently pressing on the proximal phalanx of the client's thumb in the direction of the movement. See Figure 8-20.

NECK

Note that cervical flexion and extension should be performed at the C-1 level, not with the entire cervical spine. Be sure the client is sitting up straight. Have him place a finger on each side of his head just inferior to the mastoid process (just behind the bottom of the ear). As he moves his chin up and down, his head

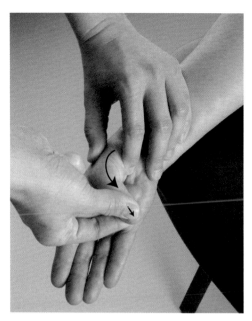

Figure 8-20 Thumb extensor stretch, therapist assisting. Client moves her thumb toward base of her little finger, with the therapist gently assisting the movement and stabilizing as necessary.

should pivot around the points he is touching with his fingers.

1. **Anterior Cervical Flexion** (8–10 reps)
   (Stretches multifidus, semispinalis, oblique capitus, and erector spinae.)
   - Begin with the client sitting up straight, with the back of her neck "long," looking straight ahead.

- Have the client tuck her chin down as close to her neck as possible, keeping her mouth closed and trunk straight (the client should not bend or lean forward).
- Stand at the side of the client and provide assistance to the stretch by using your front hand to provide a gentle pulling effort while your rear hand stabilizes client's shoulders, as shown in Figure 8-21A.
- Teach the client to perform the stretch herself, assisting by reaching up with one arm and pulling down and forward on her head.

2. **Hyperextension** (cervical extension; 8–10 reps)
   (Stretches longus colli, longus capitus, rectus capitus anterior, rectus capitus lateralis, and scalene muscles.)
   Note: If the client has been told he should not do hyperextension by his physician or chiropractor, omit this movement and have him do the posterior oblique stretches instead.
   - Begin with the client sitting up straight, looking straight forward.
   - Have the client gently tilt her head backwards, keeping her eyes open and looking up. Movement is at the C-1 level, as described above.
   - Assist the movement by gently pulling up on the client's chin and pulling down on the top of the client's head. You can also exert a gentle, superior (straight up) traction with both hands at the same time as applying the rotation. See Figure 8-22A.

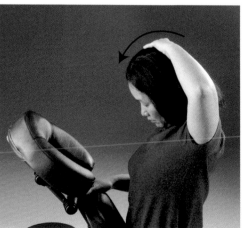

Figure 8-21 Anterior cervical flexion stretch. (A) With assistance from therapist. Note that movement occurs at the level of the C-1 vertebrae. (B) Client assisting herself in the anterior cervical flexion stretch.

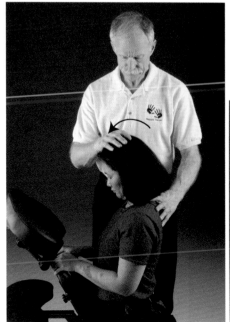

A

B

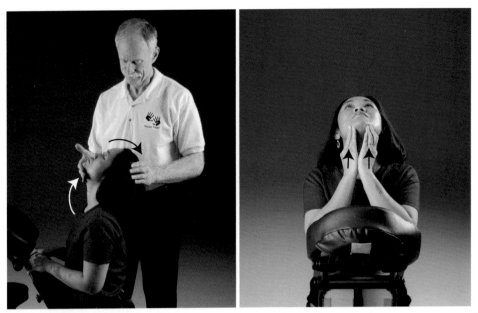

Figure 8-22 **Hyperextension cervical stretch.** (A) With assistance from therapist. Movement occurs at the C-1 vertebrae level. If client has been advised by a healthcare provider to not perform this movement, do not use this stretch. Use posterior oblique stretch instead. (B) Self-assisted. Client should be looking up with her eyes as she does the movement.

- Note the following: (1) Never cause pain or allow the client to go into pain. (2) Instruct the client to do the stretch herself, assisting herself by pushing upward on her chin with both hands, as shown in Figure 8-22B. (3) For clients with disc injuries, degenerative cervical spine conditions, or recent severe whiplash or severe trauma, hyperextension may be contraindicated. When treating clients with these conditions, do not perform this hyperextension stretch.

3. **Cervical Lateral Flexion** (8–10 reps in each direction)
   (Stretches scalene, sternocleidomastoid, and splenius capitus.)
   - Begin with the client sitting up straight, looking forward.
   - Have the client lean her head to one side, moving her ear toward her shoulder as far as she can.
   - Be sure she is isolating movement in her neck and not leaning her body.
   - Assist by stabilizing and holding down her shoulder on the side being stretched with one hand while applying gentle pressure on the client's head in the direction of the movement with your other hand. See Figure 8-23A.
   - Note the following: (1) The client can be taught to perform the stretch herself by reaching up and gently pulling on her head with her

own hand, as shown in Figure 8-23B. (2) If the client has problems keeping her shoulder down or shrugging her shoulder on the side the head is moving toward, have her grab the seat of the chair with her hands. When she assists herself, she can grab the seat on the side being stretched.

4. **Cercival Rotation** (6–10 reps in each direction)
   (Stretches multifidus, rotators, semispinalis, and sternocleidomastoid.)
   - Begin with the client sitting erect, with the back of the neck long, and looking straight forward.
   - Have the client rotate her head to one side as far as she can, also looking with her eyes to that side.
   - Guide and assist the movement with one hand on the client's temple and the other hand on the client's occiput, as shown in Figure 8-24A.
   - Note that the client may be taught to assist herself with her own hands, as shown in Figure 8-24B.

5. **Cervical Posterior Oblique** (8–10 reps in each direction)
   (Stretches anterior scalenus, sternocleidomastoid, longus colli, longus capitus, and rectus capitus.)
   - Begin with the client sitting erect and looking straight forward.

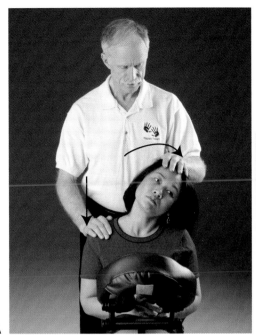

A

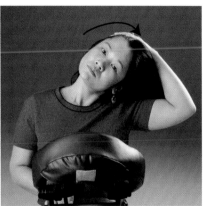

B

Figure 8-23 Cervical lateral flexion stretch. (A) With therapist assisting. Note therapist is stabilizing client's shoulder (and torso) with one hand while assisting the stretching movement with the other. (B) Self-assisted.

- Have the client rotate her head 45 degrees to one side so that her nose is centered over her breast on that side. See Figure 8-25A.
- Have the client lean her head backwards at a 45-degree angle (posterior and lateral), moving her ear toward the outer border of her shoulder blade (scapula).
- Have the client adjust the angle of rotation as necessary to obtain the best feeling of stretch in the scalene-sternocleidomastoid area.

- Assist by stabilizing the client's shoulder with one hand and providing gentle pressure in the direction of the movement on the upper side of the client's head with your other hand, as shown in Figure 8-25B.
- Note the following: (1) The client can assist herself in this stretch using her arm and hand, similar to the assist shown in the cervical lateral flexion stretch, Figure 8-23B. (2) The client may stabilize herself by grabbing

Figure 8-24 Cervical rotation stretch. (A) With therapist assisting. Client looking in the direction of the movement will enhance results. (B) Self-assisted.

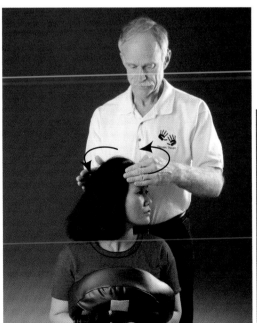

A

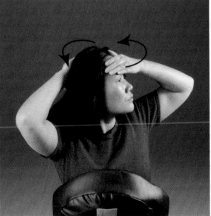

B

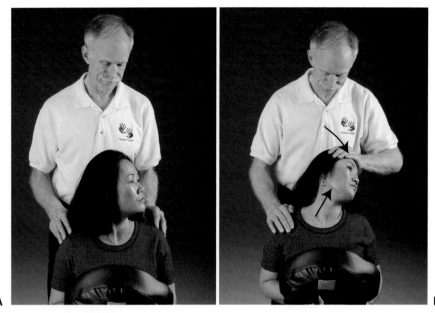

Figure 8-25 Cervical posterior oblique stretch. (A) Starting position. Client's head is rotated 45 degrees away from the side being stretched. (B) Assisted to second barrier. Client leans head posterior and lateral at a 45-degree angle away from the side being stretched. Therapist stabilizes client's shoulder while assisting to the second barrier of movement. Stretch should be felt in the scalene and sternocleidomastoid area. Note: Client can self-assist this stretch by reaching up with her left arm and pulling in the direction of the movement.

the seat bottom with her hand on the side being stretched. (3) The client should not arch her back. Instruct her to contract her abdominals to provide stabilization.

SHOULDER

1. **Horizontal Abduction** (8–10 reps in each of three positions)
(Stretches pectoralis major, pectoralis minor, and anterior deltoid.)
   • Have the client sit up erect with her arms straight down at her sides.
   • Instruct the client to lift her arms to about 45 degrees of sideward elevation, as in Figure 8-26A.
   • Ask the client to exhale and reach back as far as she can with both arms. When her movement stops (her first barrier), grasp her forearms, as in Figure 8-26B.
   • Assist the client to her second barrier, as shown in Figure 8-26C, by applying 1–2 pounds of pressure in the direction of the movement. Hold the endpoint of her movement for two seconds, release, and have her - inhale as she returns to the starting position.
   • As the clavicular fibers of pectoralis major loosen, ask the client to raise her arms to horizontal and continue the movements. The horizontal position stretches the sternal fibers.

   • Finally, ask the client to lift her arms to 45 degrees above horizontal and reach back, assisting them as in the previous two positions. See Figure 8-26D. This position stretches the costal fibers of pectoralis major and has the most effect on pectoralis minor.
   • Note the following: The client should not arch her back or jut her head forward during the stretch. Have her contract her abdominal muscles as necessary to stabilize her back. If she is jutting her head forward, make her aware that she is doing so and remind her to keep her back and neck straight.
2. **Hyperextension** (8–10 reps in each of two positions)
(Stretches biceps brachii, anterior deltoid, pectoralis major, and pectoralis minor.)
   • Have the client sit up straight with her arms at her sides, palms pointing medial, as in Figure 8-27A.
   • Instruct the client to flex her neck (bend neck forward) slightly (about 15 degrees). This prevents cervical strain during the stretch.
   • Ask the client to reach backwards and up as far as she can with both arms at once, keeping her elbows straight and without leaning forward.
   • Grasp the client's forearms just proximal to her wrists and assist the movement. Ideal

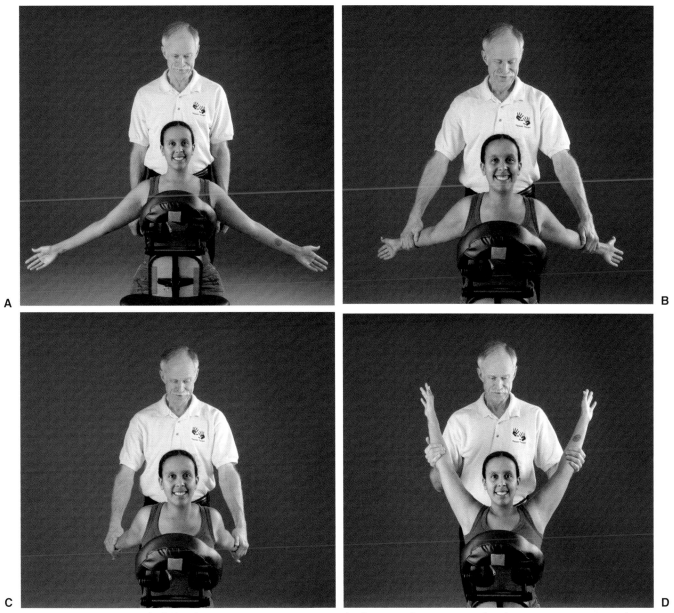

Figure 8-26 Horizontal abduction. (A) Starting position. In the first set of repetitions, client's arms are out at a 45-degree angle from her side to stretch the clavicular fibers of pectoralis major. (B) Client at her first barrier, therapist ready to begin assistance. (C) Client assisted by therapist to her second barrier. Another set of 6–10 repetitions with the client's arms straight out should be done to stretch the sternal fibers. (D) Client's arms raised to 45 degrees upward to stretch costal fibers, therapist providing assistance.

range of motion for this stretch is 90 degrees, or straight back, parallel to the floor (horizontal), as shown in Figure 8-27B. Do not go beyond this amount of movement.

- Ask the client to interlace her fingers with her palms pointing posterior (backwards), keeping her elbows locked or as straight as possible.
- Have the client again reach back and up as far as possible, as shown in Figure 8-27C, without leaning forward or arching her back.
- Assist her to her second barrier, but do not go past horizontal. This second position with

the fingers interlaced and palms pointing backwards provides a better stretch for the long head of biceps brachii.

3. **External Rotation** (8–10 reps)
   (Stretches internal shoulder rotators, including pectoralis major, subscapularis, latissimus dorsi, and teres major.)
   - Have the client sit erect with arms at her side.
   - Instruct the client to raise her arm up (sideward elevation) to parallel to the floor and to bend her elbow 90 degrees so that her fingertips are pointing forward, as shown in Figure 8-28A.

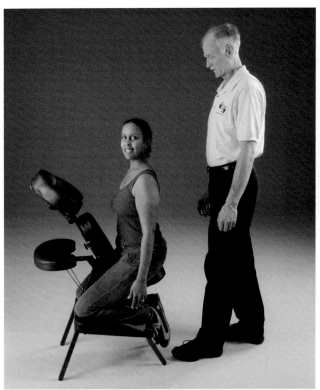

A

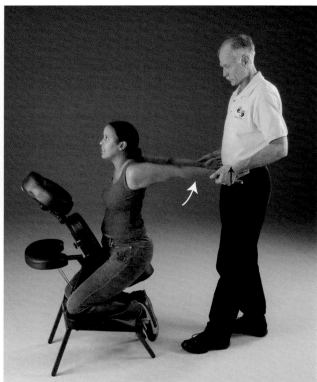

B

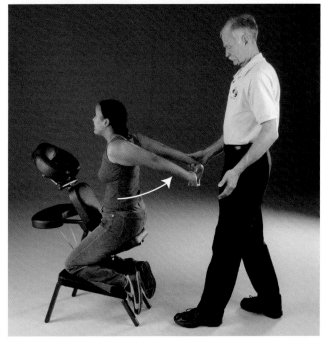

C

Figure 8-27 Hyperextension stretch. (A) Starting position. (B) Therapist assisting client to second barrier. (C) Advanced version of hyperextension stretch. Client has fingers interlaced and palms pointing posterior (backwards) while reaching up as far as she can (first barrier). Therapist will now assist client to the second movement barrier by lifting client's arm. Ideal range of motion at second barrier is 90 degrees, or parallel to the floor.

- Standing behind the client's shoulder, support her humerus (upper arm) so that it is straight out from the shoulder, not angling posterior or anterior or sagging toward the floor.
- Ask the client to externally rotate her humerus by moving her hand up and as far back as she can.

- Assist this movement with gentle pressure on the client's forearm just proximal to her wrist. See Figure 8-28B.
- Do not allow the client to arch her back or rotate her upper body in the direction of the shoulder being stretched.
- Note the following: (1) External rotation stretches the internal rotators of the shoul-

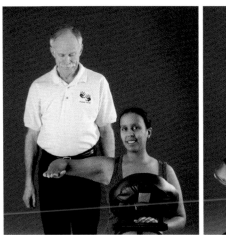
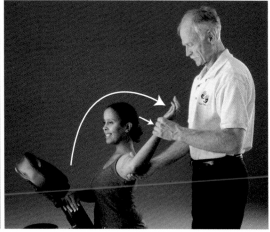

A
B

Figure 8-28 **External rotation stretch.** (A) Starting position. (B) Client assisted to second movement barrier by therapist. Note therapist is supporting client's humerus at the elbow and applying a gentle pressure in the direction of the movement on the client's wrist.

der, which are usually the tightest. This is an essential stretch for "frozen shoulder." (2) If the client experiences pain getting into this position or if she has shoulder impingement, this stretch can be performed with the elbow flexed at 90 degrees and held at the side of her body. External rotation is performed in this position by having the client move her hand lateral and posterior (reaching backwards). Hold her elbow stable and assist at her wrist.

4. **Internal Rotation** (8–10 reps; also known as "the Scarecrow")
   (Stretches external rotators of the shoulder, including supraspinatus, infraspinatus, and teres minor, the posterior rotator cuff.)
   • Have the client sit erect with arms at her side.
   • Instruct the client to raise her arm up (sideward elevation) to parallel to the floor and to bend her elbow 90 degrees so that her fingertips are pointing forward, as shown in Figure 8-29A. This is the same starting position as

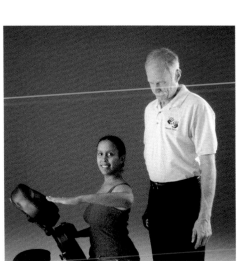
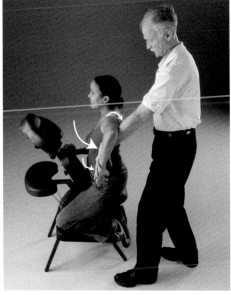

A
B

Figure 8-29 **Internal rotation stretch.** (A) Starting position. Note this is the same starting position as the external rotation stretch, Figure 8-28. (B) Therapist assisting client to the second movement barrier. Therapist's hand closest to the client is stabilizing the client's shoulder with a downward, posterior rotation pressure. Therapist's other hand is assisting the movement by pressing posterior (backwards) on the client's wrist. Note therapist's assisting arm is supporting the client's humerus.

was used for external rotation in the previous stretch.

- Stand behind the client and place your more medial hand (relative to the client) on the top of her shoulder.
- Apply a stabilizing pressure to client's scapula by pressing inferior (down) with a slight posterior rotation. If you do not do this, the scapula will move superior and rotate forward as the client does the stretch, preventing the stretch from being effective.
- Support the client's humerus with your other arm and hand by reaching under the client's humerus and placing your palm on the back of her wrist.
- While holding her shoulder down, as described in Step 4, ask her to reach backwards (external rotation) as far as possible.
- Assist the movement by applying gentle posterior pressure to the back of her wrist, as shown in Figure 8-29B.
- Note the following: Internal rotation stretches the external shoulder rotators. Stretches 3 and 4 are both very important in all rotator cuff problems.

5. **Triceps** (6–10 reps)
   (Stretches triceps brachii.)
   - Begin with the client sitting erect.
   - Ask the client to reach over her shoulder and try to touch the back side of her scapula ("shoulder blade") with the palm of her hand, as shown in Figure 8-30A.
   - Assist by pressing posterior (backwards) on the client's elbow with one of your hands, while keeping the client's hand centered over her scapula with your other hand. See Figure 8-30B.
   - After 4–6 reps, ask the client to reach more medial with her hand and try to touch her spine. Assist her in the direction of the movement as before for an additional 4–6 reps. This provides a better stretch for the lateral and more angular fibers of the triceps.
   - Note the following: (1) Be sure the client is not arching her back as you assist the stretch. If she is, have her contract her abdominal muscles for stability. (2) Have the client keep her arm close to her head throughout the movement. (3) The client can assist herself with her other arm, as shown in Figure 8-30C and D.

6. **Forward Elevation** (6–10 reps)
   (Stretches triceps brachii, posterior deltoid, and anterior serratus.)
   - Begin with the client sitting erect, arms hanging straight down at her sides, elbows locked, palms facing medial.
   - Stand behind the client, as shown in Figure 8-31A.
   - Ask the client to raise both her arms straight up as far as she can while contracting her abdominal muscles to prevent leaning backwards.
   - Assist client at the end of her movement by grasping her arms just proximal to her elbows and gently pulling straight posterior.
   - For a more precise stretch, especially for treating a problematic shoulder, only stretch one side at a time. Standing on one side of the client, stabilize her by placing one of your hands on the posterior (back) of her scapula. Assist her at the end of her movement with your other hand by applying a posterior pressure at or just proximal to her elbow, as shown in Figure 8-31B.
   - Note the following: (1) The internally rotated, head forward ("slumped") posture will restrict forward elevation. This posture may be a contributing factor in cases of "frozen shoulder." (2) The client should be able to raise her arms to straight vertical. (3) Advanced positions for this stretch are palm(s) facing anterior (forward) and palm(s) facing lateral (away from the body). (4) For best results, triceps and internal shoulder rotators should be stretched prior to forward elevation stretch. The client must be capable of 90 degrees or more of external rotation to be able to achieve maximal forward elevation. (5) The client may assist herself by assuming the lunge position in front of an open doorway, raising her arm(s), and leaning forward against the top of the door frame.

7. **Sideward Elevation** (8–10 reps)
   (Stretches teres major, latissimus dorsi, and sternal portion of pectoralis major.)
   - Begin with the client sitting erect, arm straight out to her side, elbow locked, palm facing anterior (forward). See Figure 8-32A.
   - Stand behind the client and slightly to one side.

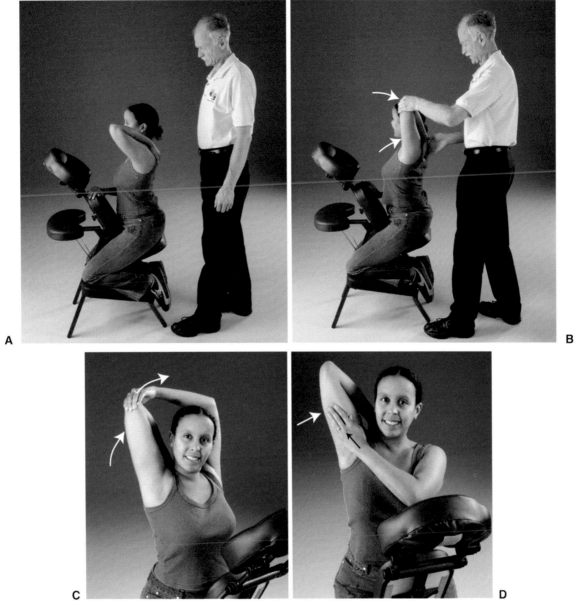

Figure 8-30 Triceps stretch. (A) Client reaches over her shoulder, trying to touch her shoulder blade with the palm of her hand. (B) Therapist assists the movement with posterior pressure on the elbow while guiding the client's hand. (C) Client self-assisting triceps stretch. (D) Alternate method of self-assisting triceps stretch.

- Ask the client to raise her arm straight up and behind her head as far as she can.
- Assist the client in the direction of the movement by gently pressing against her elbow, as shown in Figure 8-32B.
- Note the following: (1) The client may assist herself by using her opposite arm to pull in the direction of the movement from the level of her elbow. See Figure 8-32C. (2) Advanced positions of this stretch include the following: While holding the stretch, the client may lean laterally in the direction of arm move-

ment to enhance stretch of latissimus dorsi. While holding the stretch, the client may lean obliquely forward to stretch quadratus lumborum (rotate torso 45 degrees toward the side being stretched and then lean forward at a 45-degree angle, away from the side being stretched). While holding the stretch, the client may lean obliquely backwards to stretch anterior serratus (rotate torso 45 degrees away from side being stretched and then lean backwards away from the side being stretched). (3) To help free shoulder

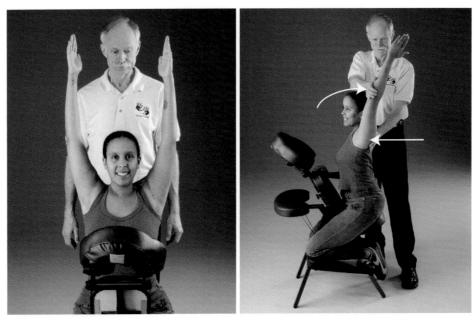

Figure 8-31 **Forward elevation stretch.** (A) Client reaching up and back to first movement barrier. Therapist can assist by pulling posterior on both arms. Be sure client does not arch back or lean backwards. (B) Alternate method: therapist assisting one side at a time, stabilizing client's scapula with one hand while applying posterior pressure on the client's arm just proximal to the elbow.

impingement, an inverted version of this stretch is helpful. Begin with the client's arm (the one being stretched) at her side, hanging straight down, elbow locked, palm facing forward. Ask her to reach behind her back as far as she can, keeping her arm straight. Assist her gently in the direction of the movement. To intensify this stretch, have her further externally rotate her shoulder until her palm faces lateral (if she can do so without pain). Use extreme caution in this position, as these tissues will be tight and easily overstretched. (4) The normal (full) range of motion for this stretch should bring the client's arm to behind the center of her head (mid-sagittal plane line). The client must have near normal forward elevation (previous stretch) to accomplish this.

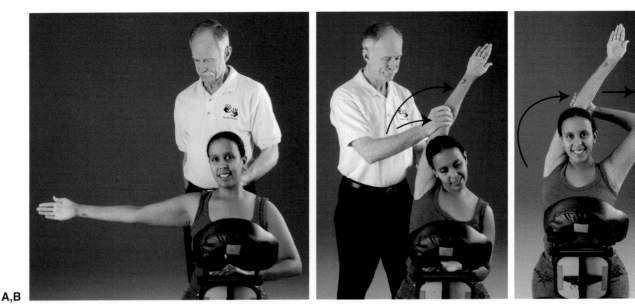

Figure 8-32 **Sideward elevation.** (A) From starting position (shown), client raises her arm straight up to her first motion barrier. (B) Therapist then assists the movement with gentle pressure applied at elbow. (C) Client self-assisting the stretch. Client shown has ideal range of motion.

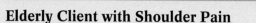

Elderly Client with Shoulder Pain

An elderly woman comes to you while you are doing massage at a Community Senior Citizens Center. She says she cannot move her right shoulder without a lot of pain.

1. How could you use stretching to assess which muscles are causing her pain and restrict her movement?
2. Which stretches would you use?
3. What would be an indication that a particular muscle is part of the problem she reports?
4. If she reports pain when doing forward elevation of her entire arm, which muscles are likely involved?
5. If she reports pain during sideward elevation at about 70 degrees through 120 degrees, what muscle/tendon might be "impinged" at the acromion process?

Athletic Client with Wrist Pain

You are contracted to provide chair massage for the employees of a local bank twice a week. In August, a 27-year-old female employee comes to you and reports she believes she has developed carpal tunnel syndrome and wants to recover without surgery. She began experiencing right wrist pain two weeks after starting her job as a bank teller, which requires counting money and operating a computer. She has been performing the job for three months and the pain is getting worse. She has not been to a physician for a formal evaluation/diagnosis. She is 5'8" tall, ideal weight, with no known health problems, no injuries, takes no medications, lifts weights, and bicycles daily. When you look at her posture you notice that her ear is about 2 inches anterior relative to her shoulder and that her hands are internally rotated with three knuckles presenting anterior instead of the normal thumb and first finger. Although she reports pain in her right wrist, she does not experience any tingling, numbness, or loss of dexterity in the hand.

1. What stretches would be the most effective to address her wrist complaint?

2. Which two or three stretches might be best to give her as homework? (Hint: What will best address the individual finger tendons, which pass through the carpal tunnel?)
3. Might her head-forward, internally rotated posture be involved in her condition? What stretches or exercises presented so far in this text would be indicated for her?
4. Could bicycling be involved in her complaint?

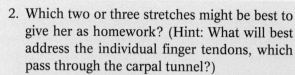

Client with Whiplash Injury

You are working with a client who sits at a computer most of the day. He has significant head-forward posture and internally rotated shoulders. Due to a whiplash accident, he has been told by his physician that he should never do hyper-extension stretches or exercises.

1. What stretches could you safely use to lengthen the front of his neck?
2. What shoulder stretches might help lessen his internally rotated condition?

SUMMARY

Stretching techniques are an important addition to seated massage. They add passive or active movement to an otherwise static experience for the client's nervous system. Correctly applied stretching techniques are sedating (relaxing) to the nervous system and contribute a deeper, longer lasting therapeutic effect from the treatment. Stretching done prior to massage techniques serve not only to elongate tissues but also as an assessment method for the therapist. Stretching done after massage techniques helps prevent the reoccurrence of trigger points and spasms, prolonging the effect of the treatment. When active stretches are used, tissue is elongated, circulation is enhanced, and the efficiency of the person's nervous system is improved.

There are four main systems of stretching: static, passive, PNF, and AIS. Done correctly, all four are effective; however, PNF and AIS are more effective than static, with passive being the least effective overall. This author prefers the AIS system, finding it quicker and easier to use in seated massage applications and more effective as a homework strategy for clients.

Regardless of which system you use, including stretching in seated massage routines will improve your overall effectiveness, give your hands a break from massage techniques, and support your clients by teaching them how to maintain what you gain for them.

> *"The patient is a victim of your knowledge, or lack of it!"*
>
> AARON MATTES (February 21, 2003)

REFERENCES

1. Mazzoni MC, Skalak TC, Schmid-Schonbein GW. Effects of skeletal muscle fiber deformation on lymphatic volumes. *AM J Physiol* 1990;259(6 Pt 2):H1860–1868.
2. Mattes AL. *Active Isolated Stretching—The Mattes Method.* Sarasota, FL: Aaron Mattes Therapy, 2000;2,5,7,9.
3. Garfin SR, Tipton CM, Mubarak SJ, et al. Role of fascia in maintenance of muscle tension and pressure. *J Appl Physiol* 1981;51(2):317–320.
4. Varela FJ, Frenk S. The organ of form: Towards a theory of biological shape. *J Soc Biol Struct* 1987;10:73–83.
5. Greenman PE. *Principles of Manual Medicine,* 2nd Ed. Baltimore: Lippincott, Williams & Wilkins; 1996:146–148
6. Schleip R. Fascial plasticity—A new neurobiological explanation, part 1. *J Bodywork Movement Therapies,* 2003;January:11–19. Part 2, *J Bodywork Movement Therapies,* 2003;April:104–116.
7. Steen EB, Montagu A. *Anatomy & Physiology,* vol. 1. New York: Harper-Collins; 1959:104.
8. Heine H. Functional anatomy of traditional Chinese acupuncture points. *Acta Anatomica* 1995;152:293.
9. McAtee RE. *Facilitated Stretching.* Champaign, IL: Human Kinetics; 1993:2–4.
10. Dirckx JH, ed. *Steadman's Concise Medical Dictionary for the Health Professional: Illustrated,* 4th Ed. Baltimore: Lippincott, Williams & Wilkins; 2001.

Notes

CHAPTER 9

Relaxation Routine

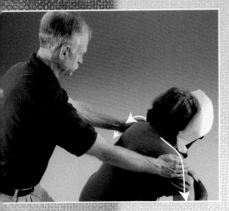

"Every now and then go away, have a little relaxation, for when you come back to your work your judgment will be surer."

LEONARDO DA VINCI

Objectives

■ Perform a general, non-specific relaxation seated massage routine in 10–12 minutes.

■ Demonstrate appropriate relaxation techniques targeted for the back, neck, shoulder, and arms.

■ Compare and contrast the techniques for a sedating conclusion versus an invigorating conclusion to a seated massage.

Key Terms

Relaxation Routine: A sequence of massage techniques assembled to be a general, non-specific treatment that will relax and sedate the client but not address any specific complaint, condition, or injury. A relaxation routine is designed to create a systemic parasympathetic response as opposed to a localized relaxation.

The preceding chapters have given you the components of seated massage. It is now time to combine them into a seated massage routine. The first routine will be a general, non-specific relaxation routine. Just like a child must learn to walk before she can run, you must learn to give a good general relaxation massage before you can give a good, therapeutic treatment. Relaxation is at the core of all massage. The beneficial effects of the parasympathetic response elicited through a relaxation massage cannot be underestimated. While therapeutic applications of chair massage are becoming more popular, the majority of seated massages performed are for relaxation and stress reduction. Therefore, you will find that an excellent relaxation routine, as presented in this chapter, is a "must have" item in your toolbox of techniques. All the therapeutic routines that will be presented in later chapters are built upon the pattern and techniques of the relaxation routine presented in this chapter. The importance of practicing this routine until you can do it smoothly and confidently cannot be overemphasized. Invest the time to master this routine before you go on to the therapeutic chapters.

The routine presented in this chapter has been developed to address the majority of the upper body in a non-specific, yet thorough manner. Legs and hips are not significantly addressed for the reasons mentioned in previous chapters. This routine will guide you to give your clients an excellent, relaxing seated massage in 10–12 minutes. It can be shortened or lengthened to meet the time period desired. As you will see, the routine is divided into sections of the body. Each step is explained in detail in the text and shown in an illustration. The explanation of each step is summarized in the caption under each illustration.

Before you attempt the routine presented in this chapter, it is suggested that you first read the entire chapter and study the illustrations. Imagine or visualize yourself performing each step as you study it. Then find a willing volunteer and begin practicing the steps in the order they are presented until you can move through the routine smoothly in 10–12 minutes. Of course it may take you quite a bit longer the first few times through. Be patient with yourself. Soon you will be able to give an awesome seated massage.

Remember, you must do the steps explained in previous chapters before you can perform the actual massage routine. These include:

1. Setting-up, and sanitizing your chair or seated support system (see Chapters 2 and 3).
2. Greeting your client and conducting your client interview (see Chapter 5).
3. Demonstrating to your client how to get onto the chair (see Chapter 5).
4. Adjusting the chair or support system to the client (see Chapter 2).
5. Establishing therapeutic communication with the client (see Chapter 5).

Having accomplished the above steps, you are ready to begin the routine presented below.

BACK

The back is the largest area of the body available for seated massage. Almost everyone loves to have their back massaged. This is the best area to begin your routine. Most people carry their tension and stress in their low back or in their neck and shoulders. Therefore, the routine begins by relaxing the large strap muscles on either side of the spine, the paraspinal muscles (erector spinae), with the client focusing on his breathing to help clear his mind of chatter and amplify the parasympathetic response achieved by your touch. The back is then treated in sections starting at the low back and working superior to the shoulders and neck. The relaxation routine for the back is described below.

Slow Paraspinal Compression with Deep Breathing

The relaxation routine begins by gently placing your hand or hands on the client's shoulders. Rest your hand(s) here as you give the client any final instructions. This initiates contact with the client in a very gentle, calming way. The first actual massage technique used will be the compression stroke, applied to the paraspinal muscles. The tempo of the stroke is coordinated with the tempo of the client's breath to promote relaxation. When you are ready to begin the massage, follow the steps below.

1. Stand behind the client in the lunge (archer) stance with your arms slightly bent at the elbows. Place both hands on his back, one on each side of the spine between the scapulas. (Do not press on the spinous processes! Each hand should be between the spine and a scapula).

2. Ask the client to take nice, deep breaths. Explain that as he exhales you will be pressing on his back and as he inhales you will release the pressure. (You should inhale and exhale along with the client.) Now ask him to take a deep breath, and inhale along with him.

3. As you and the client exhale, press into the paraspinal muscles. Your movement and power will come from your legs if you bend your front knee, keep your back straight and shoulders relaxed. Additional power can come from plantar-flexing your rear foot. Use either the palms of your hands or loosely clenched fists.

4. When you feel resistance to your compression stroke, begin to inhale and straighten the front knee to release the pressure (Fig. 9-1).
   Note: Breaths do not have to be all the way in and all the way out; just take comfortably full breaths, in the rhythm of your compression strokes.

5. Move your hands down the paraspinals (inferior) 3–4 inches and repeat. Continue the compressions at the rhythm of the breath as you work your way, a hand-width at a time, inferior to the iliums (hips) and back superiorly to your starting position between the scapulas.
   Note: Lighten up on your pressure over the low back so you do not hyper-extend the client's lumbar

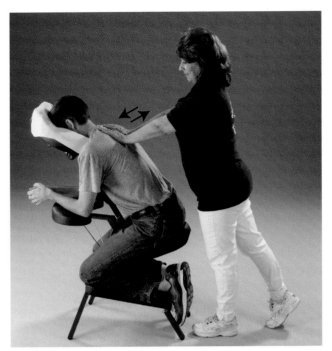

Figure 9–1 Slow paraspinal compressions. Apply the compression stroke on each side of the spine, using the palms of the hands, working in the lunge position. Exhale as pressure is applied; inhale as pressure is released and hands are moved about three inches. Begin between the scapulas, working inferior to the hips and back superior to shoulders. Try to keep wrists at a 45-degree angle of extension or less, as shown.

spine and cause pain or set off spasm in this area (Fig. 9-2).

Paraspinal Deep Friction

To intensify your treatment of the paraspinal muscles and to add movement of the client's tissues, repeat the sequence you just completed, using deep friction strokes. Circular friction is recommended, 5 to 7 circles at each hand placement. Move the client's clothes and skin as far you can without your hand sliding over the client's clothes or skin. The more movement you can create in the muscle tissue, the better. Moderate pressure is all that is required as it is the movement that does the work, spreading fibers and stimulating the nervous system. The following list explains this procedure.

1. Let the client know that he can now breathe normally, but encourage relaxed deep breaths. Suggest he focus his concentration on his breath, right at the top of his nose.

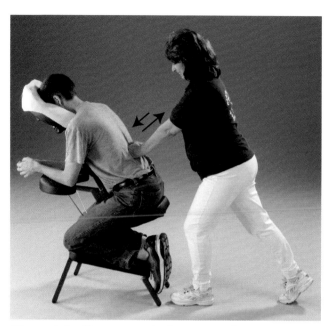

Figure 9–2 Slow paraspinal compressions. Use loosely clinched fists to apply compression to the paraspinal muscles. This allows good wrist alignment, preventing hyperextension.

2. Use the same stance and pattern of movement as with the paraspinal compressions, but use loosely clinched fists and circular movements. Move the clothes and skin over the paraspinal muscles, shifting them with a circular deep friction stroke. Again, work a hand-width at a time, moving inferiorly to the iliums and then back superiorly to the shoulders (Fig. 9-3A,B).

CLINICAL TIP

Alternatives to Circular Friction

If circular friction done with both hands (one on each side of the client's body; paraspinal muscles, mid-back) is challenging to your coordination, do four strokes of longitudinal deep friction (up and down), and then four strokes of cross-fiber friction (side to side) at each hand placement. Another option is to do circular friction when working inferior and longitudinal/cross-fiber when working superiorly. Remember, the larger your repertoire of strokes, the more success you will likely have in treating your clients.

Circular Deep Friction to Quadratus Lumborum

Many people carry a lot of tension in their quadratus lumborum (Q-L) muscles, which often becomes a source of low back pain. This is a technique to relax Q-L quickly and easily. If the client reports significant tenderness in this area, which does not resolve from the technique given below, it means more specific therapeutic treatment is indicated. The procedure for relaxing Q-L is as follows:
1. Stand behind the client and slightly to her left side.
2. Palpate for the space between the ribs and the ilium, just lateral to the spine on the client's right side.

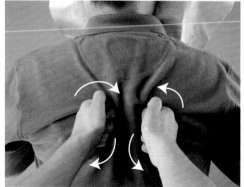
A

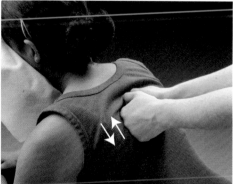
B

Figure 9–3 Paraspinal deep friction. (A) Circular deep friction. Place loosely clinched fists on the paraspinal muscles, engage skin and tissue, and move it in circles, 5–7 circles on each hand placement. Then move a hand-width and repeat. Start at scapulas and work down to hips, then back up to starting position, using moderate pressure. (B) Longitudinal deep friction (shown) moving parallel to the spine, and cross-fiber deep friction strokes, moving lateral-medial (not shown), 4–5 strokes in each direction, instead of circular strokes, treating scapula to ilium and back to scapula.

3. Use the ulnar edge (little finger side) of your right hand to apply a circular deep friction stroke to her right quadratus lumborum muscle. Press medial and anterior at a 45-degree angle into her waistline firmly enough to engage the clothes and skin. Then move your hand in small circles. Your hand should be fully open just under her ribs. You should be able to feel the 12th rib (superior), the lateral aspects of the transverse processes (medial), and the crest of the ilium (inferior) as you move your hand in a circular motion. Do 5–10 circles, starting lightly and working deeper with each circle.

4. If the client reports tenderness, stop at the tender spot and hold for 8–10 seconds; then slightly lighten your pressure and resume circular movement. Apply less pressure with each successive circle until you end contact (Fig. 9-4A).

5. Now move to the client's right side and repeat the procedure on her left quadratus lumborum (Fig. 9-4B).

Circular Friction on Mid-Back

For this routine, the mid-back is considered to be inferior to the scapula and superior to the waistline, or the lower thoracic region. Treat this area with circular friction as described in the list below.

1. Stand directly behind the client in the lunge position.

2. Begin just superiorly to quadratus lumborum on the rib cage. Use either the palms of your hands or loosely clenched fists to apply circular deep friction to the musculature over the rib cage. Treat both sides at the same time. Place your hands just lateral to the paraspinals, as you have already treated them. Move the client's clothing and skin, making 5–7 circles at a moderate tempo and pressure. Make the circles as large as you can without sliding over her clothing or skin. This will treat the serratus posterior inferior. Move superiorly a hand-width at a time until you reach the inferior angles of the scapulas.

3. Return to the starting position of the previous sequence. Move your hands laterally a hand width and repeat the circular friction sequence. This will treat latissimus dorsi (Fig. 9-5A).

4. Depending on the client's size relative to yours, it may be more comfortable (better body mechanics) for you to treat one side at a time, as shown in Figure 9-5B.

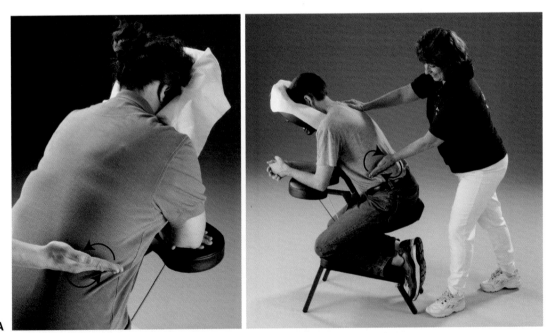

A   **B**

Figure 9–4 Quadratus lumborum (Q-L). (A) Relaxing client's right Q-L with the ulnar side of the hand, using circular deep friction strokes. Start with light pressure, gradually increasing to moderately firm pressure. Speed is 1–2 circles per second. Treating hand is between the client's ribs and ilium, just lateral to the transverse processes of his spine. (B) Relaxing left Q-L. Note therapist's right hand on client's shoulder. This is a balancing contact for both the client and the therapist.

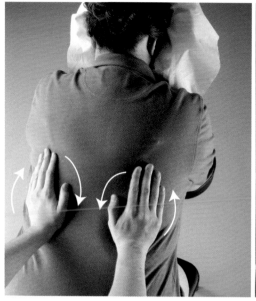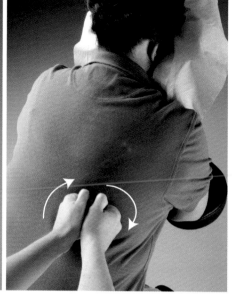

A   B

Figure 9-5 Circular friction on mid-back. (A) Treating the area between the scapulas and the waistline with circular friction, using the palms of the hands. You may treat both sides at once. Be sure to keep your wrists at a comfortable angle. (B) Treating one side of the mid-back with circular deep friction, using loosely clinched fists.

CLINICAL TIP

Watch Your Body Mechanics

If you find that treating both sides of the client's body at once, as is suggested for the mid-back and shoulder regions, is uncomfortable for you and strains your arms and shoulders, try treating just one side at a time, as this may allow you to practice better body mechanics. For example, move a step toward the side of the client and address the serratus posterior inferior and latissimus dorsi on that side. Then move to the other side and repeat. Different size clients may require you to use different positioning. If you are not comfortable, change positions, alignment, or posture. Maintaining your body mechanics is critical. It protects you from injury and allows the client to receive a better massage.

CONTRAINDICATION

FLOATING RIBS, KIDNEYS, ADRENALS

Be careful not to apply excessive pressure to the floating ribs (11 and 12) in the lower thoracic region on each side of the back as they can be easily injured, and the kidney and adrenal glands are behind them. When using the tapotement stroke, lighten up over this area.

Upper Trapezius

Many people carry excess tension in the upper trapezius. This is generally from the head-forward posture while driving or working at a desk. Nearly everybody loves to have this muscle on the top of their shoulders massaged. The seated position gives you excellent access to this muscle. The procedure is described in the list below:

1. Stand behind the client in the lunge position and place a hand on each shoulder just lateral to her neck.
2. Treating both sides at once, grasp and pétrissage (knead) her upper trapezius muscles with your hands. Using a pincer-like grip, roll, and compress the tissue between your thumb and fingers. Work lateral, one thumb width at a time, toward the acromion process until the muscle becomes too small to pick up. Then work your way back medial to the base of the neck and up (superiorly) the sides of the neck until you can no longer isolate the upper trapezius muscle between your thumb and fingers (Fig. 9-6A,B).

Another way to treat the upper trapezius is to use your forearm. This method places less stress on your thumbs and fingers. It also allows you to place more downward pressure on the client's shoulder, which adds a stretch to the muscle as you treat it. Unfortunately, this method does not allow the precise isolation achieved with the pincer grip described above.

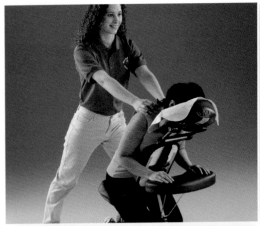

A

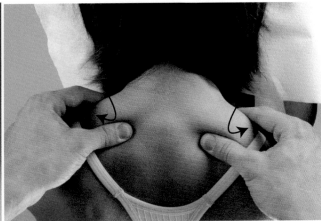

B

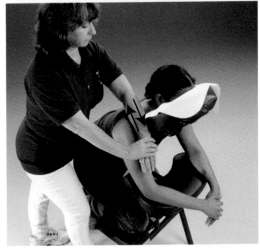

C

Figure 9–6 Upper trapezius. (A) Examining both upper trapezius muscles with pincer-grip compression and pétrissage. (B) Close-up of pincer-grip pétrissage on upper trapezius muscles. Grasp the muscles between thumb and finger(s), then flex and extend your finger(s), kneading the tissues up and down against your relatively stationary thumb. Stop and hold tender points for 10–12 seconds, then move on. Treat from the center of the muscle lateral to the acromion process and medial to the side of the neck. (C) Alternate method of treating upper trapezius, using forearm, pressing down and "sawing" back and forth (cross-fiber friction).

The alternate method for treating upper trapezius is described in the following list:

1. Stand at one side of the client and use your forearm to press into the top of the shoulder just medial to the acromion process (Fig. 9-6C).

2. Shift the clothing and skin anterior and posteriorly, "sawing" back and forth. You can also make a circular deep friction motion. Begin by using light pressure; then work your way deeper and deeper into the tissue until a firm pressure is reached or the client reports sensitivity.

3. If tenderness is reported, you should stop and hold the spot for 8–12 seconds; then lighten up slightly on your pressure and begin the sawing movement again. Gradually work your way out of the tissue, and then move over medially a few inches and repeat the sequence again. Continue until you have reached the base of the neck. Now move to the other side of the client and repeat this sequence on the other shoulder.

Posterior Cervical Region (kneading the back of the neck)

The treatment for the posterior neck will be pincer-grip pétrissage with pincer-grip static compression for tender points. As you examine this area, feel for the vertebrae, the spinous processes, the ligamentum nuchae, and the transverse processes. Be sure to stay on the posterior of the vertebra, working from the posterior of the transverse process, medial to the spinous process with your grasp. Relaxing the back of the neck can help relieve neck pain, headaches, and some motion restrictions. The following list describes this treatment:

1. Stand to one side of the client in the lunge position.

2. Use both hands to grasp the tissues of the posterior cervical area and apply pétrissage to them, kneading the tissues superior–inferior and anterior–posterior (up and down; in and out).

3. Work the entire neck, proceeding superiorly to the occiput and inferiorly to the shoulders, kneading the muscle tissues and the ligamentum nuchae (Fig. 9-7).

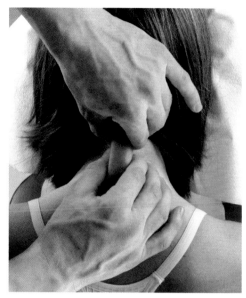

Figure 9–7 **Posterior cervical region.** Treating the posterior cervical tissues with pincer-grip pétrissage.

CONTRAINDICATION

NERVE ROOTS ON LATERAL NECK

When treating the cervical region (neck), stay in the lamina groove, posterior to the transverse processes, to avoid pressing on the nerve roots exiting the vertebral bodies on each side. If the client reports an electric, tingling-like sensation in her shoulder and arm, release pressure immediately and move to a more posterior and medial position.

CLINICAL TIP

Use Your Thumb

The thumb is a stronger and more sensitive palpation tool than the fingertips. When treating the back of the neck, as shown in Figure 9-7, it is sometimes best to go to the other side and repeat this procedure so both sides are treated equally. You could treat the back of the neck from one side and then treat from the other side as your next step, or wait until later in the treatment, as suggested in step 4 of the "Back Again" section. You will have to decide if a particular client needs this thorough (double) treatment in this area, based on your experience, the feel and sensitivity of the tissues, and the amount of time you have for the entire treatment.

CLINICAL TIP

Stop and Compress

If the client reports tenderness, you should stop and compress that area for 8 to 12 seconds, then release some pressure and resume the kneading or deep friction. Begin to use lighter and lighter pressure until you disengage and move to the next hand position. Never press on any area where you can feel the client's heartbeat!

CLINICAL TIP

Treating the Suboccipital Muscles

When treating the posterior cervical region with pétrissage, as shown in Figure 9-7, you can get more specific by treating the suboccipital muscles. This will address headaches and motion restrictions. Use your inferior (lower) hand relative to the client's head to do the treatment. If you are standing on the client's left side, this would be your right hand. At the base of the client's skull, direct the pressure of your thumb and first finger anteriorly and superiorly at a 45-degree angle in order to get between the occiput and C-1. Your finger will be treating the client's right side as your thumb treats their left side. Shift the skin laterally and medially as far as it will move by flexing and extending your thumb and finger. Start with your hand open, treating just medially to the mastoid processes. After 5 to 7 strokes, move both thumb and finger medially one inch by closing hand and treat again. Continue working medially in increments until you have the ligamentum nuchae between your thumb and fingers. Tender points can be held as described in the previous Clinical Tip. This procedure may be repeated from the other side if you feel the client needs it and if time allows

SHOULDER

The posterior shoulder and rotator cuff tendons are addressed next, using massage techniques. Stretches will be done later in the routine that will also affect the anterior shoulder muscles. The posterior shoulder muscles are usually eccentrically loaded and fatigued due to the internally rotated postures of most activities. This brief shoulder routine will increase blood flow and relax these muscles. It will also provide support for the rotator cuff tendons.

Compression on the Shoulder

Begin the treatment of the shoulder with the compression stroke at a moderate tempo. This will stimulate blood flow and warm the tissues. This technique is described in the list below:

1. Stand behind the client in the lunge position and at a 45-degree angle to his back.
2. Using the palm of your hand or a loosely clenched fist, apply compressions to the posterior scapula and shoulder joint area. You will be compressing the infraspinatus, teres major, teres minor, and deltoid muscles (Fig. 9-8).

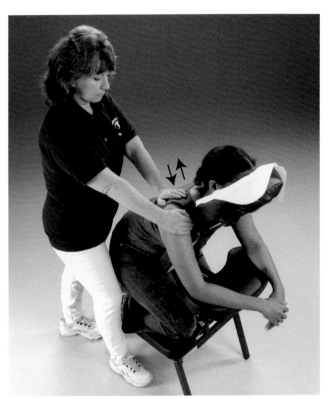

Figure 9-8   Compression on the shoulder. Apply compression to the posterior shoulder muscles. Movement should be straight in and straight out of the tissues. Treat the posterior scapula and the shoulder joint. Note the therapist's right hand providing stabilization on the anterior of the shoulder.

CLINICAL TIP

Support the Client

When treating the posterior shoulder with compression or deep friction as shown in Figure 9-8, use your more anterior hand, relative to the client's body, to support her shoulder by grasping the anterior (front) side of the shoulder joint and supporting it while doing the compression or deep friction stroke with your more posterior hand. Everyone likes to be supported!

Circular Deep Friction on the Shoulder

To provide deeper relaxation and to add more movement to the tissues, use the deep friction stroke. This can be done using either the heel of your hand or a loosely clinched fist. Circular deep friction is recommended. The muscles of the posterior scapula are fairly thick, so be sure to make 7–10 strokes in each hand placement. Use the same position you were in for the compression stroke. Massage the entire posterior scapula as well as the posterior of the shoulder joint. You are just repeating the last sequence, except this time you are using circular deep friction. Now, move to the other shoulder and treat it using the same sequence of compression and circular deep friction.

Deep Friction on the Rotator Cuff

The rotator cuff is injured in both athletic and work activities. In addition to trauma-induced injuries, the cuff tendons can sustain injury from repetitive motion. Massage helps relax this area in general and to support the health of the rotator cuff. The techniques for treating the rotator cuff are described in the following list:

1. Using the fingertips of one hand, thoroughly examine the entire rotator cuff, with either circular or cross fiber deep friction. Work all around the shoulder joint, just inferior and lateral to the acromion process. You are working through the deltoid muscle to primarily affect the rotator cuff tendons. To affect the rotator cuff tendons you must apply at least moderate pressure and make 7–10 strokes at each finger placement. This is to shift and roll the tissues around enough to affect the rotator cuff, which is the deepest layer. Your pressure should not cause pain or contraction of the client's tissues (Fig. 9-9).

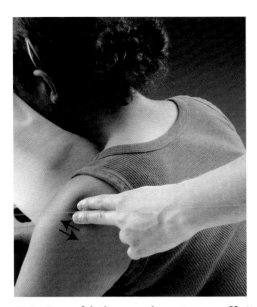

Figure 9–9 Deep friction on the rotator cuff. Use fingertips to apply deep friction to the rotator cuff tendons. Fingertips are just lateral to the acromion process, pressing on the head of the humerus. Apply 7 to 10 strokes at each finger placement. Position shown treats the supraspinatus tendon. Moving anterior to the front of the humeral head will treat the subscapularis tendon. Moving posterior about 1 inch will treat the infraspinatus tendon. Moving a second inch posterior will treat the teres minor tendon.

2. Place one of your hands on the anterior side and the other on the posterior side of the gleno-humeral (shoulder) joint. Ask the client to tell you when she feels heat in her shoulder joint.
3. Now grasp the shoulder joint between both hands using light to moderate pressure. Apply a moderate, rapid, deep-friction stroke to the entire joint area until the client feels warmth in the tissues (Fig. 9-10).
4. Remember to not slide over the client's clothes or skin. You should be moving the skin and deltoid muscle over the deeper layers either in a back and forth or circular motion. This movement generates heat from the friction between the moving layers, deep in the tissues. Most clients will find it quite pleasant.
5. Now, move to the client's other shoulder and treat it using the same sequence.

ARM

Having completed the shoulders, it is now logical to address the arms. The upper arm is not well supported in the seated position so we will treat it more generally with shaking, deep friction, and pétrissage. The forearm is nicely supported on the arm rest of well-designed chairs and can be massaged extensively. This is wonderful for people who drive, run computers, or perform other hand-intensive activities. If you are using a chair that does not provide good arm support, or a seated support system without arm rests, skip the forearm flexor and extensor steps.

Loosening up the Arm

To loosen and relax the tissues of the arm, use a combination of rapid, deep-friction, pincer-grip pétrissage, and shaking as described in the following list:

1. Gently lift the client's arm off the arm rest and allow it to hang down by her side.
2. Lightly compress her upper arm between both of your hands just below the shoulder joint and move your hands back and forth at a moderate to rapid tempo moving the tissues between your hands in a modified deep friction stroke. Do 4 to 6 repetitions, slide inferiorly a hand width and repeat. Continue until you get to the wrist (Fig. 9-11). If time allows, you can return to the top of the arm and repeat 1–2 more times.
3. To relax the biceps and triceps, allow the client's arm to continue to hang at her side and pétrissage her upper arm, being careful not to intrude into the brachial plexus on the medial side of the humerus between the triceps and

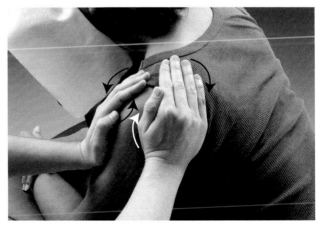

Figure 9–10 Deep circular friction on the shoulder joint using both palms. From the client's side, grasp her shoulder joint with both hands, using moderate pressure, and shift the tissues in rapid circular motions until she reports feeling heat deep in the joint (or about 20–25 circles).

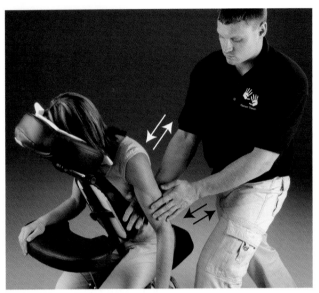

Figure 9–11 Loosening up the arm. Use rapid, light, deep friction strokes, starting at the shoulder and working down to the wrist a hand width at a time, 4–6 repetitions at each hand placement.

biceps. If the client reports an electric tingling going down her arm as you massage this area you are reaching too far around to the medial side and are hitting the nerves. Move your hands more anterior and posterior (Fig. 9-12).

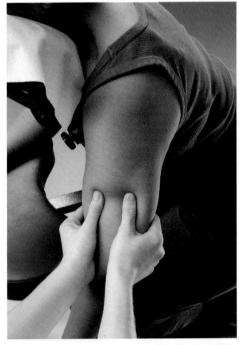

Figure 9–12 Treating biceps and triceps with pétrissage. Using pincer-grip pétrissage, massage the biceps and triceps muscles along the length of the humerus. Be careful to avoid the brachial plexus on the medial side of the humerus.

CLINICAL TIP

Arm Squeezes

When treating the arm with the loosening strokes of friction from the shoulder down to the wrist, you can incorporate a few squeezes (a form of compression) as you move back up the arm. Do not squeeze the upper third (auxiliary region) of the medial, anterior forearm, as you could compress the nerves of the brachial plexus and give the client a very uncomfortable "zinger."

4. Now grasp her hand with your hand, as if you were going to shake hands. Ask her to completely relax her hand, arm, and shoulder and just "let you have it."
5. With moderate to vigorous intensity, shake the entire arm, moving all the arm joints around for 10–15 seconds.
6. Gradually reduce the motion and gently return the forearm to the arm rest, in the palm down position. This shaking technique is utilized again at the conclusion of the arm routine and illustrated in Figure 9-19.

Forearm Extensor and Flexor Muscles

The many muscles of the forearm are often hypertonic from overuse. The following steps are effective in relaxing this area and are important to perform on any client with arm and hand complaints.

1. Stand in front of the client in the lunge position, so you are aligned with the arm you are treating. Use the palm of your hand or a loosely clenched fist to apply compression to the extensor muscles of the forearm. Begin just above the wrist and work proximally to the elbow joint, then distally back to the wrist and back proximally to the elbow, compressing the tissues three times (Fig. 9-13).
2. From the same position, use the heel of the hand or a loosely clenched fist to apply circular deep friction to the extensor muscles of the forearm. Start at the wrist. Do 4 to 7 full circles, starting lightly and working deeper into the muscles with each successive circle. Move

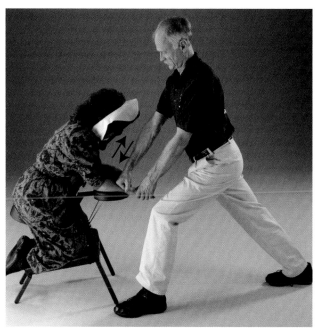

Figure 9–13 **Using loosely clinched fist to apply compression to the extensor muscles of the forearm.** Go over entire forearm three times.

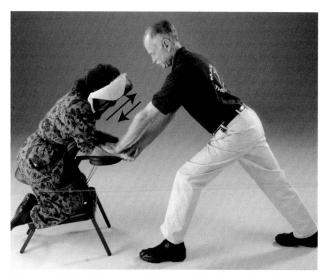

Figure 9–15 **Compression applied to the forearm flexor muscles with the heel of the hand.** Keep the rest of your hand relaxed. Go over entire forearm three times.

CLINICAL TIP

Two Methods of Compression

The compression stroke may be done in two ways. One way is to compress once and move, compress and move, etc. Work the length of the forearm from the wrist to the elbow, back to the wrist, and ending back up at the elbow. This applies three compression strokes to the entire muscle or area. The other way to accomplish the same effect is to do three compression strokes in one spot, then move a hand-width to the next spot and compress three times, etc., until you have covered the entire muscle or area. Both ways treat the tissue with three compressions. Practice both and decide which way you prefer.

toward the elbow (proximally) approximately 2 inches and do 4 to 7 circles again. Continue this to the elbow and then work your way back down to the starting position at the wrist (Fig. 9-14).

3. Roll the client's forearm palm up and repeat the compression and circular deep friction sequence on the forearm flexor muscles (Figs. 9-15 and 9-16).

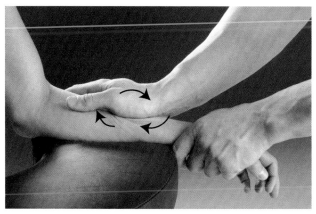

Figure 9–14 **Using heel of hand to apply circular deep friction to the extensor muscles of the forearm.** Work from wrist to elbow and back to wrist in 2-inch increments, 5–7 circles at each hand placement.

Elbow

Use rapid circular deep friction strokes to warm and relax the tendons attaching on the epicondyles at the elbow as described below.

1. Move forward in the lunge position and place one hand on each side of the elbow joint. Grasp the elbow between the palms of the hand so that the epicondyles are in the center of the palm on each side. Use moderate pressure.

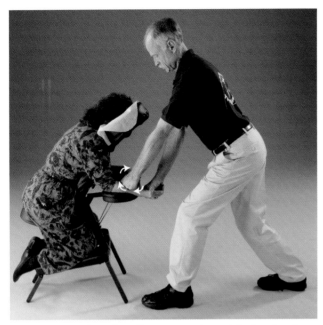

Figure 9–16 Treating flexor muscles with circular deep friction, using a loosely clinched fist. Start at wrist, work to elbow and back to wrist in 2-inch increments, 5–7 circles at each hand placement.

2. Ask the client to tell you when she feels heat in her elbow joint.
3. Moving the clothes and skin, apply circular deep friction to the elbow at a moderate to rapid tempo until the client reports warmth in the joint (Fig. 9-17).

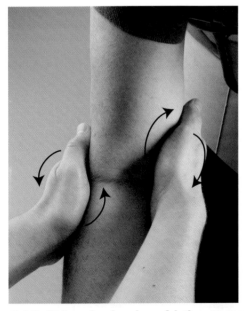

Figure 9–17 Using circular deep friction to treat the tendon attachments at the epicondyles of the elbow. Use moderate pressure with moderate to rapid tempo until the client reports feeling warmth in the tissues.

Hand

Hand massage is very relaxing. Depending on how much time you have, you may want to spend several minutes thoroughly working both sides of the client's hand. However, if time is short, 10–20 seconds is still very soothing. It will be up to you to decide what time allows in each treatment.

1. To treat the client's hand, pick it up off the arm rest slightly, holding it in the palm up position.
2. Use both of your hands to massage and stretch the hand (and digits) in a manner to relax and soothe them (Fig. 9-18).

Finishing the Arm

To complete the treatment of the arm, use shaking vibration as described in the following list:

1. Grasp the client's hand with your opposite hand, just as if you were shaking hands with her.
2. Gently, but somewhat vigorously, shake the client's arm. Keep your wrist loose as you shake the arm, causing movement in her wrist, elbow, and shoulder.
3. Move the arm laterally and medially as well as anterior and posterior. Start with small movements, working to large movements and then back to small movements.
4. Gently return the forearm to the arm rest (Fig. 9-19).
5. For a more invigorating massage, you could add tapotement as an additional finishing stroke to the forearm.

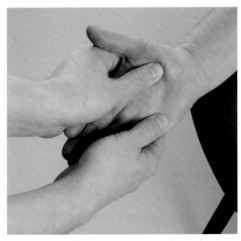

Figure 9–18 Holding and massaging the hand with thumbs and fingers.

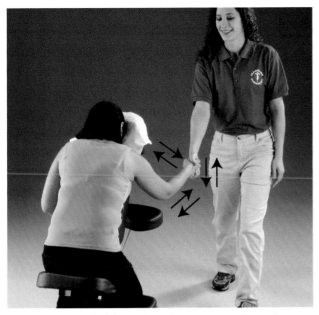

Figure 9–19 Shaking vibration to complete the arm routine. Using handshake grip, shake client's arm in all directions, up-down, in-out, back and forth. Begin gently, increase to very rapid shaking, then slow down to gentle movements, returning arm to arm rest.

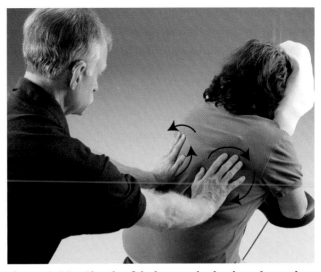

Figure 9–20 Circular friction on the back, using palms of the hands. Starting at the inferior angles of scapulas, work inferior to the iliums, treating both sides at once (or one side at a time if necessary to maintain your comfortable body mechanics). Then move medial and work up the paraspinals to the base of the neck.

Repeat the entire shoulder, arm, and hand sequence on the untreated side.

BACK AGAIN

Return to the client's back to reinforce the relaxation from the techniques done earlier in the routine. How much you do in this segment depends on the time left in the appointment. Several suggestions are described below. Use some or all of them, depending on the available time and the needs of the client.

1. Stand directly behind the client in the lunge position, using your palms or loosely clenched fists, and apply circular deep friction to the latissimus dorsi muscles. Begin just inferior to the scapulas and work inferiorly to the iliums (hips). Make 5 to 7 circles, move a hand width, and repeat. Both sides can be treated at the same time (Fig. 9-20). If working both sides at the same time causes you uncomfortable strain, treat one side at a time. This is usually a factor of your size versus the size of the client. Always work in comfortable body mechanics!

CLINICAL TIP

Working the Hips

If you feel you should work the client's hips, do not massage directly on the bony ridge of the iliac crest, as you will most likely bruise the tissues and leave the client very sore if you do. To avoid this area, skip over the iliac crest and work the tissues about 1 inch inferior to it and continue with circular deep friction around the hips. Depending on the size of the client relative to your size, it may be best to treat their hips one side at a time. You will have to spread your feet farther apart in the lunge position to maintain proper body mechanics while working on the hips. Do not hurt yourself trying to work too hard in this area; the client's muscles are stretched tight because he is in a seated position and the area is very low to the floor, making it difficult to effectively address it. Use moderate pressure with circular friction, which will improve the client's circulation and feel very good to him. You may also work about one-third of the way inferior on the lateral thigh, or as far as you can comfortably reach. Beating tapotement (loosely clinched fists) at a moderate tempo and firm pressure is also effective in this area.

2. If there is time, you might want to work back up the paraspinal muscles with circular friction, treating both sides at once, as you did at the beginning of the treatment.

3. Possibly repeat the kneading of the trapezius muscles, as well.

4. You could repeat the pincer-grip pétrissage on the back of the neck, from the opposite side you did it on previously.

5. Adjust your tempo during this sequence to more sedating (slower, lighter) or more invigorating (faster, somewhat deeper), depending on whether you want to leave the client more sedated or more alert.

STRETCHES

Stretches add dynamics and movement to the treatment. Because you have only massaged the posterior side, the anterior side is still tight. It needs to be relaxed and elongated to help the relaxation you have created on the posterior side last longer. Stretches are an efficient way to accomplish this. Several stretches are suggested and described below. You may use any stretches you feel are appropriate for the client, including AIS, PNF, or static stretches, as described in Chapter 8. Review Chapter 8 if you are in doubt about the techniques for any stretch. Try to do at least two stretches for the chest-shoulders and one for the neck. Do more if time allows. Remember, it is good to teach the client a stretch to do by herself as homework. Choose the one you believe will do her the most good. This involves the client in his therapy and helps promote future appointments.

1. Have the client slowly sit up straight in the chair.

2. Straight arm horizontal abduction stretch for pectoralis major sternal fibers and anterior deltoid can help lessen the tension between the client's scapulas. You may do both shoulders at once. Be sure client does not arch her back or lean posterior. Have her contract her abdominal muscles or support them with your hip as necessary (Fig. 9-21A).

3. Have the client bend her elbows and place her hands behind her neck. In this position do a horizontal abduction stretch. This will stretch pectoralis major costal fibers and pectoralis minor. Add a slight superior traction as you assist the stretch to more effectively address pectoralis minor (Fig. 9-21B).

4. Perform the straight arm forward elevation stretch for the shoulders (Fig. 9-22).

5. Do a lateral flexion stretch for the neck (Fig. 9-23). Optional: A posterior oblique stretch to each side.

6. When you are finished doing stretches, have the client lean forward and return to the face cradle.

You are now ready to do the finishing strokes.

FINISHING STROKES

The type of strokes you use to finish a routine depends on what effect you want to have on the client. If you want to leave the client in a more sedated state,

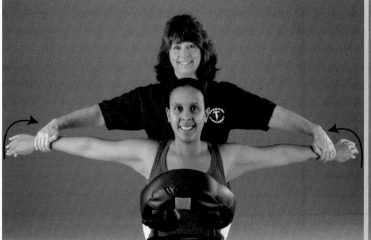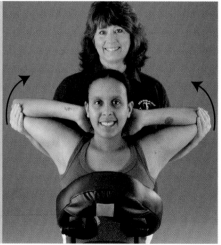

Figure 9–21 Horizontal abduction stretches. These two stretches help release tension and elongate the anterior shoulder and chest muscles. (A) Straight arm stretch for pectoralis major. (B) Hands behind head stretch for pectoralis major and minor. Assist with a posterior and superior pressure.

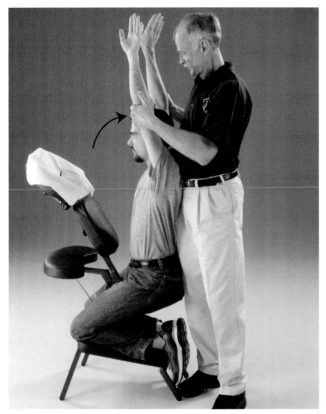

Figure 9–22 Straight arm forward elevation stretch. Client is being supported by therapist's hip to prevent arching of back. Normal movement should allow arm to be straight up.

finish with effleurage and nerve strokes on the back. If you want to leave him more invigorated, finish with tapotement and rapid nerve strokes. Some therapists like to use both sedating and invigorating strokes at the conclusion of the massage to blend the effects of the two extremes.

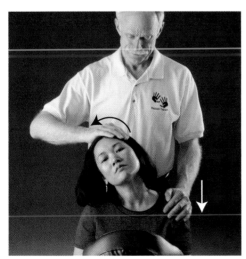

Figure 9–23 Cervical lateral flexion stretch. Ear toward shoulder, without leaning body sideways. Therapist shown assisting stretch while stabilizing opposite shoulder.

Sedating Conclusion: Effleurage and Slow Nerve Strokes

It is desirable to use a sedating conclusion when you want to leave the client in a state of maximum relaxation. This is appropriate for clients who are hyper, "stressed out," have anxiety disorders, have trouble resting or sleeping, or for the average client who is seeking the experience of seated massage. If the client is going back to a situation that requires alertness immediately after the massage, such as driving a car, operating machinery, athletic activities, or some other demanding circumstance, it is best to use an invigorating conclusion, which will be described in the next section. Techniques for a sedating conclusion are listed below.

1. Using the palms of the hands, at a pressure that allows you to slide easily over the clothes, apply long strokes to the back from inferior to superior and then from medial to lateral.
2. Finish the effleurage by sweeping from the neck lateral over the top of the shoulders and down the triceps (Fig. 9-24).

To complete the treatment, gradually lighten your effleurage strokes to nerve strokes. Use your fingertips to gently brush inferior (down) on the client's back, getting lighter and lighter with successive strokes until you are off the body (Fig. 9-25).

Additionally, you may follow the same lateral to medial and across the top of the shoulders paths used with the effleurage strokes in the previous steps. If you choose to do this, it is suggested that your final strokes to end the treatment be straight down the back on either side of the spine.

Invigorating Conclusion: Tapotement and Fast Nerve Strokes

When you wish to leave the client in a more invigorated, relaxed yet alert state, finish the massage with more bracing techniques. Increase your tempo (speed) and use tapotement, rapid vibration, and do the nerve strokes briskly. This will help bring the client back to a state of higher alertness, which is desirable if he must immediately face an intense situation such as giving a speech, driving, working out, making decisions, etc.

Tapotement

Tapotement is probably the most stimulating stroke of massage. The more impacts per second, the more stimulating it becomes. Alternating hands are more

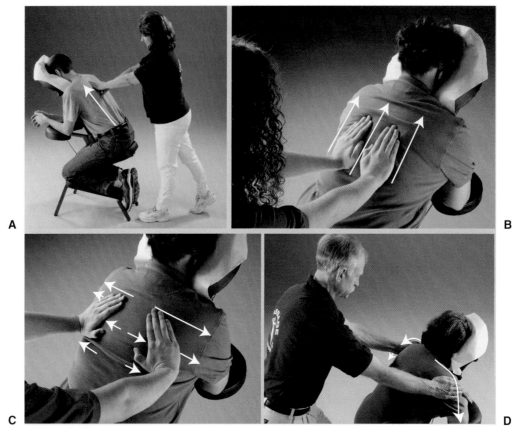

Figure 9–24 Concluding strokes: effleurage. (A) Long effleurage strokes moving up the back, using braced hands, treating one side at a time. (B) Long effleurage strokes moving up the back, using palms of the hands, treating both sides at once. (C) Light medial to lateral effleurage strokes using hands, both sides at the same time. (D) Effleurage strokes from the neck to the shoulders and down the triceps, using hands, treating both sides at once.

stimulating than synchronized hands. Synchronized hands are where both hands strike the body at the same time in virtually the same place. It has a similar effect as using only one hand. Synchronized tapotement is still stimulating, just not as much as alternating

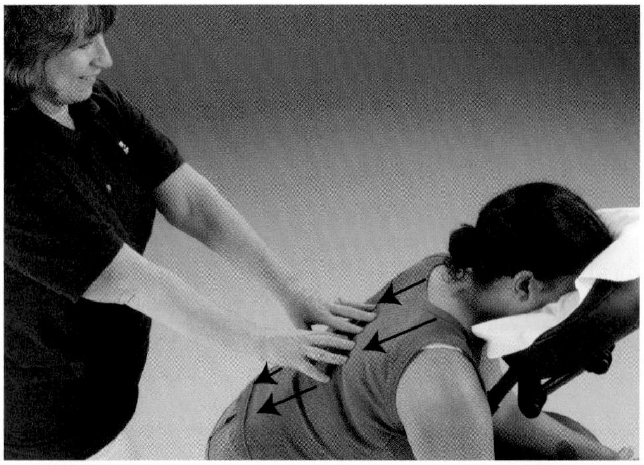

Figure 9–25 Concluding with nerve strokes. Using fingertips of both hands, lightly stroke down back from top of shoulders to hips at a slow to moderate tempo. On successive strokes, touch lighter and lighter until your last stroke is off the body.

hands. Tapotement is primarily used on the back, but can be used on the shoulders, forearms, hips, lateral thighs, and lightly on the cranium. The list that follows gives some examples of how to use tapotement in a seated massage.

1. Use hacking and beating styles to apply tapotement to the shoulders and back. Do not perform tapotement over the kidneys, quadratus lumborum, or the spinous processes. Except for these areas, cover the back thoroughly several times (Fig. 9-26A).

2. Beating style is very effective on the hips and lateral thighs. These areas are not addressed otherwise in this treatment for reasons given previously in this text. Beating tapotement is a quick and easy way to include them into the massage without compromising your body mechanics (Fig. 9-26B).

3. Treat the cranium with very light tapping tapotement with alternating hands, using just the pads of your fingertips. Direct your strokes straight in and out so that you do not mess up the client's hair (Fig. 9-26C).

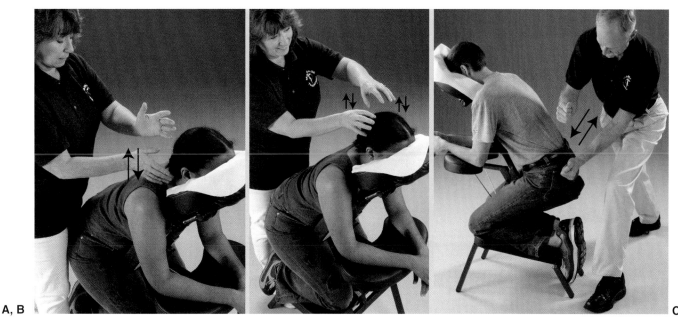

A, B
C

Figure 9–26 Tapotement. (A) Hacking tapotement on the shoulder using alternating hands. (B) Tapping tapotement to the cranium (head) using alternating hands (fingertips). (C) Beating tapotement to hips and lateral thighs using alternating hands with loosely clinched fists.

4. Finish with more alternating hands hacking and beating tapotement on the shoulders and back.

Fast Nerve Strokes

When you have completed the tapotement, it is recommended that you finish with a slightly less intense stroke. Nerve strokes are generally considered very sedating, but if done with slightly more pressure than usual and at a rapid speed, they are somewhat invigorating. Done in this manner, they make an ideal conclusion for an invigorating massage.

To accomplish this, apply fairly rapid nerve strokes, using just your fingertips, to briskly brush off the client's back, in the same pattern used previously in the sedating conclusion. Use lighter and lighter pressure until you are off the body.

Rest

Now let the client rest for 15–30 seconds or so. Then, gently ask him to sit up. Have him take a few deep breaths while sitting erect before standing up.

CLINICAL TIP

Vary Your Pace

To make a massage more sedating, work at a slower, smoother pace. To make the massage more invigorating, work at a faster pace. As a general rule, it is good to vary the tempo and provide some dynamics in the treatment. Start at a brisker tempo and slow down to a slower rhythm; then, toward the end of the treatment, increase the tempo again. Another pattern is to start slow, speed up in the middle of the treatment and slow down during the last few minutes. Remember what it is that you are trying to accomplish for your client at that moment, and adjust your tempo and choice of strokes accordingly. If someone has a headache, you might move slower in the shoulder and neck areas and work faster on the arms. This is part of the art of massage. You must consciously think about tempo and dynamics as you learn seated massage. They will eventually become second nature to you.

CLINICAL TIP

Assist the Client in Standing

Some people are unsteady after a massage or upon standing up. Be sure to be available to assist the client if necessary.

CLINICAL TIP

Hair, Makeup, and Face Massage

Be respectful of your client's appearance by not messing up her hair or makeup when giving her a massage. She may have to go right back to work or continue her day and may not have time to touch up her makeup or hair. Use tapping tapotement on the head, being careful to go straight in and straight out with your stroke, as this causes less hair movement. Deep friction strokes on the scalp move the hair less than effleurage. If she has an elaborate hairdo, ask for permission before you touch her hair or scalp. The cranium is not the most important place to work, so if she does not want you to touch there, just spend more time elsewhere.

While face massage is not covered in this text because it is seldom done in chair massage, it is acceptable to do some face massage as part of a seated treatment. Circular friction on the temples and the masseter muscles is relaxing to the jaw, and can usually be done with the client in the face cradle. She must sit up for you to massage around the eyes and on the forehead. If she is wearing makeup, ask permission before you touch the area.

CONCLUDING THE SESSION

After completing the relaxation routine, it is important that you end your session well with the client. First, ask your client to describe how he feels from the massage and address any concerns he may have. Also, remind him to drink plenty of water for the rest of the day.

Second, don't forget to collect your fee (unless you are working at a charity or promotional event, in which case, don't forget to give the client one of your business cards). In some situations, payment is handled indirectly and you do not collect from the client. Examples of this might be when you are paid a flat rate by the event promoter, or so much an hour by the employer, or your office bills the establishment for services rendered. When payment is indirect, disregard this step and move on to the next step.

Third, ask your client if he would like to schedule another massage. Suggest a date and time, possibly the same day and time next week or the same time in a few days. If the client does not want to reschedule at this time, ask when would be a good time to call him to reschedule. Don't forget to get his phone number!

Fourth, make a brief note in your client's file as to the date, time, type of treatment, and include any unusual findings. Typically this is on an HxTxCx form when doing relaxation massage (unless you are working in a clinical or medical situation, in which case you would probably be keeping some sort of SOAP notes).

Finally, sanitize your hands and equipment and prepare for your next client.

MODIFYING THE ROUTINE

The relaxation routine presented above is only a map to follow while you are learning how to perform seated massage. It is a teaching tool that helps you organize the many techniques into a learnable, useable sequence. It is an excellent treatment that can be performed in a predictable amount of time. By learning this routine well, you can go out and confidently give excellent seated massages.

However, you will rapidly find that in the real world the routine does not fit every situation. Some people want a seated massage as short as five minutes. Some would like a 20-minute massage. One client carries her tension in her low back while her neck and shoulders are fine; another has all his tension in his trapezius muscle; yet another has tight hands and forearms from carrying heavy shopping bags through the mall at Christmas. How can you help all these different people with one 10- to 12-minute routine? You learn the routine well, memorize it step by step, and then modify it as necessary. You shorten it, you stretch it, you do more of one part of it and less of another, you adapt it to each client you see.

However, if you first do not learn it well, your efforts at adapting it are likely to be quite clumsy and possibly embarrassing. So, first learn the routine and practice it until you can do it without having to think about what step is next. Then, adapt it to each client and give him the steps that will be the most beneficial for him at that moment. You will be amazed at how your subconscious and the routine mold and flow to fit each situation. Keep in mind that it takes time and many hours of practice and experience to reach that level. To help you adapt the routine to situations you may face early on in your seated massage career, the lists below give some suggestions.

Box 9–1

Relaxation Routine Outline

I. Preparing for the Client
  A. Set up and sanitize your chair or seated support system (Chapters 2 and 3).
  B. Greet your client and conduct your client interview (Chapter 5).
  C. Demonstrate to your client how to get onto the chair or seated support system you are using (Chapter 5).
  D. Adjust the chair or support system to the client (Chapter 2).
  E. Establish therapeutic communication with the client (Chapter 5).
    1. Tell me if it hurts.
    2. Tell me if it refers.
    3. Tell me when it gets better.
    4. Tell me if I am working too hard—right away.
    5. In a noisy environment, determine how client will indicate the above four communications to you (i.e., raise fingers, raise hand, etc.).

II. Back
  A. Slow paraspinal compressions with deep breathing.
  B. Paraspinal deep friction.
  C. Circular deep friction to quadratus lumborum.
  D. Circular friction to mid-back—medial and lateral.
  E. Upper trapezius—pincer-grip pétrissage and compression (alternate method: use forearm to treat upper trapezius).
  F. Posterior cervical region (kneading the back of the neck).

III. Shoulder
  A. Compression on the shoulder.
  B. Circular deep friction on the posterior shoulder, supporting anterior shoulder with other hand.
  C. Deep friction on the rotator cuff.

IV. Arm
  A. Loosening up the arm.
  B. Forearm extensor and flexor muscles.
    1. Compression
    2. Circular deep friction
  C. Elbow: circular deep friction to both epicondyles at once.
  D. Hand.
  E. Finishing the arm.

V. Back again: return to the back and re-treat mid-back, paraspinal muscles, trapezius, and back of neck as you feel appropriate for client's needs and available time.

VI. Stretches: at least two for shoulders and one for neck; more is better (Chapter 8).

VII. Finishing strokes
  A. Sedating conclusion: effleurage and slow nerve strokes.
  B. Invigorating conclusion: tapotement and fast nerve strokes.

VIII. Rest

IX. Concluding the Session
  A. Ask client to sit up and take some deep breaths.
  B. Ask client to stand up; stay by him and assist if necessary.
  C. Ask how he feels and address any concerns or questions.
  D. Suggest that he drink plenty of water during the rest of the day.
  E. Collect your fee (if appropriate).
  F. Give client your business card (if appropriate).
  G. Reschedule client (or determine where and when to contact him to do so).
  H. Complete client documentation (client's case file and accounting).
  I. Sanitize your hands and equipment and prepare for your next client.

To Shorten a Routine

- Do fewer repetitions of each step.
- For very short sessions (5 minutes), ask the client where she carries the most tension in her body. Open with the paraspinal compressions and deep frictions and then go to her tension area and work only on it.
- Only do the loosening techniques on the arm to give you more time to work on another area, such as the shoulders.
- Eliminate the "back again" steps.
- Work at a faster tempo without becoming too invigorating.
- Skip the arms completely.
- Skip any one area completely.
- Skip any two areas completely.

It is strongly recommended that you open every massage, even a 5-minute one, with the paraspinal compressions to get the client focused on her breathing and to relax the spine. Finish with either fast or slow nerve strokes on the back. In between, do whatever you believe to be the most appropriate techniques for the client in the time allowed.

To Lengthen the Routine

- Do each step twice.
- Do any one area a second time (come back to it) or a third time.
- Do two areas a second time or a third time.
- Add in one or more of the areas given in the clinical tips, such as the suboccipital muscles, the hips, and/or the face.
- Work more slowly.
- Do more stretches.

In any case, it is not recommended that you keep a client in the chair longer than 30 minutes.

CASE STUDY

Adapting the Relaxation Routine

You have been hired to provide ten, 10-minute chair massages at a bachelorette party. The party is on a tight schedule, so you cannot go overtime and must come in, set up, massage each person, pack up, and exit in 2 hours. Your normal relaxation routine is 15 minutes.

1. How would you adapt your routine to stay on time but still give a good treatment? Keep in mind that some of these people may become clients if you impress them.

SUMMARY

The relaxation routine described in this chapter is important for two reasons. First, it is the foundation for all seated massage. The therapeutic routines presented in later chapters build on this routine. You must learn this routine and these techniques before you can successfully move on to therapeutic routines. Second, the most common application of seated massage is for relaxation and stress reduction; therefore, unless you are primarily working in a clinical situation, it is quite likely that your seated practice will include more relaxation massages than therapeutic sessions. If you want to have a successful seated practice, you need to be able to give an excellent general, non-specific massage such as this routine. Practice these steps until they become second nature.

Box 9-1 summarizes the entire routine, from the steps for preparing for the client, to the conclusion. You might want to photocopy this box and keep it with your chair for referral as you are gaining experience in providing this routine for your clients.

Notes

CHAPTER 10

Therapeutic Routine for the Back and Neck

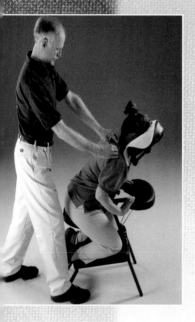

"Beware of bodywork fundamentalism. Our clients are more important than our techniques . . . their individual health problems are more important than our belief systems and agendas."

ROBERT K. KING

Objectives

▪ Perform a therapeutic seated massage routine with specific techniques for the back and neck in 10–15 minutes.

▪ Choose which muscles to examine to best address the client's complaint.

▪ Explain the approach to and goals of a therapeutic chair massage routine.

Key Terms

Lamina groove: the trough or gutter-like space formed between the spinous process and the transverse process of each vertebra (except C-1). The deep and some superficial paraspinal muscles lie in this groove.

Military neck: when the cervical spine loses its natural lordotic curve and the vertebra are in a straight line, usually at an anterior angle, presenting a straight-neck, head-forward posture.

Therapeutic routine: a massage routine that has the goal of reducing a specific soft tissue complaint by examination and treatment.

Whiplash: an imprecise term for a cervical acceleration, de-acceleration injury resulting from sudden and violent hyperextension and hyperflexion of the head and neck, as in a car wreck or fall. Such injuries include fractures, subluxations, sprains, strains, and even concussions.

In this chapter and the following two chapters, we will take the relaxation routine you learned in the previous chapter and incorporate muscle-specific techniques into it. This chapter covers the therapeutic routine for the back and neck, Chapter 11 covers the arm, and Chapter 12 covers the shoulder. The general format of the relaxation routine will be the basis of the **therapeutic routine**. If you have not studied and practiced the relaxation routine to the point that you can do it without referring back to the book, then you are not ready for this chapter. You must master the positioning, body mechanics, and basic techniques from the relaxation routine before you can effectively perform this more advanced work.

The therapeutic techniques enable you to help people with specific complaints, such as low back pain, muscle spasms, headaches, pain between the scapulas, whiplash, or almost any soft tissue condition of the posterior torso. To an even greater degree than relaxation massage, therapeutic massage is exciting work that can change peoples' lives for the better. We will be applying the principles and techniques you have learned so far, taking them to a new level of specificity. This will allow you to move from only providing relaxation and stress reduction to actually helping people with specific soft tissue complaints. While there is nothing wrong with only providing stress reduction and relaxation, the need for therapeutic massage to address soft tissue problems is widespread, even among people who come to you for relaxation massage. In many cases, it will be your job to educate your clients on how you can address their specific complaints, as most people are not even aware that massage can help them gain relief from these problems.

Effective therapeutic massage requires a thorough knowledge of anatomy. As you read this chapter, closely study the muscle illustrations provided and become familiar with them. As you practice the techniques, think of the muscle names as you touch them. Tell the client the name of the muscle you are working, especially when it is tender; this not only helps you learn the anatomy, it also educates the client. Thinking and saying the names of the muscles every day you work helps you remember anatomy terminology. More than that, it demonstrates to clients that you know what you are doing and that you care enough about them to educate them about themselves and their conditions. This builds client confidence and trust, which translates into loyalty, repeat business, and referrals.

After reading this chapter, begin practicing the routine until you have become familiar with each muscle and the techniques suggested for it. Finally, practice using these specific techniques in the time segments of your typical treatment until you can smoothly begin a session, address the main complaint, transition to finishing techniques, and complete the session in the allotted time, working from general to specific back to general. Realize that with each client your treatment will be slightly different, so do not become rigid in your routines, just comfortable within each region.

Before we begin studying the techniques, let's consider the approach and goals of the therapeutic routine.

APPROACH AND GOALS OF THE THERAPEUTIC ROUTINE

The goal of therapeutic massage can be summed up in two words: positive change. We want to facilitate change in the individual. We do this by applying stimulus to the nervous system of the body with touch and movement. This brings about a direct neurological response as well as mechanical effects that provide additional sensory information to the nervous system, resulting in reflexive effects from a variety of systems. If we correctly apply the right stimulus, the body will respond or change in the desired way. The primary change we want to bring about is a decrease in muscle tonus, resulting in improved circulation, increased range of motion, and decreased pain. We want to elicit the general parasympathetic response, initially at a systematic or overall level. This goal can be accomplished by using the opening sequence of techniques in the general relaxation seated massage routine presented in Chapter 9. However, we also want to accomplish this at localized or specific areas, which is where the sources of pain exist.

Besides stress, most people have another serious compounding factor: pain. Thus, just as the goal of relaxation massage is to alleviate stress, the goal of therapeutic massage is to alleviate pain. Pain is an alarm that tells our bodies that something is wrong and that is generally perceived as a threat by the nervous system. In fact, pain is a significant stressor, in and of itself. Most pain is ischemic in nature, meaning that there is a lack of blood in the painful area. The task, then, when dealing with local pain is to find the abnormal tissues that are ischemic and normalize them. This requires applying some stimulus to relax normal tissues and improve blood flow through them. It may also require some movement such as stretching to restore the tissues to their normal length once they are relaxed. Sometimes, the proper stretching application can also induce the desired relaxation.

Furthermore, because people are injured in very specific, small areas (an area one inch in diameter can cause excruciating pain), the therapeutic approach must include identification of painful areas. We must palpate (examine) the tissue very thoroughly and precisely to find these isolated areas of abnormal tissue. The most difficult part of a therapeutic treatment is finding the problem areas. Once the abnormal area has been located, normalizing it is usually less difficult to accomplish.

The approach for the routine, then, will be to induce a general parasympathetic response in the client with introductory or general work. Then we will begin to examine tissue, step by step, seeking to find the abnormal tissues that are the tender points, trigger points, concentrically contracted (shortened)

tissues, and eccentrically contracted (lengthened) tissues. We will carefully and precisely palpate the origins, insertions, and bellies, muscle by muscle, using deep friction strokes. Note that abnormal tissues are tender to our touch (tender points) and can cause a referred sensation to another area if they contain trigger points. When we find these abnormal areas, we will then begin treatment to normalize them, using sustained pressure as our primary technique. We will also use deep friction, petrissage, and stretching to affect abnormal tissues. At the conclusion of our treatment we will return to general techniques to reinforce the parasympathetic state. Needless to say, this requires a good understanding of anatomy, palpatory skills, and sensitivity to the client's responses.

PREPARATION FOR THE THERAPEUTIC ROUTINE

The therapeutic routine begins just like the relaxation routine, with the same sequence of preparatory steps discussed in previous chapters and summarized in Chapter 9, Box 9-1. Be sure to use the therapeutic communication techniques explained in Chapter 5. As always, be sensitive to the client's response, and avoid causing pain.

CLINICAL TIP

Avoid Causing Pain

The question often arises, how can the therapist avoid causing pain when examining tissues?

First, normal tissue is not painful when palpated with normal pressure. Ischemic tissue *is* painful, or at least tender when palpated at what should be comfortable levels of pressure. While examining tissues using normal pressure that the client reports feels good, you will often suddenly come upon abnormal tissue and the client will react in pain, either verbally or physically or both. At that moment, immediately lighten your pressure or even switch to a light, general effleurage or circular deep friction stroke using your entire hand to quickly soothe and calm the area. Then reapply your specific pressure, slowly working deeper until the client reports discomfort but not pain. There should be no tensing by their body (involuntary splinting).

At that level, hold sustained pressure until the client reports a lessening of sensation. Slowly release and move on with your examination, returning to each tender point 2–3 times in a session. Allow the body 30 seconds to a minute to "rebound" before returning to a tender point. Address trigger points that same way. This will allow you to effectively examine and treat tissue without causing pain. Remember, discomfort during examination and treatment is acceptable, but pain—so much stimulus that the client involuntarily contracts—is detrimental and counterproductive.

During your intake and interview, determine the client's main complaint and focus your therapeutic work on that area, staying general in other areas. In chair massage, there is often time to use therapeutic techniques in one area only. The main areas that can be addressed in the seated position are the cervical region (neck), shoulder region, upper extremities, thoracic region (mid-back), and lumbar region (low back). In this chapter, we discuss therapeutic techniques specifically for the back and neck.

Begin by warming the client's tissue, using the techniques described in Chapters 7 and 9, including slow paraspinal compressions with deep breathing and deep circular friction to the paraspinals. Now you are ready to proceed regionally.

CERVICAL REGION

Many clients require therapeutic massage to the cervical region because so much time is spent in the head-forward position. Sitting, driving, doing dishes, reading, operating computers, even doing massage usually has the head forward of the shoulders, putting almost constant eccentric loads on the posterior cervical muscles. These elongated muscles become hypertonic and ischemic, often aching constantly, sometimes causing headaches and occasionally restricting range of motion. Other clients may have injured their necks in **whiplash** accidents during falls, auto crashes, or athletic injuries resulting

in muscle spasms, trigger points, scar tissue, unwanted adhesions, and in the worst cases, vertebral damage. It is not unusual for one person to have a head-forward posture and an injury. Sometimes cervical pain can be the result of sleeping in a draft or a strange bed, or holding a phone under one ear for too long. When the client's complaint is in her neck or she reports a headache, the cervical region routine explained below is indicated.

Because of the interconnectedness of the body, the cervical region is functionally larger than C-1 to C-7. Muscles such as levator scapula, trapezius, and the paraspinal muscles insert at the neck but originate as far away as the sacrum. The head-forward posture also involves anterior muscles of the chest such as pectoralis major and minor, as well as anterior cervical muscles. Therefore, the cervical routine will treat and stretch the muscles of the cervical region. Stretching will be used to address the anterior muscles. Massage and stretching will both be used on the posterior muscles.

The Active Isolated Stretching (AIS) routine for the neck, along with the horizontal abduction stretches from the shoulder stretching routine, as presented in Chapter 8, support the massage routine below. The massage techniques presented for the posterior cervical region can contribute to increased head-forward posture if the shortened anterior muscles are not relaxed and lengthened. In chair massage, this is done with stretching.

It is strongly recommended that you utilize stretching in conjunction with the cervical massage techniques. Stretches may be done at the beginning or at the end of the cervical routine, depending on your preference or the client's needs and limitations. Some clients will be in too much pain to stretch first. The AIS posterior oblique stretch is probably the most universal one to use for cervical routines. See Chapter 8 for complete stretching routines and their descriptions.

We will begin with the upper trapezius, which is the most superficial muscle of the upper back and cervical spine.

Upper Trapezius

The upper trapezius is one of the muscles that is eccentrically loaded during head-forward or head side-bending postures. It becomes "tired" from holding the head up for long periods of time, and it often aches. Worse, it commonly develops trigger points that refer up into the side of the head, creating a painful arc around the ears into the temples (1). It is susceptible to injury from whiplash, usually from either head-on or lateral collisions. The upper trapezius can restrict head movement, particularly rotation and side-bending.

Begin by warming the tissues and introducing touch to this area.

1. Stand directly behind the client in the lunge position (Fig. 10-1).
2. Place your hands on the client's shoulders and begin to pétrissage (knead) the tissues of the upper trapezius muscles gently, working medially to the neck, laterally to the acromion process, and back to the center of the upper trapezius.
3. Do three strokes in each hand position, then move. This warms the tissue and introduces touch to this area.

Compressing the Tissues

The client's tissues should now be receptive to compression.

1. Now, using your thumb and fingers, grasp and compress (squeeze) the upper trapezius muscle with a pincer-like grip.
2. Hold a sustained pressure for about 7 seconds, then slowly release.
3. Move your hands and repeat. Compress the tissues a handful at a time, working both sides at the same time (bilaterally).

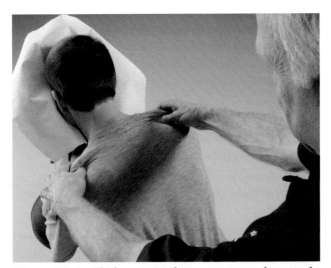

Figure 10–1 Pétrissage to the upper trapezius, working both sides at once. Knead the tissues to warm them up before performing deeper, specific examination.

CLINICAL TIP

Modify Your Approach for a Larger Client

If working on a larger person, do not compromise your body mechanics or strain yourself trying to work both shoulders at once. While working bilaterally is more efficient and saves time, it is fine to work unilaterally, examining and treating first one side and then the other. If you feel uncomfortable or strained at any time, change your positioning and method until you are comfortable.

Work medial to the base of the neck a "handful" at a time. Continue up the posterior lateral side of the neck until the upper trapezius becomes too small to grasp with your thumb and fingertips.

Work lateral a "handful" at a time to near the acromion process, where the upper trapezius again becomes too small to grasp.

Specific Examination of the Upper Trapezius Tissues

It is most efficient to examine both upper trapezius muscles at the same time, standing directly behind the client, using one hand on each side. However, when a tender point or trigger point is found, treat the affected side only, releasing all pressure on the unaffected side. Examine bilaterally, treat unilaterally.

1. To further and more precisely examine the upper trapezius fibers, grasp them between your thumb and fingertips. Place your thumbs about 2 inches inferior to the upper border of the muscle on the posterior side and position your fingers on the anterior side of the upper trapezius muscles (Fig. 10-2A).
2. Slowly flex your fingers, moving your fingertips superior and slightly posterior. You will be dragging your fingers across the fibers, kneading the tissues and feeling for tight bands of fibers (Fig. 10-2B).
3. If the client reports tenderness or referred sensation, stop the flexing movement at that point and hold the spot for 8 to 12 seconds. Ask the client if the pressure is okay. If your pressure is appropriate, the client should report the sensation has lessened in this amount of time.
4. As with the compression procedure, examine as much of the upper trapezius muscle as you can, stopping to treat any tender points and trigger

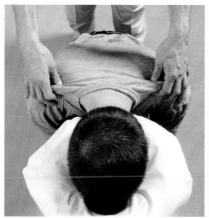
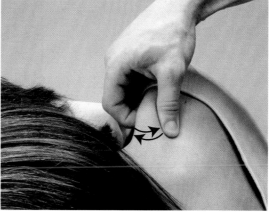

Figure 10-2   Specific examination of upper trapezius, using a pincer grip and flexed fingers to "unroll" the anterior layers of the muscle. (A) Examine both sides at once. (B) Close-up showing hand position, grasp of tissue, and indicating movement.

points you find with sustained pressure. Work medial and superior, up the side of the neck, then lateral to near the acromion process a "handful" at a time. This pétrissage movement with a pincer-like grip on the muscle allows you to feel the bands of fibers. It is very effective in locating the trigger points that cause headaches in the temporal area and restrict neck movement.

5. Try to come back and treat tender areas a second time.

CLINICAL TIP

Examine Bilaterally, Treat Unilaterally

Examining both upper trapezius muscles at once is the most efficient procedure. However, when you find a tender point or trigger point, stop your bilateral examination and only treat one side at a time. Treat the side the client reports the discomfort in (or the most discomfort in, if both sides are tender). It is overstimulation to most people's nervous system to treat two areas at once. The client's body will either tense up in reaction to the amount of sensation, or just not react perceptibly at all. Although some clients can positively respond to bilateral stimulation, most cannot, so treat one side, then the other. Then continue with your bilateral examination. When the examination of the entire muscle is complete, return to tender points and trigger points a second time to be sure they have reduced. Then move onto the next step in your routine.

CLINICAL TIP

Treat the Deltoid to Relax the Upper Trapezius

In some clients, upper trapezius trigger points will not respond to sustained pressure. They just "won't let go." The upper trapezius fibers insert at the acromion process and share a fascial connection with the fibers of the deltoid muscle. Tension from the contracted deltoid seems to prevent the trapezius from relaxing. If you examine and treat the deltoid and then go back to trapezius, it will usually respond positively to treatment. See Chapter 12 for directions on treating the deltoid.

Completion of Upper Trapezius

To complete you examination of the upper trapezius, return to the general petrissage used to warm the tissues, working from your examination pressure to a lighter and lighter pressure until you disengage the muscle. The cervical lateral flexion stretch (ear to shoulder) is suggested as part of your completion.

Middle Trapezius

The middle trapezius fibers run almost horizontal from the spinous processes of C-6 through T-3 lateral to the superior lip of the spine of the scapula and the acromium process (Figs. 10-3 and 10-4). They are inferior to (below) the upper trapezius and superior to (above) the spine of the scapula. They

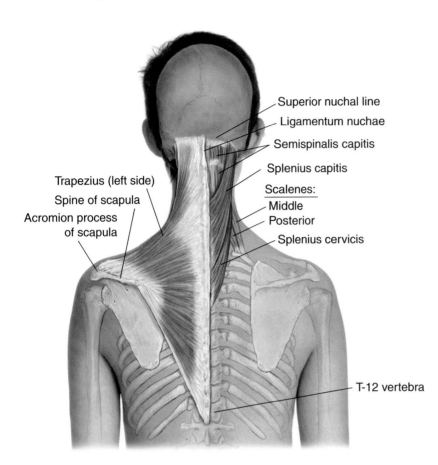

Figure 10–3 Trapezius muscle on left with underlying muscles and structures revealed on right. Reprinted with permission from Clay JH, Pounds DM. *Basic Clinical Massage Therapy: Integrating Anatomy and Treatment*. Baltimore: Lippincott Williams & Wilkins; 2003:96, Figure 3-48.

retract the scapulas and are antagonistic to the pectoralis major. Therefore, stretch pectoralis major, pectoralis minor, and subscapularis if the middle trapezius is tight or tender (see Chapter 8, shoulder section). Trigger points in this muscle contribute to pain between the shoulders and up the back of the neck to the base of the skull (1,2). The middle trapezius is typically elongated and taut due to the internally rotated posture that we sit in, drive in, and usually work in.

To isolate the mid-trapezius, your hands should not be grasping the anterior fibers of the muscle. You are picking up the middle of the flat sheet of muscle, not the superior edge.

1. Warm the tissues further with circular deep friction strokes, if appropriate. Start lightly and work to moderate pressure, moving at a moderate speed.
2. To most effectively treat the mid-trapezius, it is necessary to shorten its fibers, as they are usually elongated in the seated position. To do this, ask the client to move her hands to the back edge of the arm rest. This retracts the scapulas

slightly and significantly relaxes the middle trapezius fibers.

3. Using both hands together on one side of the spine, grasp the middle trapezius muscle and knead it between your thumb and fingers in a pincer-like grip. Shift your fingers and thumbs side to side as well as in and out without moving your hands or wrists. Start about 1/2 inch lateral from the spinous processes and work laterally a hand-width at a time until you reach the insertion on the spine of the scapula or until the muscle becomes too small to grasp (Figs. 10-5 and 10-6).
4. Stop and hold any areas of tenderness for 8 to 12 seconds. Return to tender areas twice if time allows.
5. To complete your examination of the mid-trapezius, use the palm of your hand to apply several strokes of circular deep friction at a moderate to light pressure over the entire muscle.
6. Repeat this procedure on the other side.
7. Return the client's hands or forearms to the normal position on the arm rest pad.

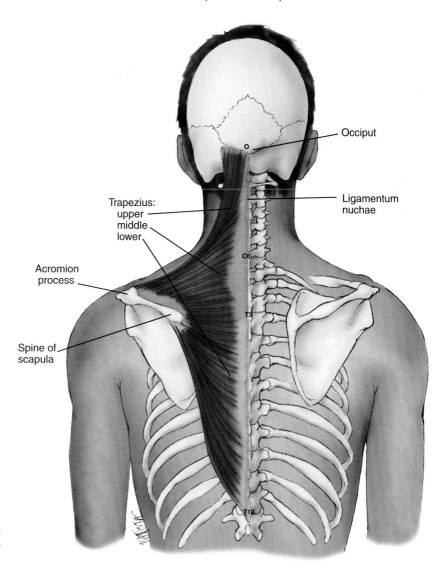

Occiput

Ligamentum nuchae

Trapezius:
upper
middle
lower

O

C6

Acromion
process

T3

Spine of
scapula

T12

Figure 10–4 Trapezius muscle indicating upper, middle, and lower sections with different shading.

CLINICAL TIP

Isolate the Middle Trapezius

Due to the fact that there are several layers of muscles beneath the mid-trapezius, it is most effective to grasp and lift it away from the deeper layers to examine and treat it. This way, if the client reports tenderness or referral, you can be fairly confident the problem is in the mid-trapezius muscle. If you just press into the muscle to examine it and the client reports discomfort, you cannot be sure if it is the mid-trapezius or the levator scapula, supraspinatus, paraspinals or rhomboids. Therefore, whenever possible, it is best to isolate the mid-trapezius by lifting and kneading it using a pincer-like grip.

Unfortunately, sometimes the mid-trapezius is very tight, adhered to the deeper tissues, or has significant adipose tissue over it, making it difficult (sometimes impossible) to lift the muscle up with a pincer-like grip. In these cases, be sure that the client's hand is as far back on the arm rest as possible, which will give you the most slack. If this doesn't help, use circular or cross-fiber deep friction, pressing into and shifting the mid-trapezius fibers around to initiate movement in the tissues. This is a great place to use a guided elbow or possibly a massage tool. Treat any abnormal tissues with sustained pressure. While not as precise, this method is still effective and is better than not examining or treating the area at all.

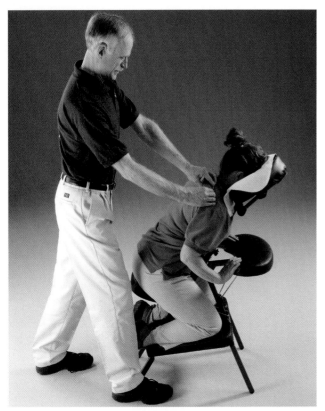

Figure 10–5 Using the pincer grip to examine and treat the middle trapezius. Working with both hands on one side makes it easier to grasp tissue. Begin just lateral to the spine and work lateral to shoulder. Note that the client's hand is on back of the arm rest of the chair to shorten and relax the mid-trapezius fibers.

The lower trapezius will not be isolated in this routine. Because of the position of the body while in a massage chair, the lower trapezius is stretched, making it very difficult to grasp, especially through the clothes. The thoracic region routine will address it

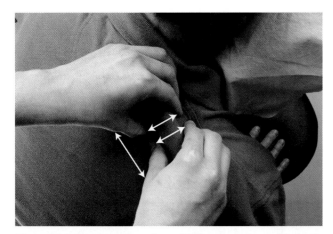

Figure 10–6 Grasping the middle trapezius with both hands, near the spine. Be careful to not reach anterior to the upper trapezius.

while working through it to examine the rhomboid and serratus posterior muscles.

Levator Scapula

The levator scapula is usually in an eccentric, taut, and elongated state due to the head-forward posture. This muscle works constantly on most people to hold the head up (cervical extension) instead of elevating the scapula. This chronic overload makes the muscle prone to trigger points that create a localized referral at the base of the neck. People with trigger points in this muscle will often reach back and grasp the base of their neck with the opposite hand. If the client indicates that this is his main or even secondary complaint, it is appropriate to examine the levator scapula very thoroughly.

The insertion points for this muscle are on the superior angle of the scapula and the transverse processes of C-1 to C-4. We will begin with the inferior attachment. (Note: In typical anatomical muscle terminology, insertion moves toward origin. Since the levator scapula can extend the cervical column *or* elevate the scapula, its origin and insertion are arbitrary, depending on which function it is performing. Therefore, in this text both attachments will be referred to as insertions).

1. Begin by examining the inferior insertion of levator scapula on the superior angle of the scapula. Stand behind and to the side of the client at about a 45-degree angle to the side you are treating.
2. Using flexed fingers, press into the tissue just superior to the superior angle of the scapula, then press inferiorly down on to the superior angle and shift the tissues lateral to medial, using a deep cross-fiber friction stroke. Adjust the angle of movement to follow the shape of the bone and examine the entire rounded area.
3. If tender, apply sustained pressure for 8 to 12 seconds (Figs. 10-7 and 10-8).
4. To better access this tissue, ask the client to place the forearm of the side that you are treating on the lumbar curve of her back. This will "wing" the scapula, and the superior angle will usually protrude and become more accessible. However, some clients cannot accomplish this arm position comfortably. If this is the case, leave the client in the standard position and move on to Step 8. (Note: This means there is some potential shoulder work for you to do in

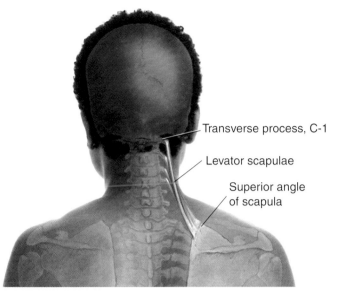

Transverse process, C-1

Levator scapulae

Superior angle of scapula

Figure 10–7 Levator scapula muscle. Reprinted with permission from Clay JH, Pounds DM. *Basic Clinical Massage Therapy: Integrating Anatomy and Treatment.* Baltimore: Lippincott Williams & Wilkins; 2003:128, Figure 4-17.

future sessions to help the client with internal rotation!)

5. Re-examine the superior angle as in Step 1. Try to hook your fingers around the superior angle and examine as much of the superior and anterior surfaces of the bone as possible (Fig. 10-9).

6. Treat for tender points and trigger points as necessary.

7. Return the client's arm to the arm rest when you're finished.

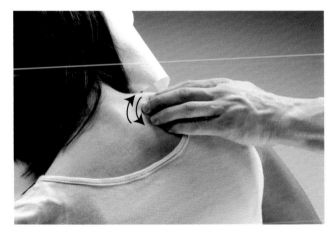

Figure 10–8 Using fingertips to "hook" into the levator scapula tendon attachment at the superior angle of the scapula. Using deep cross-fiber friction, lightly warm the tissues, increasing pressure to examine them. If a tender spot is found, apply sustained pressure using the same hand position, just stopping and holding.

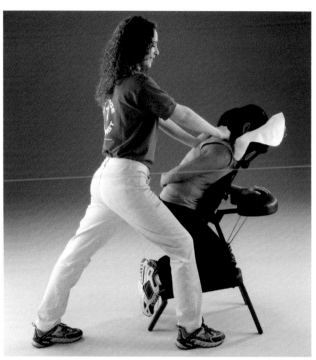

Figure 10–9 Examining the superior angle of the scapula with fingertips. Note that the client's arm is on the small of her back. Some clients will not be able to accomplish this degree of internal rotation.

8. Using the olecranon process of the ulna, guide your elbow with your other hand and examine the levator scapula belly. Start just superior to the scapula and press into the tissues, shifting them laterally and medially using a cross-fiber deep friction stroke (Fig. 10-10).

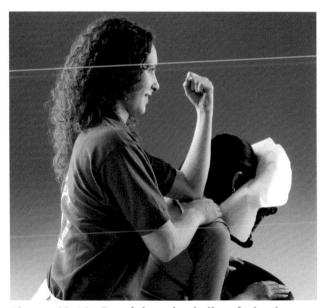

Figure 10–10 Examining the belly of the levator scapula with guided elbow, using deep friction stroke.

9. Make 5 to 7 strokes, move superior and slightly medial, and repeat.

10. Continue this until you reach the base of the cervical column. This is an area of strain and congestion in many people, so examine this entire area thoroughly. You are examining tissues of the levator scapula and also the other layers, including trapezius, paraspinals, and part of serratus posterior superior. You may use your thumbs or a massage tool instead of your guided elbow.

11. To examine the upper insertions on the posterior transverse processes of the cervical vertebrae, use the thumbs or braced fingertips. Starting at the level of C-4, engage the lateral posterior cervical tissues and apply circular deep friction strokes, starting lightly and circling deeper into the tissues until you are applying moderate pressure. *Do not* apply hard pressure in this area, as the cervical structure is relatively fragile. Be sure there is bone beneath your treating digits. You should feel for the lateral edge of the transverse processes and stay on the posterior aspect of them.

12. After 5–10 circles, move superior about 1 inch to the next vertebrae and repeat until you reach C-1. Remember that C-1 is about ½ inch wider than the other cervical vertebrae. It will typically be right at the base of the occiput (skull), about half a finger-width medial–posterior to the mastoid process.

13. Stop and apply sustained pressure to any spots where the client reports tenderness.

14. Finish treating the levator scapula with some light petrissage, light circular friction, or slow nerve strokes.

15. You may examine and treat both sides at once (Fig. 10-11A) or, for more precision, control, and possibly better body mechanics for you, one side at a time (Fig. 10-11B). Be sure to examine both sides.

16. The levator scapula may be stretched with a forward flexion or anterior oblique stretch. However, the levator is often already long due to the head-forward posture, and relief is better achieved by stretching the shortened anterior muscles opposite levator scapula (scaleni and sternocleidomastoid) with posterior oblique stretches.

Posterior Cervical Muscles

There are several layers of muscles in the back of the neck, some of which can be seen in the right side of Figure 10-3. They vary from large muscles from the torso that insert into the cervical region (such as the splenius capitis, splenius cervicis, upper trapezius, and semispinalis capitis) to small muscles that run between vertebrae (such as the multifidus and rotatores). They are primarily extensors and rotators of the cervical spine, but some have lateral movement functions as well.

These muscles are eccentrically contracted (long and taut) in the head-forward posture. They are injured in whiplash events, falls, and athletic injuries. Deep pain in the neck is often located in the small

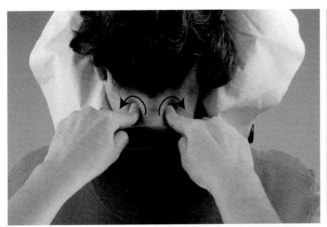
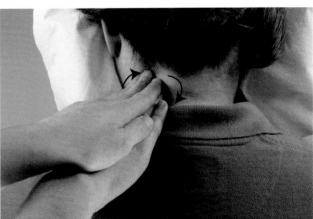

A

B

Figure 10–11 Using fingertips to apply deep circular friction to posterior aspects of transverse processes from C-4 to C-1. (A) Index fingers on each side. Remember C-1 is wider (more lateral) than the rest. (B) Using braced fingertips, examining one side at a time. Stop and hold tender points.

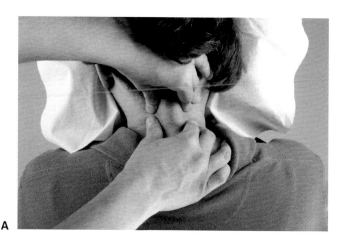

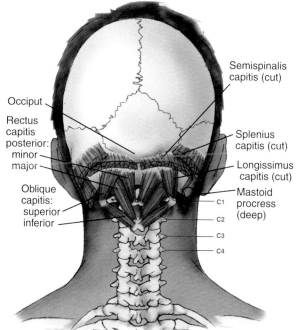

Semispinalis
capitis (cut)

Occiput

Rectus
capitis
posterior:
minor
major

Splenius
capitis (cut)

Longissimus
capitis (cut)

Oblique
capitis:
superior
inferior

Mastoid
procress
(deep)

C1
C2
C3
C4

A

B

Figure 10–12 Posterior cervical muscles. (A) Therapist examining the posterior cervical region (lamina groove) with pincer grip. Palpate from transverse processes (lateral) to spinous processes (medial). Work from C-7 up to occiput, kneading and deep frictioning. Do not go beyond the lateral sides of the vertebrae where the nerve roots exit! (B) Suboccipital muscles, C-1, C-2, occiput, and mastoid process.

muscles of the deepest layers. Splenius cervicis trigger points cause a sensation at the base of the neck, similar to those in the levator scapula. Other trigger points in this area cause headaches, neck pain, and restriction of movement. Examine the posterior cervical muscles thoroughly for all neck complaints.

1. To examine the posterior cervical muscles, move to the side of the client.
2. Using both hands at once, grasp the back of the neck with a pincer-like grip and petrissage the tissues of the ligamentum nuachae and the attachments on the spinous processes. You could think of this as grasping the "nape of the neck." Move your thumbs and fingers in and out and side to side several times. Start lightly and sink into the tissues gradually until you are applying a moderate to moderately firm pressure or until the client reports sensitivity.
3. If sensitivity is found, stop and hold with sustained pressure for 8 to 12 seconds.
4. Repeat this process several times, working superior to the base of the cranium (occiput) and inferior to C-7 (Fig. 10-12A).
5. Widen your grasp and feel for the **lamina groove**, the area between the spinous process and transverse process. Feel for the lamina

groove as you are making your grasp. Use a deep friction lateral to medial "scooping" or "sweeping" motion with your thumbs and fingers, shifting the skin over the tissues of the lamina groove with a pincer-like motion. Most of the emphasis will be on your thumb.

6. Again move up to the occiput and inferior to C-7.
7. Since your thumb is a more powerful palpatory tool, go to the other side of the client and repeat this entire sequence so you can examine the other side with your thumb. Visualize and try to feel each vertebrae as you work.

CLINICAL TIP

Position the Client's Neck Carefully

It may be necessary to adjust the face cradle to gain optimum access to the posterior cervical area, as the ideal position will vary from person to person. When doing so, be careful not to put the client into an extremely forward flexed position, as this stretches the posterior tissues and makes it very difficult to effectively sink your fingers into the tissues for examination and treatment. Try raising the face cradle and putting the client into a straight or even slightly extended position to gain better access to the posterior neck. However, this will not be very comfortable to some clients, so be sure to put the client back into a more comfortable position when you are finished in this area. Position the client so you have the best access to the tissues you are examining, but never position the client in a way that causes him discomfort or pain.

Suboccipital Muscles

The suboccipital muscles are very small muscles that initiate tilting, rocking, and rotational movements of the head. They are located between the occiput and C-2 and are the deepest muscular layer in this region. They are often injured by whiplash events and are subject to chronic strain due to the head-forward posture. If someone looks down and forward most of the time, these muscles become eccentrically overloaded. If the person has a head-forward posture when standing erect (**military neck**), these muscles will be concentrically contracted as a result of the client trying to extend his cranium and keep his eyes looking straight ahead. In either case, the person becomes susceptible to the development of trigger points. The trigger points in these muscles refer into the head, causing mild to devastatingly severe headaches. The headache pain pattern is like a hat band around the sides of the head, often reported as "my head is in a vise." Suboccipital trigger points also refer deep into the head and cause a headache that is felt behind the eye(s). They can mimic the pain of migraine headaches, causing "false migraine" headaches. The client often describes suboccipital induced headaches as "hurting all over," from the occiput to the orbit of the eye (1). It is very important to examine these muscles in all cases of headache, whiplash, painful or restricted movement of the head/neck, and for people with head-forward posture.

There are eight muscles in this group, four on each side. The muscles between the occiput and C-1, rectus capitis posterior minor, and obliquus capitis superior initiate rocking and tilting of the head. The muscles between the occiput and C-2, rectus capitis

posterior major, and the muscles between C-1 and C-2, obliquus capitis inferior, initiate rotation. Try to visualize these muscles as you examine them. Soon you will be able to feel them on most people (Fig. 10-12B).

1. Stand behind the client, slightly to one side in the lunge (archer) position.
2. Using both thumbs side by side or two braced fingertips in proper posture and with your arms almost straight but not locked at the elbows, start at the midline (mid-saggital plane) of the posterior neck at the base of the skull. Press anterior and 45 degrees superior to get up between the occiput and C-1.
3. Engage this tissue and shift it, using the deep cross-fiber friction stroke, moving medial to lateral 5 to 7 times. This is an excellent place to use the single-direction, deep friction stroke, applying pressure on the lateral movement and letting up as you return medially, then pressing again as you move lateral for 5 to 7 repetitions. Start lightly and increase pressure a little bit with each stroke until you have reached moderate to firm pressure. Remember, you are working through many layers of tissue, which must be shifted back and forth to affect the deeper suboccipital muscles (Fig. 10-13).
4. If the client reports tenderness or referral, stop and apply sustained pressure for 8–12 seconds.
5. Move the width of your treating thumbs or fingertips laterally and repeat this procedure. Work a step at a time until you feel you are rubbing up against the mastoid process at the lateral end of your deep friction stroke (Fig. 10-14).
6. Now use an inferior to superior stroke in the same space between the occiput and C-1. Make 5 to 7 strokes, then move the width of your treating thumbs medially and repeat the process until you reach the midline. You have just examined (and treated as necessary) the space between C-1 and the occiput. This has allowed you to address the rectus capitis posterior minor, the upper half of the rectus capitis posterior major, and the obliquus capitis superior. The next step is to examine the space between C-1 and C-2 to treat the rest of the suboccipital muscles, the lower half of the rectus capitis posterior major, and the obliquus capitis inferior.
7. Change the direction of your pressure to straight anterior, moving your fingertips or thumbs

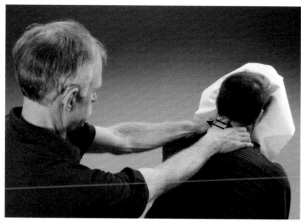
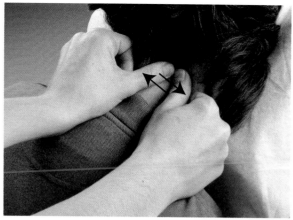

A   B

Figure 10–13 Examination of the suboccipital muscles. (A) Using both thumbs, pressing superior and anterior at a 45-degree angle between occiput and C-1, shifting tissues medial to lateral with a deep friction stroke. Start at the center line of the body. (B) After 5 to 7 deep friction strokes, move 1 inch lateral and examine again. Continue laterally an inch at a time to the medial (inside) edge of the mastoid process. Hold tender points or trigger points for 8–12 seconds.

inferior about ½ inch. Try to palpate the groove or space between C-1 and C-2. This will be easy to find on some people and impossible on others, depending on the size and muscular development of their necks. Visualize the space in your mind's eye, and after a few dozen clients you will become more sensitive and confident. However, if you cannot perceive the space, just know that if you follow the above directions you will be very close to the ideal place.

8. Examine the space between C-1 and C-2, using a medial to lateral stroke. Do 5 to 7 strokes in each thumb placement from the midline to the edge of the transverse process of C-2. When you feel the edge of the vertebrae and

you are starting to round a corner to the side of the neck, stop and change to an inferior to superior stroke (Fig. 10-15).

9. Apply 5 to 7 superior strokes and then move the width of your treating digits medially and repeat until you have reached the spinous processes at the midline of the neck.

10. Stop and treat any areas of reported tenderness or referrals.

11. Now go up to the other side and repeat this entire sequence.

12. Stretches for the suboccipital muscles could include forward and lateral cervical flexion and cervical rotation.

At this time you must evaluate the time remaining in the session. If there is very little time left, you should move on to a finishing sequence. If time remains to do more therapy, you must decide what area(s) to address. These should be the areas that are the client's secondary complaint(s).

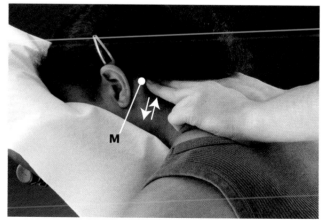

Figure 10–14 Examining suboccipital muscles using fingertips, pressing between C-1 and the occiput at the mastoid process (M). Switch from a lateral stroke to a superior stroke and work back to the midline 1 inch at a time.

THORACIC REGION

The thoracic region, or mid-back, consists of the rhomboid major and minor, serratus posterior superior and inferior, along with the paraspinal muscles (erector spinae). It could be argued that latissimus dorsi is part of this group; however, we will address it as part of the shoulder in Chapter 12. Trapezius is superficial to all these muscles, but we have addressed it as part of the cervical routine above. We will be working through it (especially its lower fibers) in this

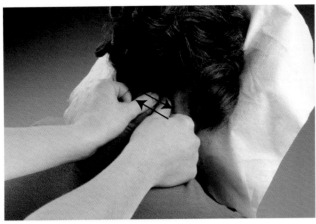
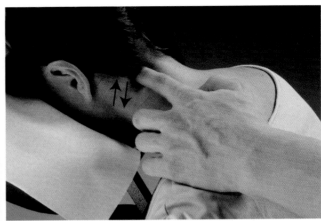

A

B

Figure 10–15 Examining suboccipital muscles between C-1 and C-2. (A) Thumbs applying pressure straight anterior, about ½ inch inferior to occiput, in the groove between C-1 and C-2. Shift tissues from medial to lateral, 5 to 7 strokes, then move 1 inch lateral and repeat. (B) Use one fingertip to examine space between C-1 and C-2, pressing straight anterior, using a superior deep friction stroke, working from lateral edge of C-2 back to the mid-line. Braced fingers are preferable.

thoracic routine, as we focus on the muscles underneath it. Since pain between the shoulders is a very common complaint reported to chair massage therapists, we will begin our routine on the rhomboids.

Rhomboids and Serratus Posterior Superior

Many people complain of pain between the shoulder blades. This is commonly caused by a head-forward and rounded-shoulders posture. Shallow breathing habits are typical of this postural pattern. While it is appropriate to work the rhomboids to address this complaint, remember that relaxing the rhomboids will allow the tight anterior muscles to pull the client further into a dysfunctional posture. Be sure to do some stretches that elongate the internal rotators (pectoralis major, pectoralis minor, and subscapularis) as part of the treatment to provide longer relief for the client.

Trigger points in the rhomboids refer into the immediate area of the upper thoracic spine. However, trigger points in the serratus posterior superior (which is beneath the rhomboids) refer through the body to the anterior chest as well as down the arm. Also beneath the rhomboids are the paraspinal muscles, which are usually working hard at this level to keep the spine erect.

1. Stand directly behind the client, but slightly toward the side you are working on to provide your body the most comfortable working position.
2. Warm the rhomboid tissues, if necessary, using the palm of your hand or a loosely clenched fist to perform circular deep friction. Start lightly at a medium tempo and work deeper into the

tissues as it warms and softens. Warm the areas from the spinous processes to the medial border of the scapula and from the superior angle of the scapula to the inferior angle (Figs. 10-16 and 10-17).

3. Examine every square inch of the area you warmed up in Step 1, using thumbs, a guided elbow, or a tool to perform circular deep friction, making 5 to 7 circles in each spot. Another method is to use cross-fiber and longitudinal deep friction to make a "+" pattern, performing four strokes lateral–medial, then four strokes superior–inferior. Then move 1 inch and repeat (Fig. 10-18).
4. Examine the origin of the rhomboids on the spinous processes in the lamina groove, using a

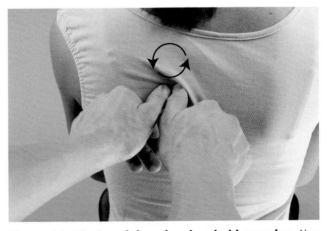

Figure 10–16 Examining the rhomboid muscles. Use both thumbs to apply circular deep friction. Perform 5 to 7 circles, then move 1 inch and repeat until entire muscle has been examined. Stop and hold tender points.

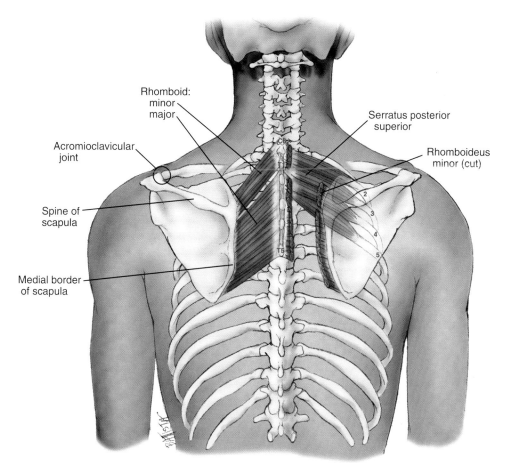

Figure 10–17 **Rhomboid (left) and serratus posterior superior (right).**

cross-fiber deep friction stroke parallel to the spinous processes. Adjust your position so that you are standing slightly posterior–lateral to the side you are treating. Your alignment should be straight toward the lamina groove on the side you are working. Use both thumbs, braced fingertips, or a tool and press into the base of the spinous processes at a 45-degree angle medial–anterior and shift the tissues superior and inferior (Fig. 10-19).

5. Examine from C-6 to T-5 and make 5 to 7 strokes on each spot. You may continue inferior to T-12 to treat the origin of the lower trapezius and serratus posterior inferior.
6. Treat tender points and trigger points with sustained pressure for 8 to 12 seconds. Treat each tender point or trigger point two or three times in the course of the session.
7. Move your treating digits lateral about ½ inch from the spinous processes and examine the paraspinal muscles in the lamina groove. You

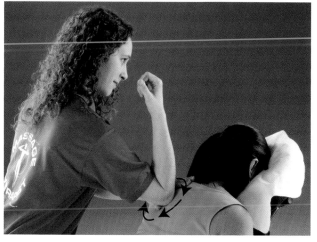

Figure 10–18 Working rhomboids with a guided elbow. Using circular deep friction, perform 5 to 7 circles as large as the skin will let you move without sliding over it. Note elbow is guided by the thumb and first finger of the therapist's left hand.

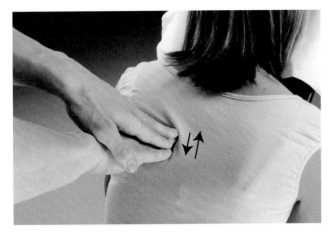

Figure 10–19 Examining rhomboid origin. Using braced fingertips, press medial and anterior at a 45-degree angle into the lamina groove, moving tissues superior and inferior 5 to 7 strokes from C-6 to T-5. Continue to T-12 to treat lower trapezius.

will feel these as vertical bands of tissue under the rhomboids. Use with the fiber and cross-fiber deep friction (up-down, left-right) strokes. Depending on the client's complaint and the amount of time you have, you may examine these muscles from T-1 to the sacrum. The largest, most pronounced band will be longissimus, about ½ to 1 inch lateral to the spinous processes (Fig. 10-20).

8. Ask the client to move the forearm of the side being treated around to rest in the small of her back, so that you can examine the insertion of the rhomboid on the medial border of the scapula. This should "wing" the scapula away

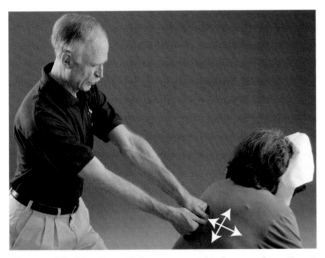

Figure 10–20 Examining paraspinal muscles. Treat these muscles in the lamina groove between the transverse and spinous processes of the vertebrae, with deep friction in two directions.

from the ribs of the back. If the client cannot comfortably reach or hold her arm in this position, have her return her forearm to the arm rest and do this procedure as best you can.

Note: For even better access to the serratus posterior superior, try grasping the shoulder joint with one hand and pulling it posteriorly and medially. Hold it there while you treat with the other hand. This can be done while the client's arm is on the small of her back to gain even better access to tissues under the scapula. You may also use this technique when the client must keep her arm on the arm rest because she cannot internally rotate her shoulder sufficiently to put her forearm on the small of her back. (Of course, this means there is some shoulder work for you to do for her in a future session. Be sure and advise her of this!)

9. Reposition yourself so you are facing the medial border of the client's scapula.

10. Examine the entire medial border of the scapula with superior–inferior strokes using both thumbs, braced fingertips, or a massage tool. Remember, the rhomboid muscles attach on the edge of the bone, not under it (anterior), so be sure to examine the edge (Fig. 10-21A).

11. Treat tender points and trigger points with sustained pressure.

12. While the client has his arm resting in the small of his back, examine the tissues under the medial edge of the scapula. Note that the serratus posterior lies under the rhomboid, inserting on ribs 3 through 5 just under (anterior to) the scapula, and tends to develop tender points and trigger points near its insertions. Use circular deep friction, pressing through the rhomboid onto the ribs, shifting the skin through the clothes as far as it will allow. It will require 5 to 7 circles to effectively address this deep layer of tissue (Fig. 10-21B,C).

13. Treat tender points and trigger points with sustained pressure, returning to them 2 to 3 times during a session.

14. Return the client's arm to the arm rest.

15. To complete this area, use circular deep friction done with the palm or loosely clenched fist at a medium to slow tempo, working lighter and lighter until you disengage. Or you can use effleurage, sliding over the clothes, working lighter and lighter until you reach nerve stroke pressure.

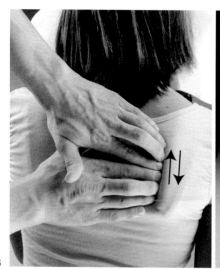
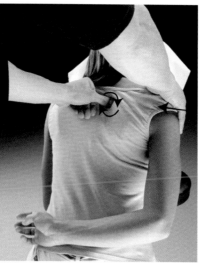
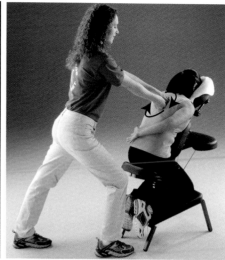

A,B　　　　　　　　　　　　　　　　　　　　　　　　　　　　　　　　　　　　C

Figure 10–21　Treating the rhomboid. (A) Use the fingertips to examine the rhomboid insertion on the medial border of the scapula with deep cross-fiber friction. The muscle attaches on the edge of the bone only. If the client can place her arm on the curve of her low back, it will raise the medial border and allow better access. (B) Working through the rhomboid to examine the serratus posterior superior. Note that the therapist's lateral hand is pulling the shoulder posteriorly and medially while the client's arm is resting on her the lumbar curve. The therapist's medial hand/thumb is working as far under the scapula as possible with pressure to the ribs. (C) Use both thumbs together to work through the rhomboid to examine the serratus posterior superior. Note that the client has her arm on her back.

Serratus Posterior Inferior

This muscle lies under the latissimus dorsi and thoracolumbar fascia. It originates on the spinous processes of T-11 to L-2 and inserts on ribs 8 through 12. Part of the abdominal wall, this muscle helps force the last of the breath out of the lungs (expiration) and is also somewhat involved in extension and rotation. A trigger point tends to form in this muscle at the level of the 10th rib and causes an annoying ache, but not a severely threatening pain (2).

1. Warm the tissues over the ribs with circular deep friction strokes, using your palms or loosely clinched fists. This area will be from the spinous processes lateral two to three hand-widths and from the inferior angle of the scapula to the 12th rib.

2. Examine the area thoroughly with circular deep friction, using both thumbs, braced fingertips, or a massage tool. Begin about two finger-widths inferior to the scapula and check every square inch of the area until you reach the 12th rib. Lighten your pressure on the 11th and 12th floating ribs, as they can be broken from excessive pressure. The client will report a sharp pain radiating outward from your treating digits if you find a trigger point, usu-

ally on the 10th rib about 2 inches lateral to the spine (Fig. 10-22).

3. Treat tender points and trigger points with sustained pressure for 8–12 seconds. Return to each point two to three times if necessary to eliminate it.

4. Complete examination of this area with large circular friction strokes with your palm or fist.

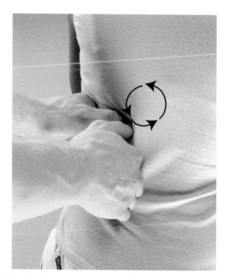

Figure 10–22　Serratus posterior inferior. Using circular deep friction with both thumbs to examine the lower thoracic area.

Examine and Treat the Serratus Posterior Inferior

The serratus posterior inferior is most often injured by coughing, sneezing, or performing a bend, twist, or lift movement. The pain from this muscle is localized to the muscle area itself. The trigger point referral pattern is a bull's-eye surrounding the trigger point, staying locally in the muscle area. If your client has a problem in this muscle, he will likely complain of low back aching pain. However, when asked to the point to the pain, he will probably point to the area on the ribs, superior to the abdominal wall and inferior to the scapula. If this is the client's area of complaint, you should treat the area with the same sequence used on the rhomboid. Examine the entire area between the inferior angle of the scapula and the 11th rib, from spinous processes to an inch lateral of the inferior angle of the scapula. Examine the entire muscle inch by inch. Lighten your pressure on the 11th and 12th ribs, as the floating ribs are fragile.

If the client has no specific complaint in this area, then treat this region as you did in the general relaxation routine, with large circular friction using palms or loosely clinched fists. You may do this bilaterally if comfortable for you, or do one side at a time as explained in Chapter 9.

Note that you will probably not have time to do a thorough examination in both the rhomboid and serratus posterior inferior areas. Specifically examine the area of the client's complaint and generally massage the other. If neither area is an area of complaint, treat both with large, circular deep friction strokes and invest your time doing specific work on the primary and secondary complaints.

LUMBAR REGION

The lumbar region is very accessible for treatment in the seated position. Quadratus lumborum as well as the superficial and deep paraspinal muscles will be addressed in the following routine.

Quadratus Lumborum

The quadratus lumborum (Q-L) is involved in the majority of low back pain complaints and can be treated very effectively in the seated position. If you become adept in treating the Q-L, you can provide many people with a great deal of relief.

This muscle originates on the crest of the ilium and the ilio-lumbar ligament (Fig. 10-23). It attaches on the 12th rib, with four individual bands of muscle fibers growing medially and attaching on the transverse processes of each of the L-1 to L-4 vertebrae. When hypertonic, the bands of fibers attaching to the vertebrae contribute to lumbar disc compression and damage. It is these insertions on the transverse processes that develop the most common trigger points in the Q-L. Along the iliac crest and at the lateral border of the Q-L on the 12th rib are the other sites where trigger points tend to form. These trigger points refer inferior to the posterior and lateral hip, sacrum, and sometimes into the abdomen.

An easy test to assess if Q-L is the source of a low back complaint is to have the client place his hands on his iliac crests at the lateral waistline and press down (1). This transfers the load of stabilizing the spine from Q-L to the hips, and the pain will diminish if Q-L was the source. Even if this test does not bring relief, examine Q-L anyway as it may have tender points or trigger points that are secondary to the main complaint.

To examine and treat Q-L, warm the muscle and then examine it with deep friction strokes, treating tender areas with sustained pressure as described in the list below.

Use the Chair for Acute Low Back Pain

The most painful movement for many people who are in acute low back pain is to get on and off a massage table or bed. However, they can usually straddle and sit down on a massage chair with minimal pain. Therefore, use the chair in your office, clinic, or on-site to work on these clients. Specifically, massage the quadratus lumborum, multifidus, and erector spinae. Once these muscles are loosened up, the client will usually be able to get onto the massage table with

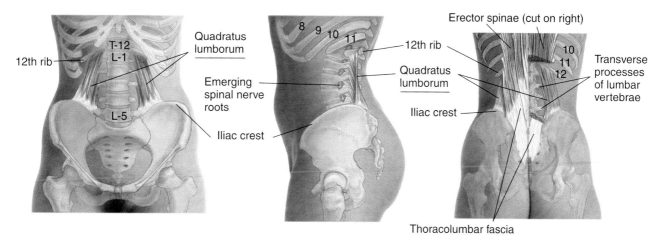

Figure 10–23 Quadratus-lumborum (Q-L): several views. Reprinted with permission from Clay JH, Pounds DM. *Basic Clinical Massage Therapy: Integrating Anatomy and Treatment.* Baltimore: Lippincott Williams & Wilkins; 2003:263, Figure 7-15.

minimal discomfort. Sometimes, in fact, the client is relieved of her pain from just the seated treatment. However, in the most severe cases nothing works predictably. Know when you are over your head and refer the client to another provider.

1. Warm the Q-L tissues as was done in the general relaxation treatment, Chapter 9. Use the ulnar edge of the hand to apply circular deep friction to the space between the ribs and ilium just lateral to the spine (Fig. 10-24A).
2. Standing at a 45-degree angle toward the side of the client's back that you are addressing, use thumbs together, or braced fingertips, to palpate the abdominal wall tissues between the ribs and ilium. Press superior and slightly anterior to contact the inferior aspect of the rib cage. Gently palpate the inferior surface of the rib cage. Feel for the lateral tip of the 12th rib (Figs. 10-24B and 10-25).

CONTRAINDICATION

RIB CAGE AND TRANSVERSE PROCESSES

When palpating the inferior surface of the rib cage, be sure your pressure is aligned with the 12th rib and on the inferior aspect of the rib itself and no deeper. Do not press anterior or up under the rib, as this could endanger the kidneys. A

similar precaution exists at the transverse process attachments of L-1 to L-4. Your pressure should be directed at a 45-degree angle medial–anterior. Do not sink your fingers in and press straight medially, as the processes are somewhat sharp and this approach may bruise the tissues. Never try to get under (anterior to) the transverse processes, as this could endanger organs and blood vessels. Stay on the lateral–posterior aspects of the transverse process.

3. Move your treating digits onto the inferior aspect of the 12th rib.
4. Using cross-fiber deep friction, engage the tissues and shift them back and forth (lateral–medial) 4 to 7 times.
5. Move 1 inch medial and repeat.
6. If the client reports tenderness or referral, stop and apply sustained pressure for 8–12 seconds.
7. Continue examining the inferior surface of the 12th rib, treating any trigger points or tender points as necessary. Move medially until you come to a hard structure that stops your medial progress. This hard structure will be the transverse process of the L-1 vertebrae. It will most likely be more lateral that you expect (Fig. 10-24C). Q-L is lateral to the erector spinae.
8. Change the angle of your pressure to a 45-degree angle anterior and medial. This will allow you to apply pressure onto the posterior lateral corner of the transverse process of L-1 (Fig. 10-26).

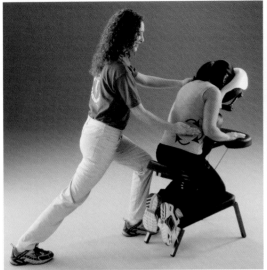

A

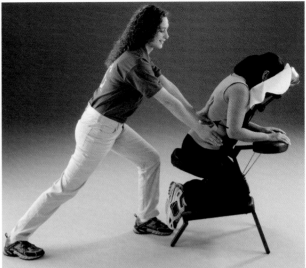

B

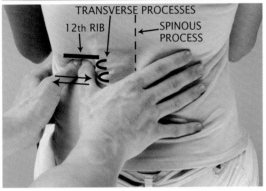

TRANSVERSE PROCESSES

12th RIB   SPINOUS PROCESS

C

Figure 10-24   Treating the Q-L. (A) Warming the Q-L using the ulnar edge of hand, shifting the tissue in a circle bordered by the 12th rib, transverse processes, and the crest of the ilium. (B) Examining the Q-L insertion on the inferior aspect of the 12th rib using a lateral to medial deep cross-fiber friction stroke. Therapist's medial thumb is against the transverse process of L-1. (C) Close-up of examination of Q-L insertion on 12th rib. Note how lateral the 12th rib and transverse processes are relative to the spinous processes.

9. Examine this attachment site with circular or cross-fiber deep friction using a circular or a superior–inferior movement.

10. Treat with sustained pressure if the client indicates tenderness or referral. Do not press straight medially on the lateral tip of the transverse process, as these structures are somewhat

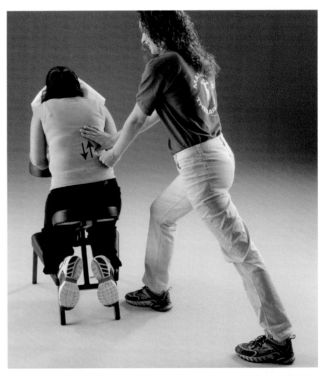

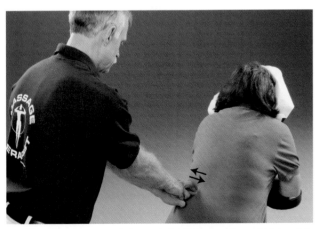

Figure 10-25   Examining 12th rib insertion of Q-L with braced fingertips using a lateral to medial deep cross-fiber friction stroke.

Figure 10-26   Examination of medial Q-L insertions. Use thumbs to apply deep friction to the posterior–lateral aspect of the transverse processes of L-1 through L-4.

sharp and you may cause trauma to the tissues being examined.

11. Move inferiorly about ¾ inch. This will place your treating digits on the transverse process of the L-2 vertebrae. Examine and treat as you did to L-1.

12. Move inferior another ¾ inch to address L-3 and continue working inferior until you reach the hard structure of the ilium. Note: Depending on the individual client, you may not get to L-4 because of the shape of the client's ilium and the degree of anterior rotation of his pelvis. Sometimes you can barely get to L-3. All you can do is thoroughly examine whatever tissue is available from the 12th rib inferior to the iliac crest.

13. Now examine the origin of the Q-L on the iliolumbar ligament and iliac crest. Change your pressure to inferior and slightly anterior. Use cross-fiber deep friction with a lateral stroke and work in 1-inch segments from medial to lateral, examining each segment with 5 to 7 lateral (cross-fiber) deep friction strokes. Treat tenderness or referrals with sustained pressure. Continue lateral to at least the mid-line of the body. This will allow you to examine not only the Q-L but also the attachments of the latissimus dorsi, the internal and external obliques and the transversus abdominis (Fig. 10-27). Note: The Q-L is the deepest layer of all these muscles. It is actually on the anterior edge of the iliac crest, so do your best to examine the anterior edge of the ilium as well as the superior surface. On some clients you may not be able to

access this area deeply, especially initially, due to tenderness or tissue mass. Do the best you can, staying within the client's pain tolerance.

14. Go back to re-examine and re-treat any tender points and trigger points.

15. Repeat this procedure on the other side.

16. Return to any tender points and trigger points on the first side a final (third) time, then a third time on the second side.

17. Conclude Q-L treatment with circular friction over the muscle using the ulnar side of your hand, like you did to warm the tissue up. Begin with a moderate pressure and gradually lighten until you lift off the body.

Multifidus

Medial and superficial to the Q-L is a large muscle group called the paraspinal or paravertebral muscles. The superficial layers of this group are called the erector spinae. The deeper layers include the multifidus and rotatories. The multifidus is very large in the lumbar region and gets much smaller in the thoracic and cervical regions (Fig. 10-28). The multifidus can harbor that deep ache in the lower back that used to be called "lumbago." When the client has low back pain, this muscle is often involved. You will be amazed at how many people with lower back complaints you can help in a short period of time when you learn to efficiently and effectively examine and treat the Q-L and the multifidus.

1. To examine the multifidus, stand to the side you want to work first and slightly behind the client. Use your thumbs or braced fingertips and find the transverse process attachment of the Q-L muscle at the L-1 or L-2 vertebrae (Fig. 10-29).

2. From this position, move your thumbs slightly posteriorly and medially. You will encounter the very thick edge of the paraspinal muscle band.

3. Press into this band of tissue at a 45-degree angle anteriorly and medially.

4. Shift the tissue superior–inferior 5 to 7 times, then anterior–posterior 5 to 7 times. Start with a moderate pressure and gradually work into the tissue as you examine it. You are pressing onto the iliocostalis to affect the deep layer of multifidus beneath it.

5. If the client reports tenderness or referral, apply sustained pressure for 8 to 15 seconds.

6. Move 1 inch inferior and repeat. Work inferior a segment at a time until you reach the crest of the ilium.

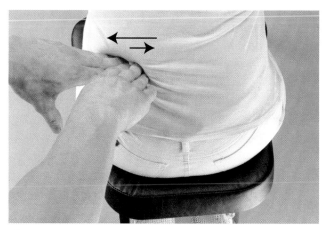

Figure 10-27 Examination of Q-L origin on the anterior edge of the iliac crest. Use deep cross-fiber friction with fingertips (or thumbs) pressing anterior–medially, treating with primarily a lateral stroke.

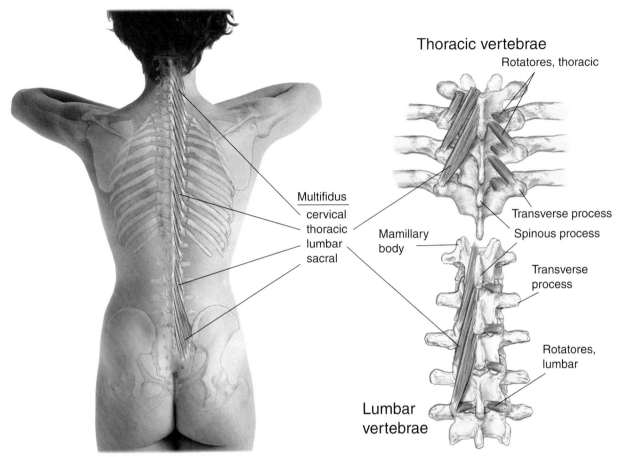

Figure 10–28 **Multifidus.** Reprinted with permission from Clay JH, Pounds DM. *Basic Clinical Massage Therapy: Integrating Anatomy and Treatment.* Baltimore: Lippincott Williams & Wilkins; 2003:242, Figure 6-18.

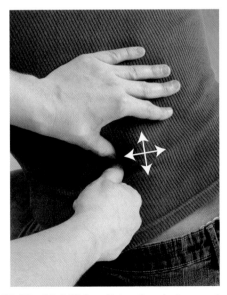

Figure 10–29 **Multifidus.** Using thumbs to examine the lateral edge of the paraspinal muscle band from T-10 to the ilium, press through the iliocostalis lumborum of the erector spinae to affect the deep, thick multifidus. Pressure is medial and anterior at a 45-degree angle. Movement is superior–inferior and anterior–posterior.

7. Return to the starting place and engage the tissue again. Re-examine this spot.
8. Move superior a segment and repeat, working superior 1 inch at a time until you have reached T-10.
9. Return to any tender points and trigger points and treat them again.
10. Repeat this procedure on the other side

Superficial Paraspinals (Erector Spinae)

The superficial paraspinal muscles, or erector spinae, consist of three muscle groups which run from the ilia and sacrum all the way up the spine to the skull. They extend and balance the spine and ribcage (2). They attach to all the ribs like a grapevine. Three muscles make up this group. From medial to lateral, they are the spinalis, the longissimus, and the iliocostalis. Each muscle is divided into lumbar, thoracic, and cervical sections along with several subsections. Trigger points in these muscles cause pain along the spine inferior into the hips and sometime through the body to the anterior chest. This treatment began by addressing these muscles with compression and circular friction. Now they will examined more thoroughly. In chair massage these muscles are best examined and treated with circular and cross-fiber deep friction and static pressure.

1. To examine the rest of the erector spinae layers of the paraspinal muscles, stand to the side and slightly behind the client. Using the fingertips of both hands held side by side and slightly flexed, engage the erector spinae tissue at the T-12 to T-10 region and shift it lateral–medial 7 to 10 times with moderate pressure. Increase pressure every few strokes until the client reports tenderness or referral or until you reach a firm pressure (Figs. 10-30 and 10-31).
2. Treat tender points and trigger points with sustained pressure for 8–15 seconds.
3. Move superior the width of your treating digits and repeat until you reach the base of the neck (C-7–T-1).
4. Then work your way back inferior in the same increments until you reach the sacrum. This technique will effectively address the spinalis and the longissimus bands of the paraspinal muscle. Note: Clients with low back pain often

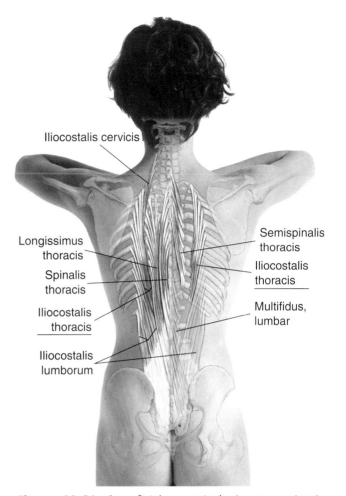

Figure 10–31 Superficial paraspinals (erector spinae). Reprinted with permission from Clay JH, Pounds DM. *Basic Clinical Massage Therapy: Integrating Anatomy and Treatment.* Baltimore: Lippincott Williams & Wilkins; 2003:234, Figure 6-6.

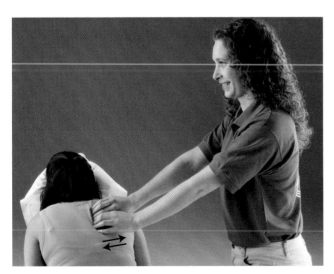

Figure 10–30 Superficial paraspinals. Using fingertips, apply deep cross-fiber friction to the erector spinae from lumbar region to C-7. Gently rocking the client is very relaxing; however, too much movement may hurt the client's neck. Ask the client if the technique is comfortable.

have tenderness on the back of the sacrum (2). This is difficult to address in chair massage because the sacrum is so close to the floor and the client's clothes are usually stretched tight over the hips. If you feel a need to examine or treat the posterior sacrum, be careful to maintain good body mechanics and not to overstrain your hands.

5. Gently rock the client side to side as you do this procedure to help relax her. However, do not rock her too vigorously. The lateral movement of the torso can put significant strain on the client's cervical spine, which cannot move laterally because her head is secured in the face cradle pillow. Excessive lateral movement in this procedure could injure clients, especially those who already have neck problems.

CLINICAL TIP

Work with the Client's Natural Rebound

The body loves rhythm. Slower rhythms are sedating, faster ones invigorating. Every person has a tempo that his or her body naturally oscillates or rocks at. To find this, stand at the side of the client and, using the palms of both hands, gently push the client away from you about 1 inch and release, letting him rebound back toward you. Note how fast he rebounds. Push again and this time, as soon as he completes the rebound, push again. Get into this natural rhythm of the client's body and do your deep cross-fiber friction strokes on the paraspinals at this tempo. This speed is the most relaxing tempo for the client. This speed will vary from individual to individual, so always establish the ideal rhythm with each person.

CLINICAL TIP

Only Perform Rocking in a Stable Chair

To perform side-to-side rocking, you need a solid, stable massage chair. If your chair is moving as you perform this technique, the client will likely not feel secure and safe and thus will not be able to relax. Either get a strong, stable chair or do not do this side-to-side rocking technique.

6. Position your fingers lateral enough so that you do not "slam" the tissues into the edge of the spinous processes at the end of your medial stroke; this could hurt the client and can bruise the tissues.
7. To specifically address the most lateral band of the erector spinae, the iliocostalis, you will need to treat "across" the client's body. Stand on the client's right side to treat her left side.
8. Place your fingertips lateral on about the line of the medial border of the scapula and examine this band of tissue using the same cross-fiber technique described in Step 1. Work inferior to the 12th rib and superior to the 1st rib (Fig. 10-32).

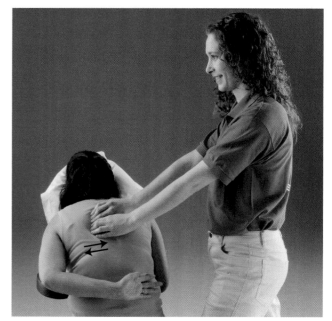

Figure 10–32   Iliocostalis. Using fingertips to examine the iliocostalis band of erector spinae with cross-fiber or circular deep friction. Better access to muscle will be gained if the client can put her arm on her back as shown.

9. To palpate the iliocostalis at the level of the scapula, it is best to have the client place her forearm in the curve of her low back to "wing-up" the medial border of the scapula, unless this position causes her discomfort. The iliocostalis will be the vertical band of tissue running right along or just under the medial border of the scapula. It will be beneath the trapezius and rhomboid muscles. A common trigger point location is just medial and inferior to the inferior angle of the scapula. This trigger point forms from the chronic strain placed on the muscle from a head-forward posture.
10. Re-treat any trigger points and tender points.
11. Repeat this entire sequence to examine and treat the erector spinae on the other side.

STRETCHING

In addition to the massage techniques covered above, stretching is an important part of any therapeutic routine. Stretching can be done at any time during a therapeutic session. You may start with stretching before you have the client lean into the face cradle, have him sit up straight at any time during the routine to stretch an individual muscle, or do an entire sequence. Some muscles can be stretched with the client forward in the face cradle, such as the external rotation stretch for the subscapularis muscle.

Even muscles that cannot be stretched directly in the massage chair can benefit from stretching related muscles. For instance, there are no stretches that effectively address the lumbar musculature or joints that can be done in the massage chair. However, do not forget that the body is an interconnected whole. A head-forward, internally rotated shoulder and arm posture puts an extra load on the thoracic and lumbar muscles. The lumbar extensor muscles (paraspinals and Q-L) have to work harder to keep the person with anterior, internally rotated posture from falling forward. Thus, stretching the cervical flexors and internal rotators of the shoulders will help you achieve longer-lasting results with your lumbar and thoracic work. Chapter 8 has stretching routines to support the therapeutic massage routines, both during the treatment and as "homework" for the client between massages.

In any case, be sure to include stretching in your therapeutic work. In some cases, the lack of stretching in a routine can actually prove detrimental to your other therapeutic techniques. For example, the powerful techniques discussed above for treating the posterior thoracic and cervical muscles will relax them, allowing the tight anterior muscles to pull the client even further into dysfunctional posture if these anterior muscles are not stretched out. So, incorporate stretching to avoid making your client's condition worse.

FINISHING STROKES

Finishing techniques to complete a therapeutic treatment are the same as for the relaxation routine given in Chapter 9. Select the sequence that is appropriate for achieving the state you want to leave your client in, whether sedated, invigorated, or somewhere in between. Effleurage and slow, light nerve strokes are sedating techniques, whereas tapotement, vibration, and faster nerve strokes are invigorating strokes.

CASE STUDY

Client With Severe Back Pain

A regular client calls you on Saturday, reporting he is in incredible back pain that suddenly started when he got out of bed this morning. He feels best crawling on his hands and knees. Getting in and out of a chair is very painful. Lying down or getting up is excruciating. To determine whether he might have a severe disc injury, you ask him whether he has any pain, tingling, or numbness going down either leg (sciatica) and whether he is leaning to one side, away from the most painful side. He responds "No" to both questions, indicating that it is likely not a disc injury. He asks you to come over and try to help him, as his pain prohibits him from driving to your office. You agree to go to his home to see if you can help.

1. What might you suggest he do for his pain until you get there? (Hint: Cold slows down nerve firing.)
2. Should you ask him not to take any analgesic between now and when you get there?
3. Should you take your massage table or your massage chair, or both? (Hint: He is a regular client in good physical shape and health with no significant lower extremity injuries or complaints.)
4. When you arrive, you ask him to put both hands on his iliac crests, one on each side and push down. You then ask, "Does that help?" He says, "Yes, that relieves the pain, almost completely. Wow, if I hold like this I can walk without it grabbing." Which muscle(s) does this indicate are likely a major cause of his back pain?
5. Make a list of the muscles you would examine and the techniques you would use to do a 20-minute chair massage for this client. What tempo would you work at? Are there any stretches that would be appropriate? Be sure to list your opening (warmup) techniques and your closing techniques. What state do you want to leave this client in, relaxed or invigorated?

SUMMARY

In this chapter we have built on the relaxation routine by adding muscle-specific techniques to allow you to address a client's complaints in the back and neck. Besides providing an even deeper and longer-lasting relaxation than the typical relaxation routine, an effective therapeutic routine can reduce the stimulus of painful ischemic tissue and trigger points.

Because there is not enough time in a typical seated massage session to examine and treat every muscle of the back and neck as presented above, you must determine the client's primary and secondary complaints and work only the tissues believed to be involved. Have him point to what he believes is the source of pain and show you the motion that makes it hurt or makes it worse. Then begin with some relaxation techniques to initiate touch with the client and smoothly transition to your therapeutic examination of tissue.

Being mindful of your time, work as many areas related to the client's complaint as possible. Avoid overtreating one spot or area, but cover it thoroughly once, returning to the tender points and trigger points a second time, at most a third. Incorporate stretching techniques into the treatment where you feel appropriate. Finally, smoothly transition to your finishing strokes.

At the end of your treatment, have the client again perform the movements that caused the pain to see how effective your work was. Give the client "homework" if appropriate (usually a stretch or two), remind him to drink plenty of water for the rest of the day, schedule the next appointment, collect fees, say good-bye, and prepare for the next client. Every session in which you use therapeutic techniques will be different from any other, and thus is never boring, either for the therapist or the client.

REFERENCES

1. Travell, JG, Simons, DG, Simons LS. Myofascial Pain and Dysfunction. In: The Trigger Point Manual, vol. 1. *Upper Half of Body*, 2nd ed. Baltimore: Lippincott Williams & Wilkins; 1999.
2. Clay JH, Pounds DM. *Basic Clinical Massage Therapy: Integrating Anatomy and Treatment*. Baltimore: Lippincott Williams & Wilkins; 2003.

Notes

CHAPTER 11

Therapeutic Routine for the Forearm, Wrist, and Hand

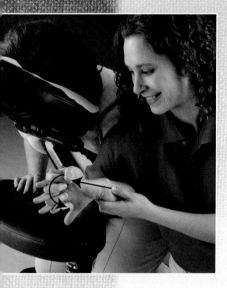

"The hands of those I meet are dumbly eloquent to me . . . There are those whose hands have sunbeams in them, so that their grasp warms my heart."

HELEN KELLER (1880–1968)

Objectives

■ Perform assessment tests to determine the presence of common arm conditions.

■ Identify the proper therapeutic technique to treat a given condition in the arm.

■ Perform a stretching routine for the arm.

■ Perform a therapeutic routine for treating the forearm, wrist, and hand.

Key Terms

Epicondyle: a projection or "knuckle" on a long bone near a joint (in this case, the elbow) which has one on each side, lateral and medial.

Herberden's nodes: little hard knobs about the size of a pea, near the distal joint of the finger. They are painful at first, but become pain-free, usually remaining for life.

Kinetic chain: the line of structures that work together to support a particular movement; in the case of the hand, the kinetic chain would include the forearm, elbow, humerus, shoulder joint, clavicle, ribs, and neck.

Median nerve: a major nerve of the forearm, passing through the carpal tunnel and innervating part of the thumb and first three fingers. Entrapment of this nerve at the wrist is called carpal tunnel syndrome.

With the prevalence of arm conditions, it is likely that many of your clients will come to you with specific complaints about their forearms, wrists, and hands. Some of the more common conditions include lateral epicondylitis (tennis elbow), medial epicondylitis (golfer's and/or Little League elbow), carpal tunnel syndrome, sprains and strains in the wrist, hand, finger, and thumb, numbness, tingling, and burning (nerve compression/entrapment). Fortunately, the massage chair allows excellent access to the arm (just as good as a table massage) and thus seated massage is an effective method of addressing these conditions. Note, however, that your chair must have a strong, stable arm rest that can be positioned to ensure proper body mechanics as you work on the client.

This chapter will equip you to therapeutically treat common arm conditions. First, it covers how to assess a client's complaint and determine the source of his pain, and presents five assessment tests that help identify some of the most common arm conditions. Second, it reviews the general relaxation massage and stretching routines for the arm covered earlier in the book, which are good to use in preparing your client for the more specific therapeutic work you will do. Finally, it provides a comprehensive therapeutic massage routine for treating the forearm, wrist, and hand.

GENERAL TREATMENT TIPS

When considering your client's arm–specific complaints, it is important to keep in mind that the hand is the end of a **kinetic chain** that begins at the neck and continues through the shoulder, down the arm. Most hand complaints that are not a result of direct trauma (bruises, strains, sprains, dislocations, and fractures) usually have causative factors somewhere up the chain. One such factor is postural distortion, such as head-forward ("military neck") posture or internally rotated ("rounded") shoulders, or both (1). Advise the client of the possibility of these causative factors and plan to do at least some general massage all the way to the neck. It will usually be necessary to do specific work in the shoulder and neck eventually, as trigger points in the rotator cuff muscles often refer pain or sensations into the forearm, wrist, and hand.

In the first few treatments, attempt to reduce the local complaint by addressing that area. This usually brings some immediate relief to the client. In the next few sessions, start working up the chain to find and reduce any distant causes. As you work, educate your client about what you are doing. He will appreciate learning about pain referral and what is causing his pain. In some cases the pain is entirely from trigger points up the kinetic chain. You will know this when you find very little abnormal tissue in the complaint area and that what little there is normalizes easily, yet the complaint still exists. If this is the case, direct your attention up the chain in the first few sessions.

If the complaint is a repetitive-strain injury (RSI), also called "repetitive-stress injury" and "cumulative trauma disorder" (CTD), which is often the case in non-traumatic forearm and wrist complaints, activity modification will be required. This type of intervention is outside the scope of this text and possibly outside your scope and training as well. If so, you may need to refer the client to an occupational therapist, a physical therapist, or some other provider who specializes in RSI treatment, including workstation assessment and movement training. In the case of athletes, they may need a coach to help them correct their form and technique. For all clients, you can facilitate their recovery by assessing their posture and working to correct any disorders in the upper body.

If the condition is caused by direct trauma, determine if swelling and inflammation are present. If either is noticeable, work above and below but not directly on the swollen or inflamed tissues. If you are trained in lymphatic drainage techniques, these may be appropriate (2). Once the swelling is reduced you may begin massage directly on the injured area. Be careful not to cause pain, as the injured tissues will often be ischemic and tender. (If inflammation is present in an RSI injury, the same precautions apply.)

Box 11-1

Carpal Tunnel Syndrome

Carpal tunnel syndrome (CTS) is one of the most common repetitive-strain injuries (RSI). This injury causes immense suffering and is very costly to businesses. On-site chair massage is an ideal program for both the treatment and prevention of this injury. Conservative treatment of carpal tunnel syndrome has been documented to be successful in the majority of cases in clients under 50 years of age who have had symptoms for less than 10 months (3). This can be a significant market for your seated therapeutic massage practice.

Carpal tunnel syndrome primarily affects people who do repetitive activity with their hands in the internally rotated, head-forward position. This position has the hands in front of the body, shoulders rounded (internally rotated), and the head forward, usually looking down. People are in this position for long periods of time, often with little significant movement. Sitting at a computer, scanning groceries, knitting, and doing massage are all examples of this type of working posture. Concerning massage, in the lunge posture we are particularly prone to being internally rotated and head somewhat forward. This is why this text stresses proper working postures and recommends exercises along with stretching to counterbalance this unfavorable position.

In the head-forward posture, the scalene muscles are shortened and elevate the 1st rib, decreasing the space between the 1st rib and the clavicle. This restricts innervation and circulation into the arm. The internally rotated shoulder posture amplifies this as pectoralis minor shortens, decreasing the space for the brachial plexus under its tendon at the coracoid process, thus also restricting innervation and circulation to the arm. This decreases the tolerance of arm, wrist, and hand tissues to repetitive activity.

Furthermore, people are especially prone to develop CTS when they begin a new repetitive activity or dramatically increase the frequency or duration of a repetitive activity, such as operating a computer, knitting, or massage. The body cannot adapt that fast and injury occurs. People need to "build up" to any prolonged or strenuous activity, whether it be work or recreational. While RSI is usually associated with the workplace, only 47% of CTS surgeries are considered to be work-related, according to the Centers for Disease Control and Prevention (1). Remember that only 14% of one's entire life is spent on the job. Non-work-related factors include obesity, pregnancy, smoking, alcohol consumption, sleeping positions, and lack of exercise.

CTS derives its name from a space in the center of the heel of the hand that contains nine flexor tendons and the median nerve. It is formed by a U-shaped cluster of eight carpal bones. The transverse carpal ligament stretches across this U-shaped channel and is the very strong "roof" of the carpal tunnel. The flexor tendons pass through and fill the carpal tunnel, encircling the median nerve. The median nerve innervates the thumb and first three fingers.

CTS occurs when the tissues around the tendons become enlarged from hypertrophy or inflammation due to persistent and repetitive strain (use), and compress the median nerve. Symptoms include reduced muscle control, impaired or lost nervous function, diminished grip strength, numbness, tingling, pain, and reduced ability to grasp, pinch, or manipulate objects with the hand (2).

Although some cases of long-term, chronic carpal tunnel injury may require surgery, CTS can usually be treated effectively with massage, stretching, and strengthening. Even when surgery is chosen, massage will help prepare for the surgery and help with the recovery afterwards. Moreover, surgery only addresses the actual injury and does nothing to correct the posture, ischemia and trigger points, and lifestyle issues that predispose the person to the injury in the first place. Therefore, it is common for the injury to reoccur after surgery once the activity is resumed.

The massage therapist can play an important role in the person's recovery by reducing the predisposing factors such as postural distortions, nerve entrapments, ischemia, and trigger points that contribute to the injury. Teaching the client AIS stretches presented in Chapter 8 for the neck, shoulder, forearm, wrist, and hand will facilitate the client's recovery and prevent reoccurrence.

ASSESSMENT TECHNIQUES

Before beginning treatment, it is important to assess the client to determine the nature of her complaint. Golfer's elbow, tennis elbow, and carpal tunnel syndrome are three of the most common elbow and wrist conditions you will encounter. Below are five assessment tests that will help you assess the client for the presence of these conditions.

Test for Golfer's Elbow

Medial epicondylitis, often called "golfer's elbow," "Little League elbow," or "pitcher's elbow," is a ballistic or repetitive-strain injury to the flexor tendons of the hand and fingers, causing pain at or just proximal to the medial **epicondyle** of the elbow. To test for this injury, provide resistance to a strong contraction of the flexor muscles.

The client's arm and hand should be straight, elbow locked. You provide resistance, preventing movement as he strongly attempts to flex his wrist. Test in three to four positions, beginning with the wrist straight, then flexed 45 degrees (shown in Fig. 11-1), then flexed 90 degrees. If pain is not experienced in these three positions, then test with client's wrist extended 45 degrees. Pain on the medial side of the elbow or just distal to it is a positive sign, especially if it matches the pain of his complaint.

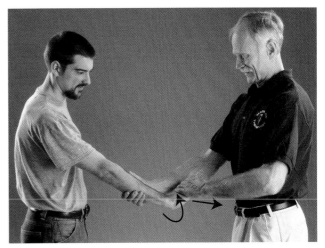

Figure 11-2 **Test for tennis elbow.** Client's arm is straight, hand flexed, resisted extension in several positions, 45 degrees of extension shown. Pain at or just distal to the lateral elbow indicates a positive test. If painful, examine and treat the forearm extensors and the lateral epicondyle.

Test for Tennis Elbow

Lateral epicondylitis, also called "tennis elbow," is an injury similar to medial epicondylitis except it is to the extensor tendons on the lateral side. The test is the same, just in the opposite direction.

The client's arm and hand should be straight, elbow locked. You prevent extension movement of the wrist as he strongly contracts. Test in three to four positions, hand and wrist straight, wrist extended 45 degrees (shown in Fig. 11-2), wrist extended 90 degrees (or at client's end of ROM). If no pain is reported in the first three positions, test with the client's wrist flexed 45 degrees. Pain on the lateral side of the elbow or just distal to it is a positive sign, especially if it matches the pain of his complaint.

Phalen's Test for Carpal Tunnel Syndrome

With the client standing or sitting erect, ask him to place the dorsal (back) side of his hands together with fingers pointed downward (in forced flexion). Ask client to try to extend (straighten) his wrists, thus pressing the back of one hand against the other. Hold the contraction in this position for 30 to 60 seconds. The test is positive if the person reports tingling or numbness in the median nerve distribution. Wrist or hand pain is not a positive sign (Fig. 11-3)!

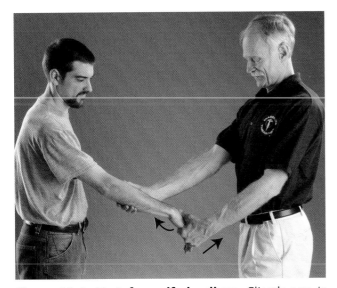

Figure 11-1 **Test for golfer's elbow.** Client's arm is straight, hand extended, resisted flexion in several positions, 45 degrees of flexion shown. If client indicates pain, examine and treat the forearm flexors and the medial epicondyle.

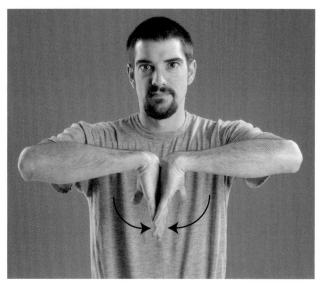

Figure 11–3 Phalen's test for carpal tunnel syndrome. The dorsal (back) side of the client's hands are placed together with fingers pointed downward (in forced flexion). The client contracts, trying to extend (straighten) his wrists. Have the client hold this position for 30 to 60 seconds. The test is positive if the client reports tingling or numbness in the median nerve distribution. Wrist or arm pain is probably not a positive sign.

Tinel's Test for Carpal Tunnel Syndrome

Supporting client's wrist, tap firmly and repeatedly with one finger over the carpal tunnel (tapotement). The test is positive if the impact produces an electric shock sensation in the **median nerve** distribution of the hand (Fig. 11-4).

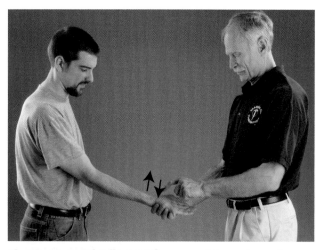

Figure 11–4 Tinel's test for carpal tunnel syndrome. The therapist taps firmly (tapotement) with one finger over the carpal tunnel. This test is positive if the impact produces sensation in the medial nerve distribution of the hand.

Sustained Thumb Pressure Test for Carpal Tunnel Syndrome

Supporting the client's wrist, press straight into the carpal tunnel with one thumb, using a moderate to firm pressure. The test is positive if the person reports tingling or numbness in the median nerve distribution of the hand (Fig. 11-5A).

If the tests for median nerve entrapment (carpal tunnel syndrome) are positive, proceed with the entire forearm routine below. Also assess the client's shoulder and neck posture and begin examination and treatment of these areas if time allows or in future appointments.

PREPARATION FOR THE THERAPEUTIC ROUTINE

Begin the specific treatment of the forearm, wrist, and hand by doing the general relaxation routine for the arm presented in Chapter 9. As a reminder, this routine is summarized below.

1. Let the client's arm hang at her side and jostle or roll the entire upper extremity between your hands (Fig. 11-6). Start just distal (below) the shoulder and move down to the wrist and back up, making several back and forth strokes at each hand width.
2. Place the client's forearm on the arm rest, palm down.
3. Standing in front of the chair, facing the client with your body aligned with her forearm, apply compression strokes to the extensor side of the forearm from wrist to elbow using the heel of your hand or a loosely clenched fist. Cover the area three times.
4. Turn the client's palm up.
5. Apply compression strokes to the flexor muscles from wrist to elbow as you did on the extensors.
6. Turn the client's palm down.
7. Apply 5 to 7 deep circular friction strokes to the extensor muscles of the forearm from wrist to elbow using the heel of your hand or a loosely clenched fist.
8. Turn the client's palm up.
9. Apply 5 to 7 deep circular friction strokes to the flexor muscles of the forearm from wrist to elbow using the heel of your hand or a loosely clenched fist.

If you are not sure of any of these steps, return to Chapter 9 and review. All of the advanced techniques build on that routine.

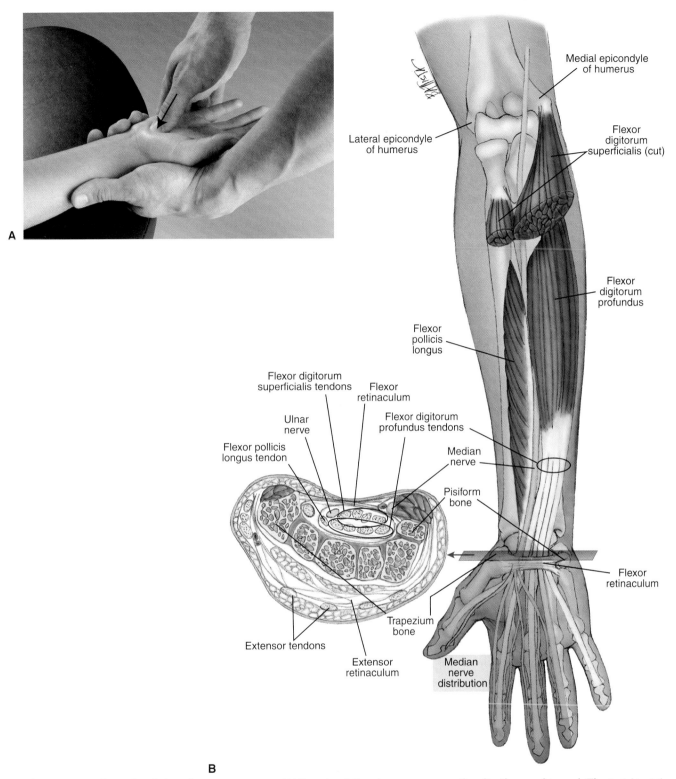

Figure 11-5 Sustained thumb pressure test. (A) Sustained thumb pressure over the client's carpal tunnel. The test is positive if the client reports tingling or numbness in the median nerve distribution of the hand. (B) Illustration of the forearm and hand, showing the muscles and tendons that pass through the carpal tunnel, the median nerve, and the medial nerve distribution in the hand (shaded). The cross section of the wrist shows detail of the carpal tunnel.

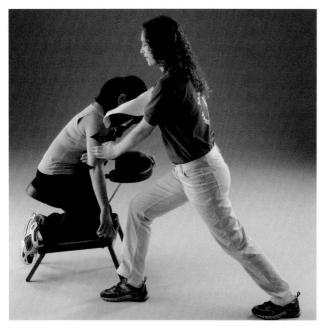

Figure 11–6 Warming the forearm. Using both hands in a back-and-forth motion, "roll" the arm between you hands at a moderately fast tempo. Move distal (down) to the wrist and back proximal (up) to just below the shoulder. Repeat this cycle 1–2 times.

Now that the tissues are warmed up, it would be appropriate to do the AIS forearm, wrist, and hand stretches from Chapter 8. These are especially important in cases of carpal tunnel and epicondyle pain. The most important homework stretches for the client are usually the flexor stretches and the individual finger stretches. If you need to review the stretches, return to the AIS section of Chapter 8.

Stretching can be done before doing any massage, between the general massage and the specific massage techniques as suggested here, or after all massage has been done. This is your decision. Base it on your experience and intuition. This author prefers to do the stretching between general and specific parts of the routine due to the assessment aspect of AIS.

As a reminder, the AIS stretching sequence for the forearm is excellent for you to do yourself, even if unassisted, to warm up before you begin giving massage and again after you have finished.

FOREARM

Now that you have assessed, warmed up, and stretched the client, it is time to begin the therapeutic routine. The primary areas to be addressed (forearm,

wrist, and hand) are each covered in detail in the remainder of this chapter, beginning with the forearm. As the major muscles of the forearm originate near the elbow and insert at the wrist and hand, to positively affect problems at either end you must address the forearm. Therefore, it is warmed up with techniques that spread fibers and relax the muscles first. Even more specific techniques are then applied to examine the forearm muscles starting at the origins on the epicondyles. The entire forearm must be examined to locate tender and trigger points in the many layers of muscles. The majority of client complaints on either end of the forearm are related to hypertonic muscles and trigger points in the forearm. This cannot be overemphasized. Finally, we will address the wrist and hand.

This routine is a step-by-step guide to help you thoroughly examine the entire forearm, wrist, and hand. It can take considerable time. The therapeutic portion of a 15- to 20-minute treatment can be spent on one arm. While this may seem unbalanced, tennis elbow or carpal tunnel syndrome in one arm makes the client feel fairly unbalanced to begin with. Bringing relief to the client's complaint is more balancing than massaging with the same number of strokes on each side. Do a quick warmup or finishing step on the other arm, which will take just a few seconds, if you feel you must do something on it.

To save time, you may omit steps not appropriate for a particular client's complaints. For example, there is no need to test for carpal tunnel syndrome if the complaint is a sore elbow. If the client has tennis elbow, you do not need to do the steps for the wrist, hand, and fingers. Carpal tunnel syndrome does not usually benefit from all the detailed massage and joint mobilization techniques on each finger. The wrist decompression steps are only necessary for wrist problems. While it is best to learn the steps in the order they are presented (and they are in a very logical and efficient sequence), once learned you can skip the ones not necessary for any particular client. We will now begin our therapeutic journey down the forearm, starting at the epicondyles.

Lateral Epicondyle

The lateral **epicondyle** is the large bony landmark (bump) on the lateral side (outside) of the elbow (Fig. 11-5B). It is the attachment site for the long extensor muscles of the wrist and hand and the brachioradialis. Examine it with deep friction and treat with static pressure.

1. Stand in the lunge position, in front of and just slightly to one side of the chair.
2. Pick up the client's arm with your hand that is more medial relative to the client.
3. Turn the client's palm up and hold it at the wrist.
4. With your other hand, grasp the client's forearm in the palm of your hand and slide proximally (up) to his elbow. Stop when your thumb encounters the large bump of the lateral epicondyle.
5. Examine the entire epicondyle with deep friction in several directions (Fig. 11-7). The epicondyle is part of the humerus and some of the attaching tendons continue 1–2 inches up the lateral side of the humerus. Examine the epicondyle and the lateral margin.
6. Then examine the extensor tendons just below (distal to) the epicondyle with deep friction, from the epicondyle to 2 inches distal to it. Use a longitudinal stroke toward the epicondyle and a cross-fiber stroke.
7. If tender areas are discovered, treat them with sustained pressure for 8–12 seconds. If either tendon or attachments are tender, it means the entire extensor side of the forearm needs to be massaged and stretched, as these tendons run distally to the hand. Treating just the tendon will not usually resolve the complaint.

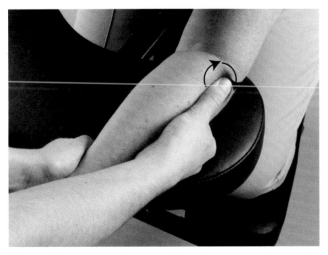

Figure 11-7 Lateral epicondyle. Examining with circular deep friction on the epicondyle. Continue examining 1 to 2 inches proximal and distal to the epicondyle. Treat tender points with sustained pressure.

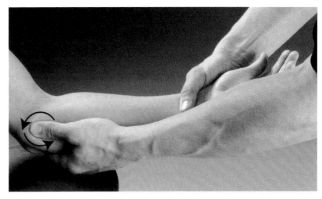

Figure 11-8 Medial epicondyle. Examining with circular friction on the epicondyle. Also examine 2 inches distal to the epicondyle. Do not go superior or posterior, as the ulnar nerve is very superficial. Treat tender points with sustained pressure.

Medial Epicondyle

The medial epicondyle is the attachment site for the long flexor muscles of the wrist and hand. Eight of the tendons which pass through the carpal tunnel originate on the medial epicondyle (flexor digitorum–superficialis and profundus); therefore, this should be the first step of a carpal tunnel syndrome treatment. It is also the site of the "golfer's elbow" injury. Most massage therapists will find this attachment site tender on themselves. If yours is, start regular massage, stretching, and exercises to prevent onset of an injury. The massage procedure for this area is described below.

Remaining in the same position you used for treating the lateral epicondyle, switch your hand positions. Your medial hand will be on the medial epicondyle, or near it. Examine the medial side the same way you did the lateral side (Fig. 11-8).

Note that the ulnar nerve may be superficial, just distal and posterior to the medial epicondyle. If the client reports intense, tingling pain down his arm as you friction this area, move anterior. *Do not* continue to treat on this nerve.

Forearm Flexor Muscles

The forearm flexor muscles flex the wrist and fingers. The longest flexor muscles originate at the medial epicondyles. Shorter ones arise along the radius and ulna. There are several layers of flexor muscles and, when well-developed, this group may be many inches thick. Both superficial and deep layers can develop trigger points that refer into the wrist and hand, mimicking carpal tunnel syndrome or just causing significant discomfort. Superficial, light massage will not

Box 11-2

Injuries to the Epicondyles

Injuries to the epicondyles of the elbow are usually from repetitive strain. Often, massage therapists will find their own epicondyles and the tendons just distal to them to be quite tender. RSIs seldom exhibit the signs of inflammation and are often a collagen deterioration from the repetitive strain, not from tearing and the inflammatory healing process. These injuries respond very well to massage, especially to deep friction techniques. See Chapter 6 for more information on RSIs. Epicondyle injuries can also be caused by sports and workplace activities that place a significant ballistic load on the tendons and periosteum of the epicondyles, causing tissue tearing (3).

For instance, flexor activities such as baseball, golf, and hammering will injure the medial epicondyle attachments, and extensor activity such as the tennis backhand shot will injure the lateral epicondyle attachments. The inflammatory response results as the body attempts to heal the torn area. When treating a client with an injury that is recent (acute) and in which inflammation is still present, use gentle stretching and massage above and especially below the area. Suggest ice and rest for the area until the inflammation resolves, as continued ballistic activity or resumption of activity too soon will keep the area in a state of irritation. Once the inflammation subsides, treat directly on the epicondyles and on the tendons just distal to them with deep friction strokes. Also work distally, examining and treating as necessary all the way to the wrist. In the case of golf or tennis injuries, the client likely needs to develop better form and technique to prevent the injury from recurring. Suggest that he get a competent instructor (coach).

or finger, to ensure better penetration. Make 5 to 10 circles of deep friction on each spot. Circle your way into the tissue far enough to affect the deep layers; however, do not push beyond the individual client's pain tolerance. He should never be tensing up. Begin on the heel of the client's hand and treat across the wrist from lateral to medial (Fig. 11-9).

4. Then move a thumb-width proximally and treat the next row of points from medial to lateral.
5. Move a thumb-width proximally again and treat across lateral to medial.
6. Continue this zigzag pattern all the way up to the elbow. Be sure to examine the flexor tendons all the way to the medial epicondyle. Thumb-saver tools may be used.
7. When tender places or trigger points are encountered, stop and hold with sustained pressure for 8–12 seconds.
8. Be sure to regularly get feedback from the client as to appropriate pressure, tender points, and any referral (trigger points) he may experience.
9. In tight or tender areas, or on trigger points, you may have the client flex and extend his wrist as you either hold a point or massage with circular deep friction. This can help stretch the tissues and increase blood flow.
10. If the client has many tender spots, and to give your thumbs a rest, every few minutes use your palm to apply a few circles of deep friction on the forearm, done at a light to moderate pressure, to soothe the area and give him relief from the intensity of the treatment. You could use moderate to slow vibration for 3–4 seconds instead of deep friction.

find or reduce these trigger points. Remember, trigger points are small, taut bands of fibers. You must examine the entire forearm, inch by inch, and melt your way into the tissues enough to affect the deep layers and find trigger points. You must massage each spot long enough for the client to respond if it is tender or referring. Being meticulously thorough will bring you results that many other therapists cannot achieve. The flexor routine is explained in the list below.

1. Place the client's arm palm up on the arm rest.
2. Stand in the lunge position facing the chair, in line with the arm being treated.
3. Examine the entire flexor side of the forearm with circular friction, using one braced thumb

Extensor Muscles

The extensor muscles, for the most part, correspond to the flexors. They are on the other side of the forearm and originate from the lateral epicondyle and the posterior side of the radius and ulna. They extend the wrist and fingers and so are antagonistic to the flexors. The extensors do not have a problematic structure like the carpal tunnel. However, they can still become hypertonic, develop trigger points, or suffer repetitive-strain injuries. For example, typing on a computer keyboard now works the extensors as hard or harder than the flexors and tendinous or tendonitis can develop from overuse. The specific examination for the forearm extensors is the same procedure as you used

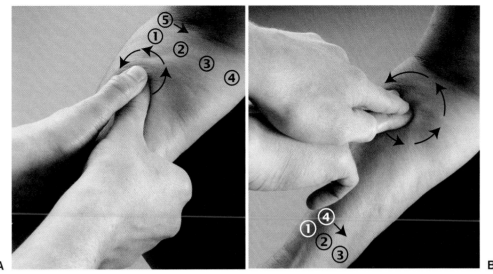

Figure 11-9 Examination and treatment of the forearm flexor muscles with circular deep friction. (A) Using a braced thumb. The numbered circles above the thumbs show the step-by-step pattern of thumb placement to examine every square inch of the forearm. (B) Using braced fingertips instead of thumbs. The numbered circles below the fingertips show the pattern with which to cover the entire forearm. Start at the wrist and work to the elbow.

on the flexors; just roll the forearm over to palm down and repeat the entire sequence. The only difference is the treatment of the supinator under the brachioradialis. The description is below.

Roll the client's arm palm down and repeat the sequence used for the flexors on the extensors. Be sure to displace and "dig" under each side of the proximal (upper) 3 inches of the brachioradialis muscle with deep friction strokes to examine the supinator muscle, which lies beneath brachioradialis and may have trigger points contributing to elbow and thumb pain. The supinator often contributes to the tennis elbow condition and can also entrap the radial nerve, causing tingling, numbness, and poor motor control in the hand (Fig. 11-10).

Be sure to examine every square inch of tissue. Make 5 to 10 circles on each spot to penetrate the deep layers and give the client time to respond. "Thumb-saver" tools are appropriate to use here.

WRIST

The wrist joint is made up of the head of the ulna, the distal end of the radius, and the eight carpal bones, all held together by a maze of ligaments. The multiple tendons and nerves that operate the hand pass over these structures and are held in place by very strong fascial bands called the flexor and extensor retinaculums. The

joint is subject to both traumatic and overuse injuries. The goal of the next treatment sequence is to normalize and stretch the retinaculums, reducing ischemia and freeing adhesions. This will be done with myofascial stretching and deep friction, accompanied by static pressure on tender points. Then, a series of manipulations are presented that can decompress the wrist using

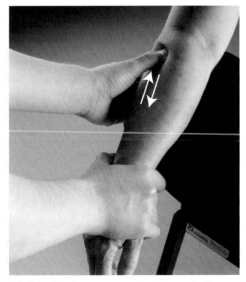

Figure 11-10 Supinator muscle. Therapist is pressing under the brachioradialis from the lateral side at a 45-degree angle while shifting the tissues with deep friction strokes to examine the lateral portion of the supinator muscle. Repeat from the medial side to examine the other half of the supinator.

traction, myofascial stretching, effleurage, and joint mobilization. This routine provides a powerful protocol to address virtually any wrist complaint, from sprains to carpal tunnel syndrome.

Myofascial Stretching of the Wrist

One type of carpal tunnel surgery involves inserting a strong probe under the flexor retinaculum and lifting anterior, stretching the retinaculum to create more space in the tunnel, thus reducing pressure on the median nerve. Such surgical myofascial stretching is effective but somewhat invasive, and beyond our scope here. This sequence is an attempt to accomplish a similar effect from the outside. The fascia will be stretched from the extensor (dorsal) side, around the left and right sides, and finally over the flexor side and the carpal tunnel, as described below.

1. Using thumbs or fingertips, perform myofascial stretching in several directions, on all four sides of the wrist.
2. Take the skin to tension and hold, feeling for the elongation of the tissue or "tissue creep." The concept here is to stretch and elongate the fascia of the wrist retinaculums.
3. Start on the extensor (dorsal) side, stretching across the fibers and then with the fibers of the extensor retinaculum, which is over the wrist joint and the carpal bones (Fig. 11-11).
4. Stretch the radial (thumb) and ulnar (little finger) sides, first across the fibers and then with

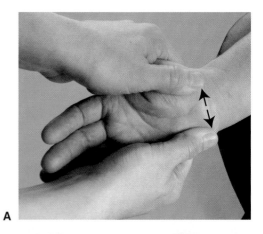

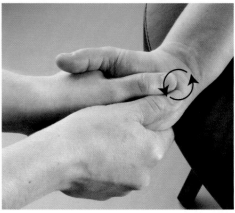

Figure 11–12   Flexor retinaculum. (A) Myofascial stretching on the flexor (palmar) side of the client's wrist, with the fibers. (B) Deep friction on flexor side of the wrist. Avoid the carpal tunnel but treat all sides of it if the client reports pain or tingling in the hand.

the fibers, working the expansion (slack) toward the flexor side.
5. Finally stretch the flexor side, first across the fibers (distally–proximally) and then with the fibers (laterally–medially). If time is of the essence, just do the flexor side (Fig. 11-12A).

Deep Friction of the Retinaculums of the Wrist

Follow the myofascial stretching with deep friction in several directions on all sides of the wrist. Again, focus on the retinaculum area all around the wrist and a thumb-width on either side of it. If time allows, repeat the myofascial stretching on the flexor side after completing the deep friction treatment. Note: If the carpal tunnel is inflamed, it will be very painful for the client if you press into the carpal tunnel. Stay on either side, above, and below the tunnel with this treatment on these clients (Fig. 11-12B).

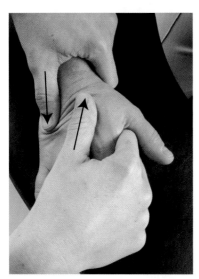

Figure 11–11   Extensor retinaculum. Myofascial stretching on the extensor (dorsal) side of the client's wrist, across the fibers. Hold and feel for the "tissue creep." Stretch in 3–4 places, then stretch with the fibers.

Check for Extensor Tendinopathy

If you are working with a person who has been diagnosed with carpal tunnel syndrome (CTS) and he is spending a lot of time operating the keyboard of a computer, be sure to perform the CTS tests provided in this chapter. It is quite common that the client has extensor tendon pain or extensor tendinopathy that may have been diagnosed as CTS. Have the client point to where he feels the pain. If he points to the dorsal (back) side of his wrist, he probably does not have CTS.

Computer keyboards are now so sensitive that they require little downward pressure to activate a key (flexion). The computer operator expends more energy picking his fingers up off the keys (extension) than pressing them down, which thus leads to extensor tendon pain. Thoroughly examine the extensor muscles and their attachments at the lateral epicondyle of the elbow, as described in this chapter. Stretches should be given with emphasis on hand and finger flexion to stretch the extensors. Once the condition is reduced, strengthening exercises for the extensors should be given. Several good extensor exercises are given in Chapter 6.

Wrist Mobilization

The repetitive contractions of the flexor and extensor muscles compress the carpal bones and wrist joint. This series of manipulations serves to decompress and mobilize this important area. It is done in two parts. The first sequence uses traction and effleurage to stretch the fascia on all four sides of the wrist. The second sequence uses traction with shearing and rotational movements to mobilize the wrist joint. See the contraindication noted below before proceeding.

CONTRAINDICATION

ACUTE WRIST INJURIES

In cases of acute wrist injuries, the wrist mobilization sequence should not be performed if there is significant swelling or if the possibility of a fracture exists. Refer the client to a physician for diagnosis.

1. Kneel or sit down by the massage chair, facing the same direction as the client. (It is unlikely this sequence can be effective with other seated support systems.)
2. Place your humerus over (anterior to) the client's humerus, with your elbow just medial and somewhat anterior to the client's.
3. Place the palm of your hand against the palm of the client's hand and interlace fingers with the client (Fig. 11-13A).
4. Lift the client's arm, flexing her elbow to approximately 45 degrees.
5. Then move your hand into extension, pressing distally into the heel of the client's hand, which moves the client's hand into flexion. This movement should create a stretch between the client's elbow and hand, decompressing the elbow and, more importantly, the wrist joint. Note: If your forearm is longer than the client's, place your elbow further medial, away from the client's elbow, thus creating a larger triangle. If your forearm is shorter than the client's, place your elbow against the client's anterior humerus. In some cases it may be necessary to place a towel or pad of some sort on the client's forearm to further elevate the therapist's humerus.
6. Maintaining the traction, use the thumb of your other hand to effleurage across the client's wrist joint, starting 2 inches proximal to the wrist and finishing 2 inches distal to the wrist. Imagine decompressing the carpal bones and the wrist joint during this procedure (Fig. 11-13B).
7. Go over the entire extensor side of the wrist several times. Lubrication is not required, but pressure will have to be adjusted to be able to slide across the skin, pressing firmly but without causing skin burn or pulling hair.
8. Maintaining the traction and flexion of the client's wrist, tip her wrist toward the little finger side of her hand (ulnar deviation) and effleurage the lateral (thumb) side of the wrist, moving distally from 2 inches proximal to the wrist until you reach the first knuckle of her thumb (Fig. 11-13C,D).
9. Gently release the traction on the client's wrist by returning both wrists to neutral.
10. Release the client's hand, but keep your elbow and forearm in the same place (medial to the client's forearm).
11. Rotate the client's hand so the dorsal (back) side of her hand is against your palm.

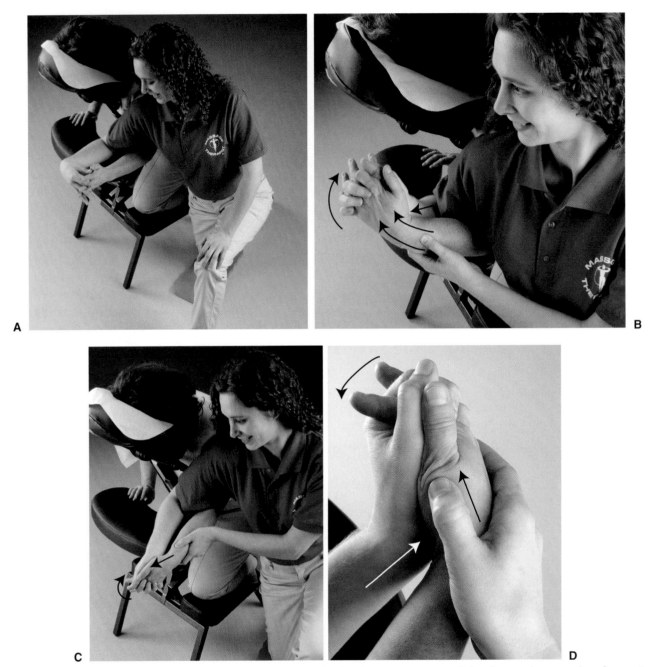

Figure 11–13 **Wrist mobilization.** (A) Position 1: kneeling by the client, your arm medial to hers, palms together, fingers interlaced. (B) Position 2: treating the extensor side with the client's wrist in flexion and traction, performing effleurage from 2 inches proximal to 2 inches distal to wrist. (C) Position 3: treating the radial (thumb) side of the client's wrist. Maintaining flexion and traction, add ulnar deviation; then effleurage distally across the wrist joint to the first joint of the thumb. (D) Close-up of Position 3.

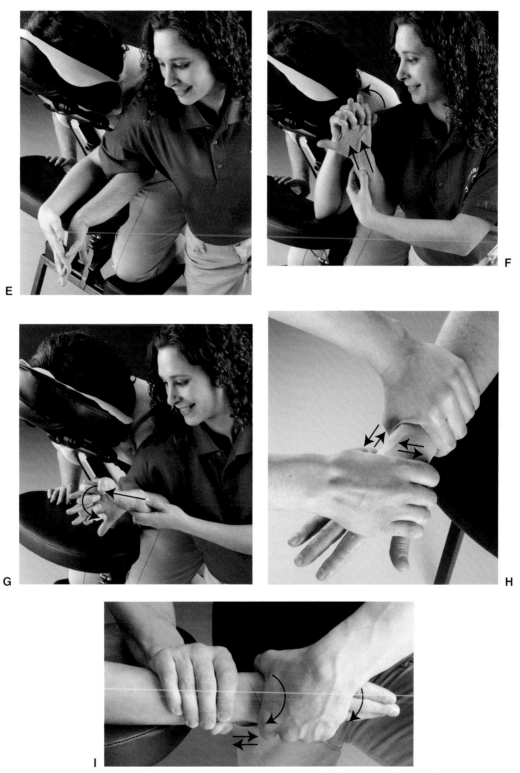

Figure 11–13 *(cont)* (E) Position 4: Reposition so that your palm is against the dorsal (back) side of the client's hand, fingers interlaced. (F) Position 5: Treat the flexor side. (G) Position 6: treat the ulnar (little finger) side. Maintaining flexion and traction, add radial deviation; then effleurage distally across the wrist joint to the first joint of the little finger. (H) Position 7: traction and shearing. While tractioning the wrist joint apart, stabilize the client's forearm; then move the client's entire hand straight lateral and medial 5–6 times, then anterior–posterior (floor to ceiling in this position) 5–6 times. (I) Position 8: traction and torquing. Maintaining distal traction, stabilize the forearm and rotate the client's hand counterclockwise. Hold the stretch for 6–10 seconds. Then rotate the hand clockwise and hold for 6–10 seconds.

12. Interlace your fingers with the client's again (Fig. 11-13E).

13. Move your own wrist into extension, taking the client's wrist into extension as well.

14. Using the thumb of your other hand, effleurage from 2 inches proximal to 2 inches distal to the wrist on the flexor (anterior) side of the client's wrist, just as you did on the extensor side (Fig. 11-13F).

15. Go over the entire flexor side of the client's wrist 3 to 5 times.

16. Then, maintaining the extension and traction, tip the client's wrist toward the thumb side (radial deviation) and treat the little finger side of the wrist (Fig. 11-13G). Note: Be aware of the interlacing grip and do not squeeze the client's fingers together. Grip with your fingertips, not by squeezing the phalanges of your fingers together, as doing so becomes very uncomfortable for the client.

17. Release the extension and deviation and let go of the client's hand.

18. Have the client shake out her wrist. It should feel looser and more mobile.

The final procedure of wrist decompression is to traction the wrist joint apart and mobilize the joint with shearing and rotational motions. A shearing motion is one that is perpendicular to a straight line drawn through the axis of the joint when the joint is in its neutral position or "straight."

1. Stand at the client's side, facing her wrist. Place her palm down and grasp her wrist with both of your hands on the dorsal (back) side of her wrist and arm. Place one of your hands just distal to the wrist joint and the other hand just proximal to the joint.

2. Traction the joint straight apart with a firm stretch.

3. Maintaining this stretch, move her hand straight back and forth sideways (lateral–medial) 4 to 6 times, holding her forearm still. This is a tiny movement between the carpal bones of the hand and the radius and ulna of the forearm (Fig. 11-13H).

4. Continuing the traction (stretch), move her hand anterior–posterior 4 to 6 times. This is *not* flexion or extension (no bending of the wrist joint occurs); one side of the joint is moved parallel to the other side of the joint.

5. Maintaining the traction on the wrist and not allowing her forearm to move, rotate the

client's hand counterclockwise, and hold for 6 to 10 seconds at the end point of her movement, feeling for the tissue "creep" as it elongates (Fig. 11-13I).

6. Then traction and rotate clockwise and hold for 6 to 10 seconds.

7. Release the wrist.

8. Have the client shake out her wrist, move it through its range of motions, and ask her how it feels now.

Note: Be sure to keep the grip on the wrist very close to the joint on each side and always apply traction before doing shearing or rotational movements. This is an excellent technique sequence for preventive maintenance of the wrist as well as for restorative therapy.

HAND

The intrinsic muscles of the hand can become hypertonic due to stimulation from nerve entrapment in the forearm or carpal tunnel. Relaxing these muscles helps reduce residual ache and pain. Clients with various hand injuries or with arthritis may report hand pain, stiffness, loss of fine movement control, and other uncomfortable conditions. Trigger points can form in the hand muscles and mimic conditions such as arthritis. Unless the client reports specific complaints in his hand or fingers, there is no reason to perform the detailed steps given in the following sections. However, if you work in a salon, this hand routine would be a wonderful treatment prior to a manicure. Use these hand techniques when you feel that they are appropriate. A hand massage is almost always appreciated.

Metacarpal Spaces

The technique described in this section is primarily aimed at the interosseous and lumbricale muscles that lie between the metacarpal bones and provide fine motor skills, especially at the metacarpophalangeal joint. The best access to these muscles is on the dorsal side. There are also palmar side interosseous muscles. On the palmar side you will also affect the pollicis muscles and other intrinsic muscles of the hand. The interosseous muscles can develop trigger points that refer into the palm, web of thumb, and the first and little fingers. They can mimic arthritis pain and are associated with a tender nodule on the distal interphalangeal joint called **Herberden's nodes** (4). Because the space between the metacarpal bones is relatively small, use your little finger or a small massage tool to get deep between the bones, as described below.

1. Place the client's arm on the arm rest, palm down.
2. Stand in front of the client, facing the chair, aligned with the forearm on the side of the client that is being treated.
3. Using one fingertip, apply deep friction to the tissues between the metacarpal bones on the dorsal side of the hand. Friction the tissues in a direction parallel to the metacarpal bones, beginning at the web of the fingers and moving proximally in ½-inch segments until reaching the carpal bones. Do this between each finger and between the first finger and thumb (Fig. 11-14).
4. Rotate the client's hand palm up and repeat this sequence on the palmar side of the hand.

Fingers

The finger treatment is for clients with damaged or sore, aching fingers. It can also help improve movement of the fingers. While time-consuming, it can be very beneficial for people with hand complaints. Use only light to moderate pressure while performing the techniques listed below.

CONTRAINDICATION

DEGENERATIVE ARTHRITIS AND OSTEOPOROSIS

Do *not* perform the wrist and finger mobilization techniques on clients who have degenerative arthritis, without their physicians' permission. Also be particularly careful and sensitive when mobilizing the finger joints of seniors who may have severe osteoporosis.

1. Apply 4 to 6 deep longitudinal friction strokes to all four sides of each joint capsule of each finger, including the metacarpal–phalangeal joint (Fig. 11-15).
2. When working the little finger, continue proximally up the ulnar side of the hand along the 5th metacarpal bone. This tissue is the abductor digiti minimi muscle. You may also pick it up in a pincer-like grip and examine it. A trigger point in this muscle can refer pain into the entire length of the little finger (4).
3. Mobilize each finger joint just as you did on the wrist joint by holding the finger on either side of a joint.
4. Traction the joint apart and move each side of the joint in opposite directions. Do this shearing

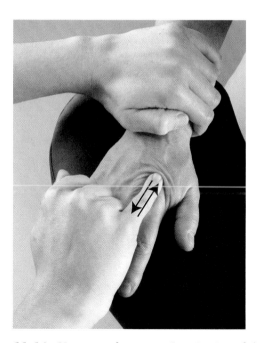

Figure 11-14 Metacarpal spaces. Examination of the extensor (dorsal) side of the hand with longitudinal deep friction, using the little finger.

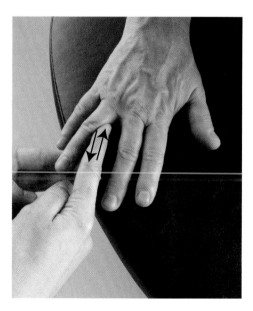

Figure 11-15 Finger. Treatment of the joint capsule with 4–6 strokes of deep friction. Treat all four sides of each finger joint. Support the opposite side of the joint being treated. Note improper support shown.

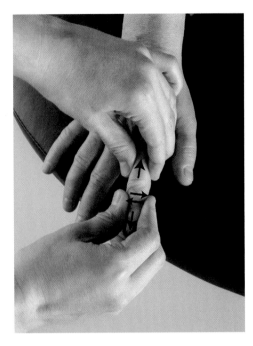

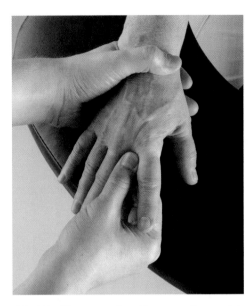

Figure 11–17 Finger webs. Compressing and kneading the web between each finger with a pincer-like grip.

Figure 11–16 Mobilization of finger joints. Finger joints are mobilized with traction while shearing lateral–medial (shown) and anterior–posterior, and rotating (twisting). Repeat at each joint capsule.

movement in both lateral–medial and anterior–posterior directions. Be sure to maintain the traction (Fig. 11-16).

5. Continuing to hold the finger as above, traction and rotate (twist) each finger joint. Work from the distal joint to the proximal joint (metacarpal–phalangeal joint). Rotate (twist) counterclockwise, then clockwise while applying traction. Hold the stretched position for several seconds.

Note: Remember to do these steps to the thumb as well!

Finger Webs

Continue the treatment of the fingers by examining the web of tissue at the proximal end of each finger. Compress and knead this web of tissue with a pincer-like grip. Treat with sustained pressure if tender (Fig. 11-17).

Thumb (Pollicis)

Everyone uses their thumbs to do an incredible amount of work, especially massage therapists. The following sequence is for clients with thumb pain. Be sure to incorporate the AIS thumb stretching sequence from Chapter 8.

1. Compress and petrissage (knead) the entire web of the thumb with a pincer-like grip.
2. Apply deep friction all around the base of the thumb, examining the area thoroughly.
3. Examine the thenar eminence (the pad of the thumb) on the palmar side of the hand. Press into it using circular deep friction. Then try to pick it up, compressing and kneading it with a pincer-like grip,
4. Apply sustained pressure to tender and trigger points if any are found. Trigger points in the pollicis muscles of the hand refer locally into the thumb region (4) (Fig. 11-18).

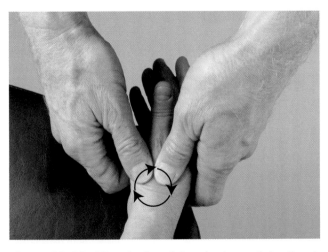

Figure 11–18 Thumb. Examining the base of the thumb with circular deep friction.

CONCLUDING THE ROUTINE

Finally, to wrap up the therapeutic routine for the arm, perform the following

1. Go back and re-examine any tender points and trigger points found during the examination.
2. Review any stretches that the client will be given as "homework."
3. Repeat any stretches that were previously restricted or painful.
4. Remove the client's arm from the arm rest and let it hang down by his side.
5. Using both hands, roll the tissue of his arm back and forth, moving up and down the arm, as you did at the beginning of the treatment, concluding at the hand.
6. Grasp the client's hand in a handshake grip and shake his arm out with moderate intensity, moving in all directions to "loosen everything up." Gradually reduce shaking movements and return his arm to the arm rest (shaking vibration).
7. For a more invigorating conclusion, you could also do tapotement; however, do not apply tapotement over areas where you found trigger points, as it can cause them to re-form.
8. For a more sedating conclusion, roll and shake the arm with less intensity, then finish with some light, slow effleurage strokes, transitioning to slow, light nerve strokes.
9. Repeat part or all of the above routine on the client's other arm if appropriate for his complaint and if time allows.

Note: When time is limited and both of the client's arms are problematic, do the above therapeutic routine to the arm with the most serious degree of complaint and do the general routine to the other arm.

CASE STUDY

Tennis Elbow

Your chair massage practice is at the largest fitness center in your city and it is hosting the city open tennis tournament, a three-day event. You are given permission to set up in a high-traffic area near the tennis courts. You want to be well-prepared for this opportunity.

1. Design a chair massage routine to assess and treat tennis elbow.
2. Practice this routine until you can do it in 15 minutes or less.

CASE STUDY

Hand Pain in the Elderly

You are doing volunteer chair massage for the residents at an assisted-living facility. Several seniors have enlarged distal finger joints and hand pain.

1. What techniques would be appropriate for these seniors?
2. What contraindications might apply?
3. How could you find out if a particular client has contraindicative conditions? (Hint: Is there a nurse station?)

SUMMARY

Forearm, wrist, and hand injuries are very common, and chair massage can address these complaints as well as table massage could. The therapeutic routines for the forearm are built upon the techniques of the relaxation routine in Chapter 9. The same general beginning (warmup) and concluding techniques are used. In between are routines for each area to thoroughly examine, virtually inch by inch, each region, looking for tender and trigger points and treating to normalize them when they are located.

Assessment tests for epicondyle injuries and carpal tunnel syndrome can help you identify the source of a client's complaint. Tennis elbow is an injury to the lateral epicondyle attachments of the long hand extensor muscles. Golfer's elbow is an injury to the medial epicondyle attachments of the long hand flexor muscles. Carpal tunnel syndrome is a repetitive-strain injury causing entrapment of the median nerve in the carpal tunnel, resulting in hand pain and dysfunction.

The AIS routine from Chapter 8 provides both assessment and treatment in one routine. Use AIS stretching for range of motion and movement pain assessment, therapy, and as homework for clients. It also provides valuable support for your own forearms.

Based on the client's complaints, you must decide which of the routines or parts of the routines given are appropriate for each massage. There is no need to do the finger and thumb routines for someone with carpal tunnel syndrome. Likewise, there is no need to do the wrist and hand routines for a client with tennis elbow. Each routine is a separate tool in your toolbox to use as you feel appropriate, based on time available and the main complaint(s) of your client.

REFERENCES

1. Academy of Orthopedic Physicians. "Cumulative trauma" claims driven by job happiness, financial incentives. *Academy News*. The Annual Meeting Edition of the AAOS Bulletin, March 22, 1998.
2. Tortland PD. Nonsurgical management of carpal tunnel syndrome. *Techniques in Orthopedics*, 2003;18:23–29.
3. Lowe WW. Condition on focus–Medial epicondylitis. *Orthopedic & Sports Massage Reviews*. Issue 38, January/February, 2001.
4. Travell JG, Simons DG, Simons LS. Myofascial Pain and Dysfunction. The Trigger Point Manual, vol. 1. *Upper Half of Body*, 2nd ed. Baltimore: Lippincott, Williams & Wilkins; 1999.

Notes

CHAPTER 12

Therapeutic Routine for the Shoulder

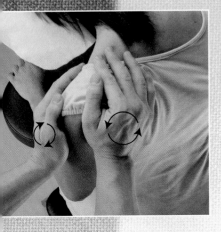

"All labor that uplifts humanity should be undertaken with painstaking excellence. There are no substitutes for expertise and compassion."

MARTIN LUTHER KING

Objectives

■ List some of the common conditions that would indicate therapeutic massage for the shoulder.

■ Perform the AIS stretching routine for the shoulder.

■ Warm up the tissues of the shoulder in preparation for the therapeutic routine.

■ Perform a therapeutic routine treating each of the various muscles of the shoulder.

Key Terms

Angina (pectoris) pain: constricting pain, tingling, numbness, and ache radiating from the chest down the arm, classically from myocardial ischemia (heart attack). However, "false angina" pain may arise from trigger points in the shoulder girdle, commonly the pectoralis major and minor, serratus anterior, and subclavius.

Bursa: a sac lined with synovial membrane and fluid, usually formed in areas of friction where a tendon or muscle passes over a bone.

Bursitis: inflammation of a bursa, usually from too much pressure from the tendon passing over it or from overuse.

Fossa: a depression or indentation below the level surface of a bone or part.

Glenoid fossa: the hollow in the head of the scapula that receives the head of the humerus to make the shoulder joint.

Glenohumeral joint: The shoulder joint.

Tubercle: a slight elevation or nodule on a bone providing an attachment site for a muscle.

If a client's complaint involves the shoulder, you may want to invest the time in a thorough examination and treatment of each muscle of the shoulder girdle. Fortunately, the seated position allows virtually the same access to these tissues as do the prone and supine positions on a table, with the exception of the subscapularis, which cannot be addressed as completely and effectively in the seated position.

Some of the common conditions that call for a specific therapeutic routine for the shoulder include:

- Rotator cuff injuries that do not require surgery.
- Rotator cuff injuries that may or have required surgery.
- Frozen shoulder.
- Movement restrictions of the shoulder joint.
- Pain complaints in the shoulder area.
- Carpal tunnel syndrome.
- Golfer's and tennis elbow.
- Rounded (internally rotated) shoulders.
- Head-forward postures.
- High or low shoulder.

The shoulder routine presented below will address these complaints very well and will usually bring about reduction of the complaint(s). It will require most of the time in a typical seated session, so advise the client that you may not have time to address other areas, such as the low back.

This chapter first reviews the Active Isolated Stretching (AIS) routine for the shoulder and provides instruction on warming up the tissues of the shoulder. Then, the therapeutic routine for the shoulder is presented, categorized by individual muscles.

PREPARATION FOR THE THERAPEUTIC ROUTINE

The Active Isolated Stretching (AIS) routine for the shoulder(s), which is covered in detail in Chapter 8, is a great way to begin a therapeutic treatment of this region, as this will provide an excellent assessment of which muscles are too tight or may have trigger points in them. For instance, restricted motion during stretching indicates a muscle that is hypertonic or in spasm (too tight) and may indicate a trigger point. Pain indicates spasm and ischemia. Referred pain indicates trigger points or possible nerve entrapment.

Unfortunately, some clients may be too tense or too injured to withstand the stretching routine to begin with. For these cases, begin with massage and then either do the stretches at the end of your massage routine or do a particular stretch for each muscle after you have examined and treated it.

Below is a review of the general AIS protocol for the shoulders. If you need descriptions of the individual shoulder stretches, refer to the Active Isolated Stretching—Shoulder section in Chapter 8.

1. Have the client sit up straight in the chair.
2. Advise him to contract his abdominal muscles during the stretches to prevent arching his back, to exhale as he does the stretch, and to inhale as he returns to the starting position.
3. Assist him to the second movement barrier when his movement into the stretch stops (first movement barrier). Remember, the client should perform the movement; you just assist

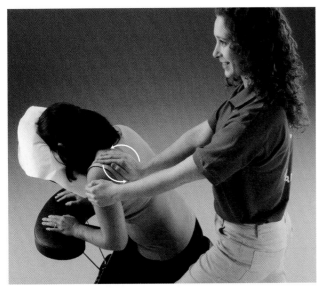

Figure 12–1 Warming the posterior shoulder. The therapist is using circular deep friction with the palm of the hand. Note that the therapist's left hand is supporting and stabilizing the client's shoulder.

with 1 to 2 pounds of pressure at the end of the movement.

After completing the stretching routine, you may further prepare your client for the therapeutic routine by warming his tissues, following the steps below.

1. Stand behind the client and on the side of the shoulder to be treated.
2. Support the anterior of that shoulder with your hand that is further away from the client.
3. Use your other hand to apply circular friction with the palm or a loosely clinched fist over the entire posterior scapula and the posterior side of the shoulder joint (Fig. 12-1).
4. Apply circular friction to the lateral aspect of the shoulder joint with your hand that is more lateral in relation to the client.
5. Move more to the side of the client, grasp the shoulder joint with both hands, and apply circular friction to the anterior and posterior aspects of the shoulder joint. Ask the client to tell you when they feel warming (heat) in the joint and continue until they tell you it feels warm (Figs. 12-2 and 12-3).

INFRASPINATUS

The infraspinatus covers most of the posterior scapula. It originates in the infraspinatus fossa of the scapula and inserts on the greater tuberosity of the humerus. The superior–medial portion is covered by the trapezius. The infraspinatus is the primary external rotator of the arm, working in conjunction with the teres minor and the posterior deltoid. It also stabilizes the humerus on the glenoid fossa during movement.

Clients with infraspinatus problems will report difficulty and pain reaching behind their backs. Athletes will say shoulder pain is limiting their strength. The infraspinatus can cause some clients so much pain when they are trying to sleep that they have to sleep sitting up. Side-lying sleep postures either compress the infraspinatus or elongate it. Sometimes even lying supine is uncomfortable. Trigger points in this muscle can develop anywhere but most commonly appear along the spine and medial border of the scapula, referring into the deltoid, rhomboid, and down the arm into the hand, mimicking the pain of median nerve entrapment (carpal tunnel syndrome) (1).

Massage is very effective in treating this muscle but must be done inch by inch over the entire muscle, with enough time and intensity to penetrate to the deeper fibers. The muscle is often over 1 inch thick. Internal rotation stretches this muscle. In chair massage, it is best to warm and examine the infraspinatus with circular deep friction strokes, as described below.

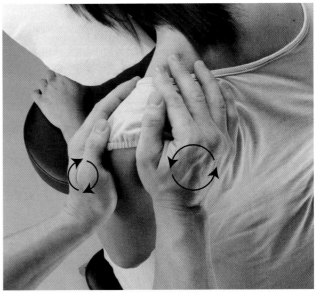

Figure 12–2 Warming the shoulder capsule. The therapist stands at the side of the client, using both hands to apply deep friction to the anterior and posterior of the shoulder joint.

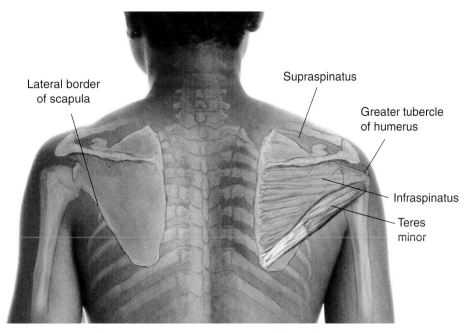

Figure 12–3 **Shoulder showing the three posterior rotator cuff muscles.** Reprinted with permission from Clay JH, Pounds DM. *Basic Clinical Massage Therapy: Integrating Anatomy and Treatment.* Baltimore: Lippincott, Williams & Wilkins; 2003:142, Figure 4-42.

1. Locate the scapula and find its inferior angle, its lateral and medial borders, and the spine of the scapula. The spine is the bony ridge running horizontally from the acromium process to the medial border. The infraspinatus is below the spine, as its name implies.
2. Stand behind the client and slightly to the side being treated.
3. Beginning at the medial border of the scapula just inferior (below) to the scapular spine, engage the tissues with thumbs or fingertips and apply circular friction (Fig. 12-4). This muscle is about 1 inch thick at the base of the scapular spine, so it requires 5 to 10 circular strokes to affect the deeper layers.
4. Move a thumb-width lateral and repeat. Continue until you reach the lateral border of the scapula.
5. Then move a thumb width inferior and work back to the medial border.
6. Continue this zigzag pattern until you have examined the entire posterior scapula.
7. Be sure to isolate and examine both the teres minor and teres major origin attachments. They are on the posterior surface, just medial to the lateral border of the scapula. The lateral portion of infraspinatus is quite thick and, when you move off of its lateral side, it will almost feel

like you are dropping off the edge of the scapula bone, but you are not. There is a "shelf" or "ledge" just lateral to the infraspinatus where the two teres muscles attach. Examine this quite thoroughly with deep circular friction. These attachments are often quite tender and

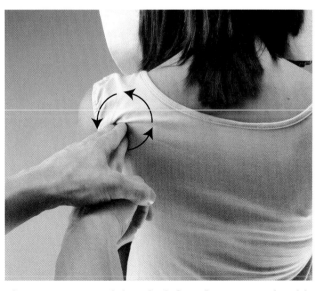

Figure 12–4 **Examining the infraspinatus muscle with deep circular friction, using braced fingertips.**

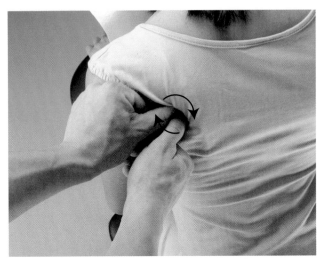

Figure 12–5 Examining the teres minor origin on the lateral scapula with deep circular friction, using thumbs. The site is lateral to the infraspinatus, on the posterior aspect of the lateral border.

commonly refer into the shoulder joint and upper arm (Fig. 12-5).

8. Finish the infraspinatus and teres muscles with general deep circular strokes, using the palm or loosely clinched fist of your hand.

SUPRASPINATUS

The supraspinatus is located superior to the spine of the scapula in the supraspinatus fossa of the scapula. Its tendon proceeds under the acromion process and attaches at the upper aspect of the greater **tubercle** of the humerus. The supraspinatus abducts (raises) the arm (in conjunction with the deltoid) and prevents downward displacement of the humerus when the arm is carrying loads.

The muscle is often injured while carrying briefcases or luggage; thus, it is a good muscle to check in clients if you are working in an airport. Pain in the supraspinatus is felt strongly during abduction and as a dull ache at rest (1). Trigger points can form in the tendon on the humeral head or in the belly of the muscle and refer primarily to the deltoid area, often mimicking the pain of subdeltoid **bursitis** (inflammation of the **bursa**), and sometimes to the lateral elbow and into the forearm.

Massage and stretching are very effective for treating this muscle. A good stretch is to have the client put his arm on the small of his back and reach as far as he can toward the other side. Try a PNF (proprioceptive neuromuscular fascilitation) CRAC (contract-relax,

antagonist-contract) stretch to increase range of motion. Examine the muscle as described below.

1. Again locate the spine of the scapula. The supraspinatus will be superior to the scapular spine in a deep channel of the bone called the supraspinatus fossa. The supraspinatus lies deep to the mid-trapezius, so you must examine through the mid-trapezius with thumbs or fingertips, using deep friction strokes in multiple directions.

2. Start at the medial border and examine in thumb width increments until you encounter a V-shaped structure that stops your lateral progress. This is the "V" of the acromioclavicluar joint. The muscle goes deep under this "V," emerging on the superior aspect of the head of the humerus.

3. As this is sometimes difficult for the therapist to reach and still maintain proper body mechanics, you may examine this with the olecranon process of your elbow, guided with the first finger and thumb of your other hand (Figs. 12-6 and 12-7).

Note that you may find it easier to access this muscle by standing slightly to the side and in front of the client, facing the chair.

LATISSIMUS DORSI

The latissimus dorsi, "the wood-chopping muscle," originates from the spinous processes of T-8 to L-5

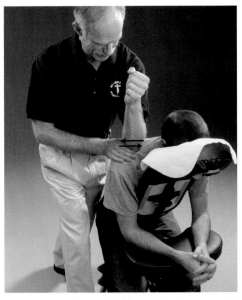

Figure 12–6 Examining the supraspinatus with deep friction, using a guided elbow.

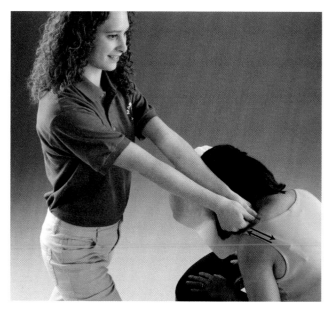

Figure 12–7 Examining the supraspinatus with deep friction, using thumbs. Standing in front of the client may give you better body mechanics. You may use with the fiber, cross-fiber, or circular strokes.

and the sacrum as well as the anterior crest of the ilium, actually growing out of the thoracolumbar fascia. It is the most superficial muscle of the lower torso. Its insertion is with the teres major on the medial aspect of the bicipital groove of the humerus (2). Along with the teres major and minor, it forms the posterior border or "web" of the armpit.

The latissimus extends, adducts, internally rotates, and depresses the humerus. When one swims the crawl stroke or chops wood, this muscle pulls the arm down. It can also depress the shoulder. Its lower fibers are involved in supporting the torso when one walks on crutches. Typically, clients who experience pain in the latissimus report that the pain only manifests when they reach up or far out in front and when they engage the muscles, as in pulling down or in. Then pain may be felt in the muscle or shoulder and down the arm. It can be the source for a mid-thoracic backache, which is sometimes constant. Trigger points can form at the level of the inferior border of the scapula that refer into the mid-back and down the arms, occasionally as far as the ring and little fingers (1). A lower trigger point at about the 11th rib causes pain in the lateral abdominal area.

Forward and sideward elevation stretches are effective in treating this muscle. The latissimus dorsi can be involved in the "frozen shoulder" condition, along with the teres major and the subscapularis. The latissimus is accessible for you to examine in the posterior "web" of the armpit and along the side of the chest, as described below. Depending on the therapist's height relative to the client's, it may be necessary to kneel or sit down in order to maintain proper body mechanics while addressing this area.

1. Stand (or kneel or sit) posterior and to the side of the shoulder being treated and place your fingertips on the lateral border of the scapula.
2. Move your thumbs slowly into the client's armpit and, using a pincer-like grip, apply compression and petrissage to examine the entire "web" of the posterior armpit. Start at the center of the posterior "web" and examine in thumb-width increments, moving superior until you reach the humerus.
3. Then angle your thumbs superiorly and proceed as far superior as you can up into the armpit. Eventually you will feel a band of tissue running horizontally. This will be the long head of the triceps.
4. Work back inferior a thumb-width at a time, re-examining the tissues until you reach the inferior angle of the scapula.
5. Continue your examination inferior in thumb-width increments on latissimus dorsi from the inferior angle of the scapula as far inferior as the muscle remains available to pick-up and knead between your thumbs and fingertips (Figs. 12-8 and 12-9).

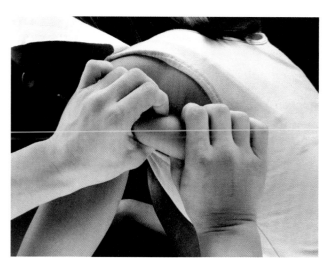

Figure 12–8 Examining the latissimus dorsi and the teres major and minor with both hands in a pincer-like grip on the posterior "web" of the armpit. Place fingertips on the lateral border (edge) of the scapula, bring thumbs under, and examine thoroughly all along the scapula.

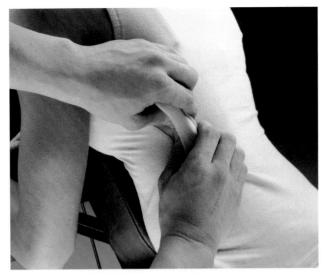

Figure 12–9 Examining the latissimus dorsi on the lateral chest wall with a pincer-like grip, compressing and kneading the tissues. On a client with a well-developed latissimus, you can grasp it as shown. On some clients, it is too small to grasp just inferior to the scapula.

6. Treat tender and trigger points with sustained pressure. Stretch the muscle after treatment.

CLINICAL TIP

Check for Frozen Shoulder

The latissimus dorsi and the subscapularis are the two primary muscles involved in the complaint of "frozen shoulder." Secondary muscles are the teres major and sometimes the teres minor, with occasional involvement of the deltoid. Check all of these for this condition. Trigger points are very commonly associated with the frozen shoulder complaint. Massage and stretching will usually reduce this complaint and restore functional movement.

CONTRAINDICATION

BRACHIAL PLEXUS IN THE ARMPIT

The armpit or axilla is made up of the bellies of four muscles that need to be examined. However, the brachial plexus, a bundle of major nerves and blood vessels, passes through this area. Be extremely cautious in this area and do not intrude into the nerves or vessels. While the specific mus-cles are safely available as described, if you are slightly off you could contact the plexus. Should you feel a pulse, let go immediately and reposition. Should your client suddenly report a tingling, electric, shock-like, or other painful sensation going down her arm, release immediately. Gently rock and soothe the area. Then carefully check your positioning and try again. The catch is that trigger points in these muscles can also refer down the arm. However, direct stimulation of a nerve is almost always a more electric, tingling, and intense sensation. Be aware, be precise, and be in close communication with your client when working in the armpit and medial humerus area.

DELTOID

The deltoid forms a cap over the shoulder joint and initiates most shoulder movements. It is innervated in three sections (anterior, middle, and posterior), with the anterior and posterior being antagonistic to each other. The anterior section originates from the lateral third of the clavicle, the middle section from the lateral edge of the acromion process, and the posterior from the spine of the scapula. All three sections insert on the deltoid tuberosity, a bump on the lateral shaft of the humerus.

The anterior deltoid flexes (raises) the arm forward; the lateral deltoid (along with the supraspinatus) abducts the humerus (sideward elevation); and the posterior deltoid extends the humerus. Trigger points typically form in the anterior and posterior sections and refer locally in the shoulder joint area (1). Trigger or tender points in the deltoid are often mistaken for bursitis (2). Injury often comes from sudden impact trauma to the deltoid during a fall or athletic activity. Clients usually complain of pain in this muscle when moving the shoulder or when sleeping on the affected side. Swimming, throwing, and racquet sports often cause strain and soreness in this muscle, as well. Examine this muscle thoroughly, as described below, for any shoulder complaint.

1. Warm-up the deltoid muscle with deep friction strokes, using one hand or both.
2. Examine the entire deltoid muscle, by picking the tissue up between your thumbs and fingertips and rolling it (petrissage) (Fig. 12-10).
3. Then isolate each of the three sections of the deltoid, anterior, posterior and lateral using

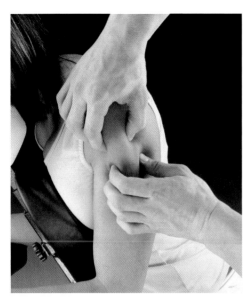

Figure 12–10 Examining the anterior deltoid. Using a pincer-like grip, lift, compress, and knead the fibers along their entire length.

pincer compression and petrissage. It is most efficient to stand posterior–lateral to the client to examine the anterior deltoid. Then stand anterior–lateral to examine the posterior deltoid. The middle deltoid can be examined from either position (Fig. 12-11).

4. Place the fingertips of both hands along the anterior deltoid fibers and apply deep cross-fiber friction at the edges of the muscle. Remember, the anterior deltoid runs from the deltoid tuberosity of the humerus to the lateral third of the clavicle.

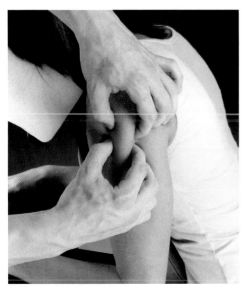

Figure 12–11 Examining the middle deltoid with a pincer-like grip, using compression and petrissage.

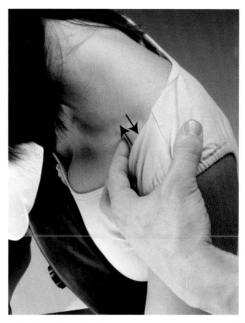

Figure 12–12 Examining the origin of the deltoid on the lateral third of the clavicle with one finger, using deep cross-fiber friction. Examine the anterior clavicle; then continue around the edge of the acromion process to the spine of the scapula.

5. Grasp the anterior deltoid fibers and lift them away from the bone. Lift them to tension and then give them a little tug to release them from adhesions to the deeper tissues.
6. Work along the anterior deltoid fibers in this manner, then the posterior deltoid, and finally the lateral fibers.
7. Use thumbs or fingertips to examine the deltoid insertion on the deltoid tuberosity of the humerus with circular friction.

Note that you may want to examine the origins of the deltoid along the acromion process and the lateral third of the inferior clavicle with deep friction (Figs. 12-12 and 12-13).

This should be done if the deltoid is tender or contains trigger points. Other reasons to examine the deltoid origins are local pain reported in these areas, an auto accident when restrained by a shoulder belt, falls, collisions, and contusion injuries to this area.

CLINICAL TIP

The Deltoid–Trapezius Connection

If the deltoid will not respond to pressure and relax, examine the upper and mid-trapezius. Likewise, if the trapezius will not relax, examine the

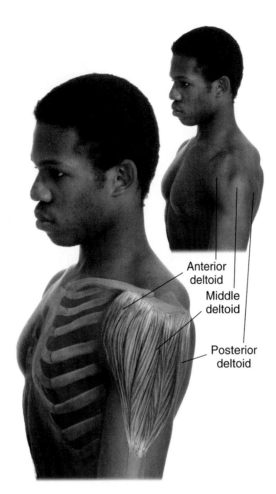

Anterior
deltoid

Middle
deltoid

Posterior
deltoid

Figure 12–13 Deltoid muscle. Reprinted with permission from Clay JH, Pounds DM. *Basic Clinical Massage Therapy: Integrating Anatomy and Treatment.* Baltimore: Lippincott, Williams & Wilkins; 2003:136, Figure 4-31.

deltoid. The fibers of these muscles have fascial interconnection at their mutual attachment on the acromion process.

ROTATOR CUFF

The rotator cuff is a group of tendons that attach to the superior head of the humerus and that provide both movement and stability to the **glenohumeral (shoulder) joint**. These tendons are injured through overuse, strain, and direct trauma. Massage can be beneficial to help repair these tissues when they are injured and to help prevent overuse and strain injuries. These tendon attachments should be examined on all of your clients who actively use their

shoulders in either occupational or recreational settings. These tendons are often referred to as the SITS tendons, being composed of the supraspinatus, infraspinatus, and teres minor on the posterior side and the subscapularis tendon insertion on the anterior (Fig. 12-14). We will examine them in the order just listed. As they are covered by the deltoid muscle, we must use deep friction to examine them. If tenderness is reported by the client, treat with sustained pressure for 8–12 seconds.

1. Position the client properly. In the typical seated massage position, if using a massage chair, the shoulder is comfortably internally rotated and the humerus adducted (elbow at her side), with the forearm resting on the arm rest of the chair. This is the ideal position to examine the posterior tendons of the rotator cuff.
2. Find the "V" of the acromioclavicular joint. Move laterally across the acromion process until you drop off the process onto the head of the humerus.
3. Apply deep friction with thumb or fingers in a front-to-back (anterior–posterior) direction. This will apply cross-fiber friction through the deltoid to the supraspinatus tendon.
4. Move posterior and inferior about a thumb-width, where you will find the infraspinatus tendon.
5. Apply deep cross-fiber friction here to treat the infraspinatus tendon. Move another thumb-width inferior until you are at the posterior aspect of the head of the humerus. This will be the teres minor tendon (Fig. 12-15).
6. Press anterior and apply deep cross-fiber friction through the posterior deltoid, shifting the tissues superior–inferior.
7. Now move the client's forearm lateral to the edge of the arm rest, which will rotate the arm externally.
8. Examine directly on the anterior aspect of the head of the humerus to treat the subscapularis tendon.
9. Press posteriorly through the anterior deltoid tissue and apply deep friction in an inferior–superior direction (Fig.12-16).

PECTORALIS MAJOR

The pectoralis major is a fan-shaped muscle consisting of three groups of fibers originating on the medial two-thirds of the clavicle, the lateral border of the

Figure 12-14 Rotator cuff tendons (SITS Tendons) of the shoulder joint. The supraspinatus is superior, the infraspinatus is 45 degrees posterior–inferior, the teres minor is 90 degrees posterior, and the subscapularis is anterior. Note the "V" formed by the acromioclavicular joint. This is a landmark used to locate the supraspinatus tendon, which is straight lateral from the "V."

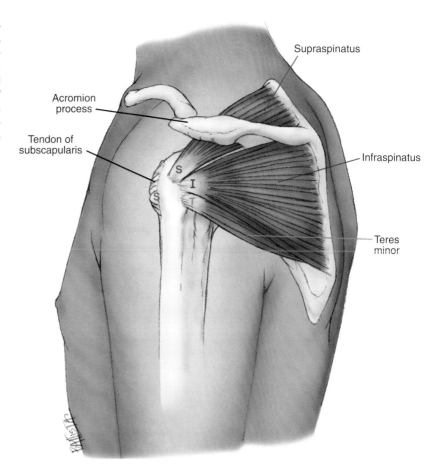

Figure 12-15 Posterior rotator cuff tendons. The therapist examines the teres minor tendon of rotator cuff with cross-fiber deep friction, using thumbs. The direction of pressure is almost straight anterior onto the posterior aspect of the greater tubercle of the humerus. If you move approximately one thumb-width superior and pressing anterior–inferior, you will be examining the infraspinatus tendon. Another thumb-width superior should be the supraspinatus tendon, which is directly on the superior aspect (top) of the greater tubercle of the humerus, just lateral to the edge of the acromion process.

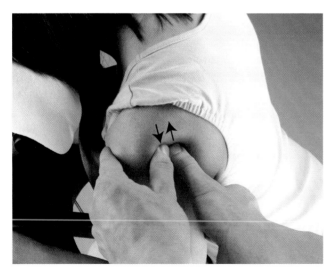

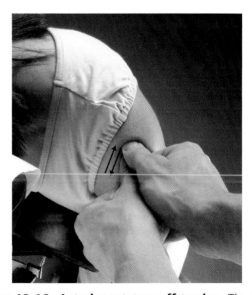

Figure 12-16 Anterior rotator cuff tendon. The therapist examines the subscapularis tendon on the lesser tubercle of the anterior humerus with cross-fiber deep friction (circular deep friction may also be used). Best access is gained if the client externally rotates her arm to at least the edge of the arm rest.

sternum, and the costal cartilages of ribs 2–7. There are also fibers that merge into the abdominal wall muscles of the abdomen. All three sections insert on the lateral lip of the bicipital groove of the humerus.

This muscle performs a variety of movements, primarily adduction, movement of the arm across the chest, and internal rotation. Trigger points can form in all three sections and refer into the breast area, deltoid, and down the arm to the middle fingers. This muscle plays a large role in the round-shoulders, head-forward, "poor posture" condition and must be massaged and stretched in such cases (1,2). You should examine the pectoralis major muscle when clients report or exhibit the following:

- Chest pain
- Arm pain
- Anterior rotated shoulder/arm posture
- Restriction of movement in the shoulder/arm
- Desire to enhance shoulder movement and function

To examine the anterior shoulder muscles, you may need to kneel or sit on a chair or stool facing the side of the client, just slightly anterior (forward) of her shoulder. Keep your back straight, your head up, and your hands in proper alignment.

1. With the client in the standard chair position, grasp her humerus (upper arm) just proximal to the elbow and hold so that the humerus is coming straight out from her shoulder joint and parallel to the floor.
2. With your other hand, reach in and grasp the pectoralis major muscle (which makes up the front web of the armpit), using a pincer-like grip.

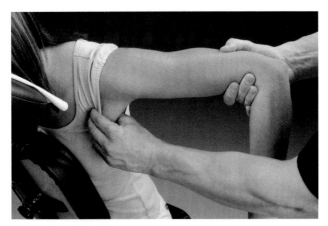

Figure 12–17 Examining the pectoralis major. Using a pincer-like grip, compress and petrissage the anterior "web" of the armpit. Support the client's arm as shown. It may be better for your body mechanics if you kneel down or sit on a stool. Stay lateral or superior to breast tissue on female clients.

3. Compress and petrissage as much of the muscle as you can without compressing breast tissue (on a female) (Fig. 12-17).
4. Hold tender points 8 to 12 seconds.

Note that you can also compress and hold the muscle as you move the humerus posterior and/or superior, thus elongating the muscle. The pectoralis major is a strong internal rotator of the humerus. It can develop trigger points that refer into the chest, breast, and down the arm. If these are on the left side, they can mimic **angina pain**, which is the pain experienced during a heart attack.

PECTORALIS MINOR

The pectoralis minor is beneath the pectoralis major. It originates on the medial tip of the coracoid process and divides into three heads that insert on the 3rd, 4th, and 5th ribs. It is a primary contributor to upper-body postural distortion and is very involved in the anterior–internal shoulder posture. Once shortened, the pectoralis minor can entrap the brachial plexus, which passes under it. This can lead to a condition called thoracic outlet syndrome, also known as brachial plexus entrapment syndrome. Furthermore, this muscle is often injured in auto accidents on the side of the body restrained by the shoulder belt. It is also likely implicated with carpal tunnel syndrome. This author and others have found that shortening of the pectoralis minor and scalene muscles is a predisposing factor for carpal tunnel syndrome. Finally, in the "round shoulders" posture, the client will not be able to raise his arms straight up over his head (forward elevation), and this restriction can be the beginning of frozen shoulder.

EXPERIENTIAL EXERCISE

Shoulder Posture and Range of Motion

Sit up straight. Take in a nice deep breath and let it lift your sternum and clavicles up. Make the back of your neck long. In other words, get into good posture. Now raise your arms straight up in front of you (forward elevation). How far can you raise them? You should be able to raise your arm up until it is beside your ear and aligned on the coronal plane.

Lower your arms, exhale, let your sternum fall into your abdomen, and let your shoulders internally rotate until you assume a round-shouldered, head-forward posture. Now try to raise your arms up in front of you. How far do they go now? What happened?

Trigger points in this muscle refer into the chest and down the arm in much the same pattern as in the pectoralis major, sometimes mimicking angina pain.

Examine this muscle when the client complains of:
- Shoulder and/or arm pain
- Tingling, coldness, or numbness of the arm
- Carpal tunnel syndrome
- Golfer's elbow
- Tennis elbow
- Restriction or pain during shoulder movements
- Internally rotated shoulder posture
1. Holding the client's arm out from his body without stretching the pectoralis major too tight, reach under the pectoralis major with two or three fingers (Figs. 12-18 and 12-19).

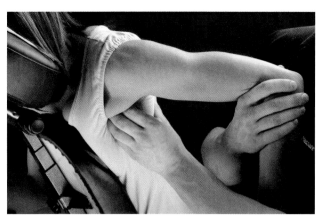

Figure 12–18 Examination of the pectoralis minor. Gently slide your fingertips beneath the "web" of pectoralis major in a superior–medial direction as far as you can while supporting the client's arm as shown. Then, flex your fingertips against the client's ribs and slide laterally. You should feel a layer of tissue over the ribs that you drop off of as you move lateral. This layer is the pectoralis minor. Treat gently with the fibers (superior–inferior) and across the fibers, applying sustained pressure to tender points. This muscle can be extremely tender; be gentle and move slowly.

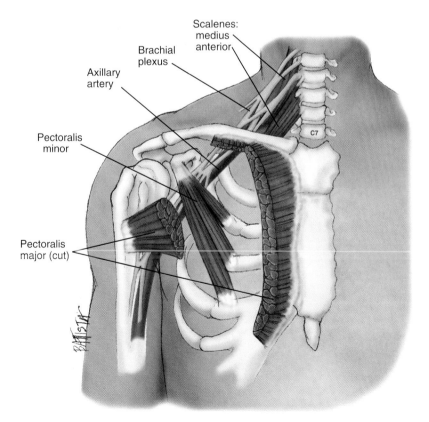

Figure 12–19 Pectoralis minor muscle, with brachial plexus and structures. The pectoralis major is cut away. Note potential entrapment sites along the path of the brachial plexus between the clavicle and 1st rib, then beneath the pectoralis minor.

2. Point your fingertips anterior–superior and place them on the lateral chest wall at about the 5th rib (about the level of the nipple).

3. Gently slide your treating fingers anterior and medial, displacing the pectoralis major, lifting it anterior off the ribs and moving under it as far as the tissue will let you go.

4. Then flex your fingertips, pressing medially against the pectoralis minor fibers on the ribs, and move your fingertips lateral–medial (deep cross-fiber friction), shifting the skin. If the client is extremely sensitive, use a superior–inferior, with the fibers stroke, as this will be less painful. Feel for a somewhat fibrous layer of tissue running more or less vertically. As your fingertips move laterally, you will drop off this layer onto the ribs.

5. Make 3 to 5 cross-fiber friction strokes, then move your fingertips superior and medial about 1 inch and repeat. The pectoralis minor can be very tender, so be gentle.

6. Repeat this procedure again.

7. Continue examining in 1-inch increments until you reach the coracoid process or until you cannot move any further superior due to tissue tension.

8. If tender points or trigger points are discovered, hold with sustained pressure for 8 to 12 seconds. In some cases this tissue will be so tender

it will not respond. In this case, ask the client if he can tolerate three strokes in four places (or whatever you feel is appropriate). If he agrees, do exactly what you agreed upon, as he will be counting every stroke. Do not betray his trust or break your agreement. Let the muscle rest and/or perform the external rotation stretch. Then re-treat it two more times during the session. This muscle will respond very rapidly to massage and stretching.

SUBSCAPULARIS

The subscapularis is the anterior muscle of the rotator cuff. It originates on the anterior surface of the scapula in the subscapular fossa and inserts on the lesser tubercle of the humerus. It is the internal rotator of the rotator cuff, also assisting in adduction and stabilization of the humerus in the glenoid fossas. It is typically short and strong (hypertonic) from internally rotated postures and working positions (such as massage, typing, knitting, driving, etc.). When hypertonic, it can restrict raising the arm overhead and thus contributes significantly to the frozen shoulder condition. Trigger points in the subscapularis refer down the arm and into the wrist, sometimes mimicking the feeling of carpal tunnel nerve entrapment (Fig. 12-20).

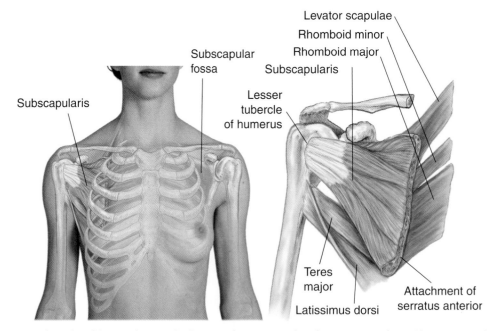

Figure 12–20 Anterior shoulder: subscapularis muscle. Reprinted with permission from Clay JH, Pounds DM. *Basic Clinical Massage Therapy: Integrating Anatomy and Treatment.* Baltimore: Lippincott, Williams & Wilkins; 2003:144, Figure 4-44.

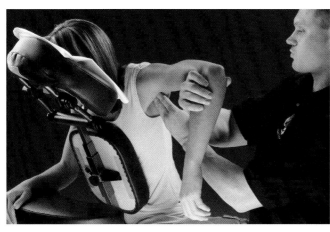
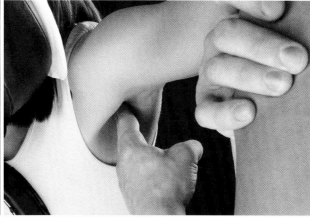

A   B

Figure 12–21 Examination of the subscapularis muscle. (A) With fingertips using gentle cross-fiber deep friction. Support the client's arm, tractioning it lateral and anterior to bring the scapula more lateral. Press medially into the center of the armpit with fingertips until you touch the ribcage, then flex your fingers posteriorly onto the anterior surface of the scapula. Examine with deep friction strokes in several directions. Examine superiorly to the humerus and inferiorly until the scapula becomes inaccessible due to the ribs. Treat tender points with sustained pressure. (B) Close-up view.

Examine and treat the subscapularis when clients complain of wrist pain, shoulder pain, restricted shoulder movement, frozen shoulder, recurring anterior dislocations ("trick shoulder"), and carpal tunnel syndrome.

Access to this muscle is limited at best and is marginal in the seated position, but worth the effort due to the relief it can bring from the above conditions. External rotation stretches will improve the results of your massage techniques.

1. Hold the client's arm away from her body as was done previously with the pectoral muscles.
2. Place two or three fingertips gently into her armpit, with the pad of your fingertips facing posterior (Figs. 12-21 and 12-22).

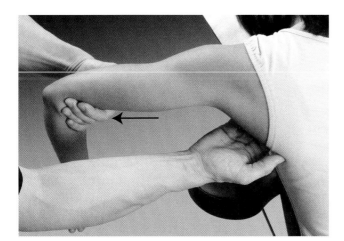

Figure 12–22 Examining the subscapularis muscle: posterior view.

3. Gently press straight into her body (medial) until your fingertips touch her ribs.
4. Traction her arm-scapula lateral and slightly anterior.
5. Move your fingertips slightly medial and posterior, trying to get between her scapula and ribs.
6. Now press posteriorly, flexing your fingertips into the subscapularis muscle on the anterior (front) side of the scapula bone.
7. Examine and treat with deep friction and sustained pressure.
8. Move superiorly in finger-width increments along the scapula to the humerus. The tissue should become more fibrous as you move superiorly and reach the tendon. Also work inferiorly to as near the inferior angle of the scapula as is accessible. If the subscapularis is very tender, you may need to ask the client to agree to only three or four strokes in three or four places, as was explained for the pectoralis minor.
9. Use external rotation stretches to elongate the subscapularis after treating it.

COMPLETION

Go back to any trigger points or tender points and re-treat, especially those directly related to the main complaint(s). As the shoulder is a working unit, it is important to try to do this entire routine for clients with shoulder problems. Time often does not allow this, so you can initially focus on the main complaint.

For example, if you only have time to massage the posterior muscles, at least stretch the anterior muscles. However, educate your client on the need to examine and normalize the entire shoulder and probably the other shoulder as well.

Complete the shoulder treatment with whatever stretches you feel are appropriate, and with gentle, broad circular deep friction to the entire area, followed by some gentle shaking vibration of the entire arm. Tapotement could also be used to leave the client more invigorated.

CASE STUDY

Shoulder Pain

You are doing chair massage on Tuesday morning at the major accounting firm in your town. The owner, a 50-year-old athletic man who has never received a seated massage before, comes by, looking very tired. He asks if a massage might help him relax his shoulders. You assure him it might and ask him to fill out a client intake form. As you interview him, he yawns deeply. You comment that he seems to be very tired today. He then tells you that he has not been able to sleep for two nights because his shoulder ached so badly after playing tennis for the first time this season that he has had to sleep in his recliner chair. He could not get comfortable in bed on his side or on his back.

1. What muscle is likely involved in this complaint, probably with trigger points?
2. Which stretches would be appropriate for his complaint?
3. Since he has to go back to work after the massage, what type of conclusion would you do for him, relaxing or invigorating?

CASE STUDY

Frozen Shoulder

On a cold winter morning you are working at a health and fitness center when a 70-year-old woman stops by your chair massage space to ask if you can help her with her shoulder pain. She reports that she feels fine until she reaches up to get her tea out of the cupboard at home or to do the lat pull-down exercise on the circuit. It has been getting worse lately and now is affecting her tennis serve. Her doctor has told her she is getting frozen shoulder and that nothing can be done for her until it gets bad enough to operate.

1. What muscles are involved in "frozen shoulder" that would cause pain when raising the arm in forward elevation and external rotation?
2. Which stretches would be appropriate to use during your massage on her?
3. What stretch or two would be appropriate to give her to do as homework?
4. Create a 15- to 20-minute routine to address this condition and practice it.

SUMMARY

The shoulder joint is susceptible to a variety of injuries, many of which have postural components to them. Muscles, along with the nervous system, control posture, especially the posture/position of the shoulder joint.

Chair massage is an excellent format to address shoulder complaints, as the shoulder is as available for massage in the seated position as it is on a massage table, except for the subscapularis. An advantage to the seated position is the ability to perform all shoulder stretches that cannot be done with the client on a massage table.

The primary muscles of the shoulder joint are the rotator cuff muscles, known as the SITS muscles/tendons. The infraspinatus, supraspinatus, teres minor, and subscapularis are the SITS muscles. Their tendons form a cuff on the humerus and stabilize the humerus on the glenoid fossa and provide the primary movements of the joint. They are injured by repetitive activity, especially in athletics, and in direct trauma events, such as falls. Secondary muscles to the shoulder joint include the deltoid, which forms the cap over the joint; the latissimus dorsi and teres major, which power the down-stroke movement; the pectoralis major, a powerful internal rotator and abductor that can contribute to postural alignment; and the pectoralis minor, a postural muscle that anchors the scapula to the chest and has the potential to entrap the brachial plexus, which passes beneath it. Trigger points in the shoulder muscles refer into the joint area and often down the arm to the hand. The referred sensations can be mistaken for arthritis, bursitis, tendonitis, and even carpal tunnel syndrome.

Examine the shoulder thoroughly, step by step, muscle by muscle. Evaluate your client's posture and range of motion. Incorporate stretching from Chapter 8 into your routine. Conclude your routine with broad, general strokes to "tie the shoulder back together," and end with either sedating or stimulating techniques.

Practice the shoulder routine until you are confident with your palpatory skills. You will soon be able to help most people with shoulder pain.

REFERENCES

1. Travell JG, Simons DG, Simons LS. Myofascial Pain and Dysfunction. In: The Trigger Point Manual, vol. 1. *Upper Half of Body*, 2nd ed., Baltimore: Lippincott, Williams & Wilkins; 1999.
2. Clay JH, Pounds DM. Basic *Clinical Massage Therapy: Integrating Anatomy and Treatment*. Baltimore: Lippincott, Williams & Wilkins; 2003.

CHAPTER 13

The Business of Chair Massage

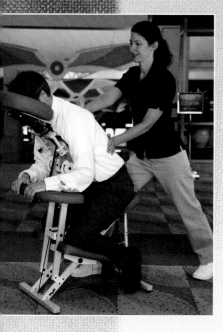

"You are not born a winner or a loser—you are born a chooser. Choose now to be successful."

Objectives

- Identify your primary desires for your practice.

- Write mission and vision statements for your career and goals to accomplish them.

- Describe the advantages and disadvantages of being an employee versus being self-employed.

- List and briefly describe the common business entity options.

- Identify your target market and list several promotional strategies for reaching that market.

- List the three levels of government to contact regarding permits and licenses when starting your own business.

- Describe key considerations to take into account when setting rates and establishing contracts with clients and independent contractors.

- List some strategies for maintaining a professional practice and retaining clients.

Key Terms

Accounts receivable: money that is owed to you (your business) by another individual or business for goods or services provided by you. They are amounts you are to receive, usually due in 10 or 30 days from the date provided.

Corporation: a separate legal entity with perpetual life, governed by state law, which shields its investors (shareholder-owners) from personal liability, provides anonymity, gives tax advantages, and allows transfer of ownership through the sale of stock.

"C" corporation: the primary corporate structure that is used by most businesses and international companies.

General partnership: a business entity made up of a number of individuals known as "members." In insolvency there is no protection for the individual members of the partnership. The individual partners or members are fully liable for all the partnership debts and liabilities if the partnership cannot meet them. A partnership ends when one partner pulls out, dies, or becomes bankrupt.

Independent contractor: an individual or business who makes a contractual agreement (preferably in writing) to provide services, usually involving labor, to another business, but does not become an employee of that business.

Joint and several liability: implies that all members (of a partnership) are individually liable for the partnership debts in full or in part, usually dependent on their ability to pay. Thus a creditor or creditors can "go after" the member with the most assets first, then other members, and so on until all debts are satisfied or until all partners are made bankrupt.

Limited Liability Company (LLC): a relatively new business entity that combines the limited liability of a corporation with the pass-through income flow of a partnership. In some states, LLCs may apply for "S" corporation status. Good for individuals or a few owners, LLCs can provide an alternative to the professional corporation.

Marketing: presenting products or services to potential customers in such a way as to make them eager to buy.

Mission statement: a statement of purpose and function for your business.

Personal services corporation: also called a professional corporation; it is an IRS designation placed on a "C" corporation formed by a professional in the field of healthcare, veterinary services, law, engineering, architecture, accounting, performing arts, or consulting that taxes all income at 35%. This is not a desirable entity. Alternatives to this are the "S" corporation and the LLC.

"S" corporation: a "C" corporation that has filed IRS form 2553 applying for "S" election with the IRS. An "S" corporation becomes a pass-through entity to the owners (shareholders), who are limited in number. It can be an alternative to the personal services corporation for professionals such as massage therapists.

Shareholders: owners of a corporation who own (hold) shares of stock, which are ownership units. The shareholders can write and adopt resolutions that direct how the corporation operates. Usually one share gives its holder one vote. One person can own all the stock in a corporation, or many people may own shares. The shares can be freely bought and sold.

Sole proprietorship: a simple business entity (structure) in which your personal assets and liabilities and your business' assets and liabilities are one and the same, even if you use a business name. Unless you set up a formal structure, you will be considered a sole proprietorship if you are self-employed.

Vision statement: a statement of your preferred future, based on your desires.

Beyond being a health profession, seated massage is also a business. To be successful in this field, you not only have to master the techniques and routines covered earlier in this book, but you also need a good grasp of some basic business concepts. The purpose of this chapter is to provide you with a grounding in these business concepts and to equip you to succeed in your massage career, no matter what your particular goals are.

Specifically, this chapter will guide you through the process of determining what you want from your career, establishing mission and vision statements, and setting goals. It also presents the primary business structure options that you may choose to utilize in your career. Next, it covers various marketing strategies you can use to promote your own business. Then the practical matter of obtaining the proper permits and licenses is addressed, along with the financial considerations of setting rates and establishing contracts. Finally, it conveys some tips on maintaining your practice in the long term, including finding a mentor, practicing professionalism, and retaining clients.

It is suggested that you read the entire chapter first and then go back and begin the desire and goal setting exercises. Then you can begin to make your business plan and, finally, implement it.

EXPLORING VALUES AND SETTING GOALS

Before embarking on your career in chair massage, it is important that you clearly identify what you desire to gain from it and to set some realistic goals to achieve those desires. This initial planning will guide the decisions you make in setting up your practice and, thus, is a critical factor in your success.

Desire: The Starting Point for All Achievement

"There is one quality which one must possess to win, and that is definiteness of purpose, the knowledge of what one wants, and a burning desire to possess it. Through some strange and powerful principle of 'mental chemistry' which she has never divulged, nature wraps up in the impulse of strong desire, 'that something' which recognizes no such word as 'impossible,' and accepts no such reality as failure."

NAPOLEON HILL

Most successful people have a burning desire to do what they love and to achieve success by doing it. Whatever you desire, you can achieve; otherwise, you would not desire it. It is only the limits you put on yourself that prevent you from reaching your full potential. If you believe you cannot do something, you are probably right; however, if you believe you *can* do something, you are probably right. You must go deep into your mind and your heart to find those desires that really resonate with your entire being. You may have many desires in many areas of your life, and the process for fulfilling any of them is the same. However, for the moment, just focus on your desires for your massage practice.

This is about *you*, not other's desires for or about you. Do not allow what others have said you cannot do to hold you back or limit your desire(s) for a successful massage practice. If it is your burning desire and if your intentions are honest and ethical, follow your heart and do not allow what others think to influence you. Determine what you truly desire and write it down.

What Do You Want from Your Career in Massage?

What does success mean to you? What do you need to be satisfied and feel successful? These questions should be the starting point of your career planning because your answers will help you determine what kind of practice you will set up. As you answer these questions, be sure that it is *your* definition of success that is guiding you, and not someone else's. Remember that it is perfectly fine if success for you is different from what success means to another therapist.

For instance, consider the time commitment involved in a massage practice and staffing considerations. One of the wonderful things about this profession is that you can participate in it at any level that you desire. You do not have to put in a 40-hour week. In fact, some therapists only want to work a few hours a day, such as a mother who only wants to work while her kids are at school. For her, success might be doing massage for four hours a day, four days a week. She may have no desire to subcontract or employ other therapists and create a large business. Her desire is for a given level of supplemental income for the family budget and to be able to spend time with her kids when they're home. Success for her is completely different from that of someone who desires a substantial income from a large clinic with

10 therapists on staff in-house and dozens more doing on-site seated massage throughout the city. However, for either of these people to be successful, each must clearly understand what she desires and create a plan to achieve it. While their goals are vastly different, they can both be successful.

Thus, it is important that you take time during the next several days to find a quiet place where you will not be disturbed, and contemplate what you desire for and from your career. To simply want to do massage on people is not specific enough. Ask yourself the following questions:

- Do you want to do seated massage or table massage or some of both?
- Do you want an on-site practice, an office practice, or a combination?
- Do you want to work in a medical setting such as a clinic or a hospital, or do you want to work at or from your home, or from another situation?
- How many clients do you want to see per day and per week? How much income do you need to be comfortable?
- Do you want a general massage practice, where you work with anyone for whatever reason they come to you?
- Do you just want to work with athletes, or the elderly, or clients with fibromyalgia? (Note: If it is your goal to have a 100% chair practice at golf tournaments, you may have to start with a general chair practice until you can get enough tournaments scheduled, but clearly set your ultimate desired goal.)

Until you clearly know what you desire and can articulate it verbally, write it down, and say, "Yes, that is exactly what I desire!" you cannot attain it. Just as when driving a car, if you do not have a clear destination when you set out, you will probably not like where you find yourself. Success is strongly linked to (even defined by) achieving your desires, so until you clarify these desires, you cannot be successful.

"All of us could take a lesson from the weather. It pays no attention to criticism."

UNKNOWN

Establishing Vision and Mission Statements

Now that you have clearly determined your desires for your massage therapy practice, you must create a plan to achieve these desires. The first step in this plan is to establish a clear **vision statement**. A vision statement is a concise description of the end result you desire. For example, your vision might be "To be the sole owner of an on-site seated massage practice that sees eight clients per day for 15 minutes per client, five days per week (40 clients per week) at a rate of $1.00 per minute, thus earning $600 per week."

The next step is to create a **mission statement** (a statement of purpose) for the practice that you envision. It should be short and clear enough that you can memorize it and repeat it every day. Your mission statement should focus on serving the needs of others.

Your mission statement could be the following: "To supply high-quality, professional, on-site seated massage for relaxation and soft tissue pain relief to 40 individuals each week in a manner that exceeds their expectations and improves the quality of their lives."

Setting Goals

Now you must develop a plan to accomplish your mission statement. This requires setting specific goals and timelines. Without deadlines, procrastination becomes a major saboteur. You must determine what needs to be done, in some logical order, to achieve your desires. Goals are like the road map to get from where you are now to where you want to be. Your goals might look something like the following:

- Goal 1: Research and select the best massage school I can find and enroll by January 1, 2XXX.
- Goal 2: Complete massage school and graduate in the top 10% of my class by December 1, 2XXX.
- Goal 3: Have business cards, logo, flyer, uniforms, and business entity structure in place by December 1, 2XXX.
- Goal 4: Acquire a massage chair with travel bag and sternum pad by February 1, 2XXX.
- Goal 5: Take and pass certification and licensing exams by February 1, 2XXX.
- Goal 6: Take advanced training in seated massage, learning all therapeutic techniques and routines by April 1, 2XXX.
- Goal 7: Make a list of all possible businesses that may be interested in seated massage and that I would want to work with, and begin making sales presentations to two prospective clients per day, four days per week beginning April 15, 2XXX.
- Goal 8: Have contracts signed for 10 clients per week by May 1, 2XXX.

- Goal 9: Have contracts signed for 20 clients per week by July 1, 2XXX.
- Goal 10: Have contracts signed for 30 clients per week by October 1, 2XXX.
- Goal 11: Have contracts signed for 40 clients per week by December 30, 2XXX.
- Goal 12: Take a 5-day "Success Party" at the Health Spa Retreat Center, December 31–January 4, 2XXX, to celebrate my success and reward myself for my accomplishments.
- Note: You may also want to develop several steps and sub-timelines for each goal.

You now have a destination with a plan to get there. You can measure if you are on schedule or not. Of course, you may have to make adjustments to the schedule, as things don't always happen as quickly as we'd like. But keep in mind that you have not failed if you do not make a particular deadline, as long as you are still working and making progress toward the goal. Accept the reality of obstacles, adjust your timeline reasonably, and continue working toward the goal and the ultimate fulfillment of your desire. Chart your progress and reward yourself in some reasonable but significant way each time you accomplish a goal.

EMPLOYMENT CONSIDERATIONS

One major consideration to take into account as you are planning your career and setting goals is how you will be employed—as an employee or self-employed. There are pros and cons to both, and these must be weighed as you make this decision.

Box 13-2

Note to Experienced Therapists

Although much of the information in this chapter is geared to new massage therapists about to enter the workforce (many of whom will be starting their own businesses), any therapist, no matter how established, can benefit from assessing his desires and goals for his practice. In particular, if you would like to grow your practice, offer different types of service, or make any other significant changes to your business, start by reviewing your vision statement (or creating one). Quite often, your vision changes as your career evolves. Maybe you do not want to see 40 clients per week anymore, or maybe you want to see 50. You may want to start developing a table massage practice and hire other therapists to do half of your on-site chair accounts. Maybe you want to start doing less relaxation massage and do more specific therapy. It is important to re-evaluate your vision and mission statements regularly and keep them tied to your current passion. Once your mission statement is updated, write new goals to accomplish it. This will often put new life and enthusiasm into your practice.

Often, such changes are necessary for your practice to continue to thrive.

You must constantly be generating new customers and adapting, learning new skills—if not massage techniques, then business and investment skills. If you are not satisfied with where you are and what you are doing, you must change if you want your business to. Re-invent yourself and move to the next level.

Box 13-1

Business Planning Tools

To have a successful massage practice, you must plan it out carefully from the beginning, making sure that you have clear direction and goals. The tools listed below will help you in this planning process.

- Vision statement: written down, memorized, and repeated daily.
- Mission statement: written down, memorized, and repeated daily.
- Goals with deadlines.
- A plan to accomplish the mission and goals.
- Regular monitoring, evaluation, and updating of progress.

Another consideration for those who choose to be self-employed is which type of business structure to adopt. By accident or design, a business will be structured. It is best to do it by design. This process is sometimes called "entity planning," since a business is a legal entity. There are several forms your business can take; these are discussed below. Whichever form of business entity you choose, you should have professional counsel. If you are a sole proprietor, this may be no more than tax help at the end of the year. If you plan to set up a more formal structure, you will need help from an attorney, accountant, or banker. There are two reasons for this. First, you need this professional guidance to be sure the structure is set up and maintained correctly. Second, accountants, lawyers, and bankers are potential clients and may become a regular source of income for you!

In any case, you should at least have a tax advisor, who does not have to be a Certified Public Accountant (CPA) but should have some credentials and experience doing business tax returns. It is also a wise idea to develop a working relationship with a lawyer who works in corporate and business law, even though you may not use his services regularly, in case a lawsuit appears at your door. Establishing a relationship with an officer at your bank is another excellent idea and will come in handy when you need a loan, have a banking problem, or need some financial advice. As you get to know these people, they can become references for you and your business as well as potential clients.

Employee

Perhaps one of the most basic questions you must ask yourself when planning your career is, do I want to work for myself or for someone else? As an employee, you are hired by another individual or a business who pays you, sets your hours, makes the rules, and pretty much controls what you do, how you do it, and when. Your income will be reported on a W-2 form and taxed through your 1040 form as earned income. Your employer must withhold Social Security, Medicare, income tax, etc., from your paycheck, which makes it easy for you, the employee, but has the least tax advantages. As an employee, you are really not in business. You are in someone else's business; you have a "job."

For some, this is a good fit. If it is your desire to be an employee for someone else, that is what you should be. It is also appropriate to be an employee for someone else as a step toward the goal of having your own business, if that is your plan. You can learn a lot by working for a successful business before starting your own.

If you are an employee, you do not need to worry about business structures. However, you still need to keep accurate records of any expenses and investments you make that enhance your abilities to perform your job. Many of these can be tax deductions. This can include continuing education seminars, investments in equipment, business mileage (not commuting mileage), and others. Keep all receipts, a mileage log, and your schedule book for tax time. Consult with your tax advisor for specific advice.

When applying for employment at a hospital, clinic, or with another massage therapist, explain why you want to work with them. Address the following questions: Do you believe in their mission and their public image? Do you want to help them become more successful? How can you help them? Why will hiring you benefit them? Why should they choose you as opposed to some other therapist?

If you would like to work with a specific market but do not want to run your own business, consider approaching an established massage practice and proposing, if you are hired, to expand their business in that particular market. For instance, consider the following scenario: You want to reach the accounting firms in your town with seated massage, but do not want to run your own business. Your uncle is known as one of the best accountants in town, and so you have connections with this market. Additionally, you have excellent training in seated massage. You decide to approach the XYZ Massage Services Corp., a group of therapists who specialize in providing seated massage at conventions and other events, and offer to help them diversify by reaching accounting offices. You can do this because of your skills and the fact that your uncle is well-respected as an accountant in town and likes your seated massage. You can eventually generate more work than you can do by yourself and will be able to provide work during the week for their convention therapists, who usually work on weekends and evenings. Now you have presented the XYZ Corp. with a good reason to hire you, a mutually beneficial plan.

If you are unsure as to what specific market to focus on, network in your community and find out which types of work are conducive to conditions or injuries that are treatable with massage. These problems could include a high incidence of carpal tunnel syndrome (or other repetitive-strain injuries), low back injuries, or other computer-related injuries. Alternatively, you could approach a spa or clinic that does not yet offer soft tissue therapy. Once you have done your research, you can tailor your proposal to benefit to them.

You may become an employee either by finding a job that is vacant or by convincing an employer to create a job for you, as discussed above. Your other option is to be self-employed.

Self-Employment

If you decide you do not want to be an employee, or you cannot find an acceptable employment opportunity, you can join the majority of massage therapists who are self-employed. This means you must start your own business. It may sound scary and intimidating to start your own business, but actually it is relatively easy. In fact, starting a business is the easiest part—just do it! Maintaining and growing it is more challenging than starting it. However, you will find that having your own business provides you many advantages over being an employee, a major one being more options to control your taxes. Being your own boss can be much more rewarding than being an employee, financially as well as in terms of satisfaction and pride of ownership. You will have to decide how you will structure your business and if you and your new business will work directly with you clients or if you will work as an independent contractor. These options will be discussed below.

Independent Contractor

As an alternative to being an employee, consider being self-employed and working as an **independent contractor** (sometimes called an independent subcontractor). This gives you many tax advantages and allows you more options to grow your own business. As an independent contractor, your business works on a contractual basis for another business. While this is similar to being an employee in that you are working for someone else and are partially under their direction, it is very different legally, as you are your own independent business. In this situation, you avoid most of the investment, the overhead, the liability of having a facility (office, equipment, etc.), and managing and promoting the business, yet you still enjoy the benefits of being self-employed. The business you contract with pays your business and therefore you are not on their payroll, thus saving them all the payroll accounting, Workmen's Compensation, unemployment, and payroll taxes. This can be a win-win situation for both parties if done correctly and respectfully. Of course, as an independent contractor you are responsible for paying taxes, Social Security, and insurance yourself. With increased freedom comes increased responsibility and the need for self-discipline.

As an independent contractor you can promote your business (your practice) and may contract with several different massage businesses. You might contract with a salon for two days a week, contract with a chair massage business that does conventions and special events on weekends, and have your own practice under your name one day a week, or whatever arrangement you desire and can negotiate.

As an independent contractor, you show up to do the mutually agreed-upon task at mutually agreed-upon times, much like a janitorial service would show up every day to do the agreed-upon cleaning and maintenance during a certain time period. However, when you show up to do massage, there is a third party involved (the client) who pays someone for the service (massage) provided. This money is then split between you and the business you are contracted with. This exchange complicates the situation legally and tax-wise. If you just show up, do what you are told, when you are told, and receive so much an hour for it from the company you are contracting with, you are really no different than an employee and the IRS will rule that you are an employee. This is especially true if you only work at one place and are there most of the time, as if it is a "job." If the IRS rules you are actually an employee after an independent contractor agreement has been in operation for several years, the tax and penalty consequences can be devastating. Therefore, it is important to conduct a subcontractor relationship properly.

Because some companies have labeled employees as independent contractors simply to avoid payroll, tax, and other liabilities, the IRS has established strict regulations that define the independent contractor status. Accordingly, there are three main factors that determine a worker's status:

1. Behavioral control
2. Financial control
3. The type of relationship the parties have

It is worthwhile to note these distinctions, detailed below, so that you will be apprised of your rights when working for someone else (1).

BEHAVIORAL CONTROL

You are probably an employee when the business owner directs and controls you or has the right to direct and control you. This may include:

- If you receive instruction from the owner (or his/her representative) as to how to perform your work.
- If the owner trains you on required procedures and methods.
- If the owner specifies what tools or equipment to use.
- If the owner provides the tools, equipment, and supplies used.
- If the owner specifies how, when, or where to do the work.

Of course, an independent contractor must be given some direction as to how the job is to be done, so use discretion when considering these guidelines.

FINANCIAL CONTROL

An independent contractor has the right to control financial aspects of the business. This may include the following:

- If a worker has a significant financial investment in the facilities and/or equipment he uses in working, he may be an independent contractor.
- If the worker is not reimbursed for some or all of the operating expenses or supplies, he may be an independent contractor.
- If the worker has the opportunity to realize a profit or incur a loss, he is probably an independent contractor.
- Who collects (controls) the money? If you collect the money from the client and then pay the business you are contracted to a percentage or fee, you are more likely to be considered an independent contractor than if they collect the money and pay you.

RELATIONSHIP OF THE PARTIES

A contractual relationship should exist between an independent contractor and the person and/or firm that contracts with them for services. A written contract should show what both parties intend. It is always best to have a "work for hire agreement," sometimes called an "independent contractor agreement." These are available as standardized forms in office supply stores or on computer programs such as *Family Lawyer*.

As an independent contractor, you are a business and you will have to select a business structure.

SELECTING A STRUCTURE FOR YOUR BUSINESS

If you decide to become self-employed, you will have to select a legal structure for your business. The most common business structures or "entities" are described in the next sections. These include sole proprietorship, partnership, corporation, and limited liability company. Each has advantages and disadvantages, and you will have to decide which one is right for you. Most therapists begin as a sole proprietorship, or possibly a partnership, and as their practice grows they adopt a more formal structure such as a corporation.

Box 13-3

Employee vs. Independent Subcontractor

If you work for someone else, it is important that your type of employment be accurately classified so that your rights are protected and to avoid legal problems with the IRS. Below are lists of factors indicating whether you should be classified as an employee or independent contractor.

Factors that may indicate you are an employee include:

- Required uniforms.
- Required hours.
- You do not handle your own sales receipts or collect money.
- You do not make your own appointments.
- Business owner provides training.
- Business owner provides towels, lubricant, and/or other supplies.
- You receive health insurance and/or other benefits from the business owner.

Factors that may indicate you are an independent contractor include:

- You have a "key to the shop" or accessibility to the business at all times.
- You set your own schedule.
- You purchase your own products, or at least some of them.
- You have your own phone number.
- You have your own liability and health insurance.
- You pay your own Social Security and estimated taxes.
- You have your own business entity established (1).

Sole Proprietorship

Sole proprietorship is the most basic business entity or structure and is more or less the default setting if you do not select a more complex entity. As a sole proprietorship, you may chose to become an independent contractor for another business, such as a spa or an on-site chair massage business. In this case, your business (your sole proprietorship) contracts to provide services to another business, as described above. However, you may work alone or hire staff or even independent contractors. With having your own employees, however, comes the added responsibilities of setting up Workmen's Compensation and unemployment programs and doing the necessary payroll withholding from your employees' paychecks. It is highly recommended that you have professional help in setting up these employee programs. If done incorrectly, you can be liable for penalties, fines, and damages.

Regarding income taxes, your income from business activity and all business-related expenses are reported on Schedule C tax forms. This is a real advantage, as you have control of your expenses. Expenses are subtracted from income on the Schedule C tax form and what is left is your taxable income, which goes to your 1040 form. This is the simplest one of several types of "pass-through business entities" that pass the net income (which is the money left over after expenses) onto your 1040 personal income tax form. In other words, the business entity of your sole proprietorship pays no taxes; it handles the money and reports what is left to be taxed at your personal income tax rate. Any expense or purchase that is directly related to conducting your business can be deducted from the gross income of the business. This includes continuing education, massage chairs, face cradle covers, a travel bag, advertising, promotions, printing, a business website, dues, subscriptions, uniforms, possibly some of your home expenses such as rent and utilities if you have a dedicated space for your business, and more. Be sure to keep every receipt and a travel log of all business driving and travel, along with your schedule book, for tax time. Consult a business tax advisor for specific advice regarding your situation.

On the down side, as a sole proprietor you are personally liable for any debts or consequences of your business. You and your business are one and the same, even if you use a DBA ("doing business as") name. Should someone sue your business, it is the same as if you are sued. Likewise, if someone sues you personally, your business is sued at the same time. Everything you own and everything your business owns are up for grabs in the event of a lawsuit against either you or the business or your spouse, if you are married. This is not a problem if you do not have many assets for someone to pursue. However, once you are successful and have assets and property worth suing for, it is best that you structure your business to isolate it from your personal property and wealth. This structuring can also be beneficial in further reducing tax liabilities, depending on your level of income (2).

Partnership

There are several forms of legal partnership entities. The most common is a **general partnership**. When you agree (verbally or in writing) to do business together with another person or persons, you are acting in partnership. A general partnership is just like a sole proprietorship, except with more exposure to liability. Each partner is responsible for everything each partner owns, owes, does, and has done. You have **joint and several liability** with your partners. This means you are completely liable for everything, whether you are involved directly or not. You are liable for their acts even if you were not involved. If the partnership has debts, you can be held liable for the entire debt. You are jointly liable with your partners *and* you are individually liable. The several partners can each be held completely liable. How this works is that creditors go after the partner that has the most ability to pay, then the next and the next until they collect the entire debt or all partners are bankrupt. A partnership is a simple business entity, but before you enter one, be sure you have more to gain from the partnership than to lose to it (2).

The partnership ends when one or more partners pull out, die, or become bankrupt. In the case of the death of a partner, you may become partners with their heirs (spouse, child, parent, or estate). A general partnership is another pass-through entity and, like a sole proprietorship, pays no taxes. The net income, the money left after the partnership expenses, is passed through to each partner according to their percentage of ownership. Each partner then pays personal income tax (1040) on their share of the profits (net income). Your personal business expenses (those not paid for or reimbursed by the partnership) may be deductible on your 1040, but not as advantageously as on a Schedule C in a sole proprietorship. Check with your tax advisor as tax law changes often.

If you think you want to form a partnership, get good professional legal and accounting advice. *Never* enter a partnership without a written partnership agreement that you have had reviewed by an attorney. Even if you are going into business with your best friend or a relative (sister, cousin, etc.), have a written agreement. Written agreements (contracts) keep friends as friends. The agreement should spell out each partner's responsibilities and obligations, as well as how the partnership can be altered or terminated.

A general partnership is not a very desirable form of business structure due to the liability exposure. It may work for you, but it is recommended that you consider a more formal structure, such as a Limited Liability Company (LLC) or a corporation.

Corporation

Corporations are the most sophisticated business structure. Corporations offer ease of ownership transfer (via shares) and provide tremendous liability protection to shareholders, directors, and officers. A corporation is a separate legal entity from its owners and is governed by state law. Owners are called **shareholders** and can own various percentages (shares) of the corporation. Shareholders are not individually liable for actions, debts, or liabilities of the business. The business is not liable for actions of its shareholders. Likewise, the individual shareholder's personal wealth is well-protected even when the individual is an officer or director of the corporation. This means if the business is sued, your personal wealth is protected. Likewise, if you are sued, the business is shielded. Of course, lawyers attempt to "pierce the corporate veil" when they sue either the business or the individual, but they are seldom successful if all the procedures and paperwork isolating the individual from the corporation are done correctly. Care must be taken to be sure all corporate formalities, flow of activity, and paperwork are done properly so as to maintain the business as a separate legal entity. The corporation must not be just an alterego of its stockholder(s). (This is a very good reason to have professional advice to make sure you run your corporation properly.)

Directors and shareholders (who may be one and the same) make the bylaws and policies. Officers run the corporation. You may be the shareholder, officer, and director of your corporation, all in one. There are two types of corporations, the "C" and the "S."

The "C" Corporation

The **"C" corporation** is the premier wealth-building entity in the United States. Wealthy individuals and major businesses use "C" corporations to control wealth and to protect it. It is a very formal structure and offers many tax and benefit advantages. Often, multiple corporations are intertwined to protect an individual's personal wealth and property, with each corporation providing another layer of protection. The corporate structure is allowed by law to provide better tax-free benefits such as retirement programs, health care, and insurance, and has more options as to how it compensates it employees, officers, and shareholders. However, due to certain IRS rulings, a "C" corporation is difficult for an individual massage therapist, or even several therapists, to maintain if the primary business is providing services such as massage. The IRS will require filing as a **personal services corporation** (a PSC), which is a corporation that provides personal services such as healthcare veterinary services, law, performing arts, consulting, etc. The PSC has its own flat tax rate of 35%, which makes this a very undesirable business structure if you want to get much of the money you earn. If you move beyond just providing services (massage) and start selling a significant number of products, promoting educational classes, managing property, etc., a "C" corporation may work well for you. Until then, the "S" Corporation is probably best. Consult with your tax advisor or attorney for your specific case.

The "S" Corporation

An **"S" corporation** is a "C" corporation that has filed IRS Form 2553 requesting an "S" election. The "S" corporation now becomes a pass-through tax entity similar to the ones discussed above, but still provides the asset protection of a corporation. The "S" corporation pays no taxes. Profits not held within the business (the amount that can be held as profits without tax penalty is limited by law) are passed on to the shareholders according to their percentages of ownership and taxed at their personal income tax rate (1040). You can solely own an "S" corporation, or several therapists can go in together and own the corporation. There are limits on the number of shareholders an "S" corporation can have; however, this is not usually a problem with massage therapists. If your business becomes so successful that you have the need for many stockholder therapists or you decide to go public, you can upgrade to full "C" status.

The "S" corporation is a viable alternative to the professional services corporation and its high tax rate. The "S" corporation allows more creative tax planning and benefit options than other pass-through entities and still maintains the separation and protection desired of a corporation. The personal tax savings of this structure are well worth looking into and more than offset the expenses of setting up and maintaining the "S" corporation.

Limited Liability Company

A **Limited Liability Company (LLC)** is a relatively new form of business structure that is becoming very popular, especially with those who want to move beyond a sole proprietorship or a general partnership. It is another pass-through entity that pays no taxes itself; therefore, accounting is relatively simple. It can be set up similar to a corporation and can be structured to give most of the advantages of a small corporation ("S" corporation) with less formality and fewer accounting procedures. There is even an "S" election available in some states for LLC structures that make them essentially the same as an "S" corporation but with a less formal structure. There can be multiple owners, each owning shares (membership certificates) in equal or varying percentages of the business, making an LLC a better structure for several massage therapists to work through together than a partnership. There are more tax strategies available in the LLC than in a sole proprietorship or a partnership. In an LLC the business becomes an independent legal entity, isolating and protecting the owner/member(s) from personal liability for the business and from the other members, much like a corporation. This means your personal assets (home, car, possessions, money) cannot be taken by creditors to make good on business obligations or to pay lawsuit judgments against the business. LLCs provide very good personal asset protection for the individual practitioner, such as a massage therapist. LLCs do require more accounting procedures than do sole proprietorships and, if not done correctly and in a timely manner, can invalidate the desired protection. Nevertheless, the tax advantages and asset protection far outweigh the cost and effort to maintain the structure. Again, the laws on LLCs are evolving, so check with professional counsel for current advice (2).

MARKETING

Because its purpose is to create a customer, a business has two functions and only two functions: Marketing and Innovation. Marketing and Innovations produce results, all the rest are costs.

CHERI S. HILL, *The Magic of Compound Marketing*

Once you have successfully set up your business, your next concern should be how to get the word out to potential clients about your practice. This process of promoting your business to attract potential clients is call **marketing**. Because there are many choices (therapists) for the potential massage client to choose from, you must ask yourself, "Why should they choose me?" Here are some very good reasons:

- You are highly proficient.
- You are professional.

- You are dependable.
- You are honest.
- You help them.

Beyond simply announcing the existence of your business, you need to clearly communicate to your market the benefits that you can offer them.

Identifying and Reaching Your Target Market

Before you begin promoting your business, however, you need to clearly identify who your market is. One of the wonderful things about the massage profession is that you can create your very own, unique practice. You can gear your services to a general market (relaxation) or to a very specific market (golfers). You may have to accept a more general clientele when starting your practice, but the focus of promotion can be toward developing the specific client group you prefer to work with.

For example, if the desired target market is chess players, your promotion should be aimed at explaining how seated massage can benefit chess players. Examples of possible benefits include more accuracy in computation skills, as proven by research (3), enhanced alertness, less back and shoulder pain, and enhanced health by reducing stress, thus improving immune system functioning. These results may appeal to other clientele groups as well, such as accountants, so in the beginning you may need to work with whomever is attracted to your promotion. After you become more established, however, you might well have enough clients who are chess players that you can focus on this group exclusively. Of course, you may also be faced with the reality that there are not enough chess players in your area to solely support your practice at the client load you desire. In that case, you will always need clients from the broader market. However, you can still focus on chess players, possibly helping them promote chess in your area, which would only increase the number of chess players you could provide massage to!

To reach chess players, you could place your business card, brochure, or flyer at all local chess emporiums. Get to know the leaders of the chess community in your locale. Attend the major chess events in your city. Ask chess players about their muscular–skeletal complaints and create chair routines to specifically address these. Try to arrange a presentation to the local chess club about how massage can benefit chess players on several levels (mentally, physically, emotionally). Try to find one of the better-known chess players in your community and offer them a slight discount in return for their endorsement.

The point of this example is that you should develop a clear understanding of whom you want to primarily work with and what your message to them will be. Then go out, find those people, and communicate this message to them.

Self-Promotion

One of the tests for any promotional materials you produce is, do they stimulate the desire for your services in the intended population? If your promotional messages awaken the desire for your services in the target population (lawyers, for example), that is good. If they awaken the desire for your services in the general public, so much the better. Below are some simple yet effective means of promoting your services to your target market.

Business Card

A business card should clearly state who you are, what you do, and your contact information. The importance of clarity in a business card cannot be overemphasized; avoid esoteric professional terminology. The public will likely be unfamiliar with many specialty modalities but will know what massage is. Additionally, the look of your card should convey you as a professional, ethical therapist. Keep it simple: your name, your business name (if different from your name), what you do ("Chair Massage Therapist"), and your contact information. It is now appropriate to have an e-mail address or website address along with a phone number. You should have no more than two phone numbers or else your card becomes cluttered, hard to read, and confusing, causing potential clients to wonder which number to call. If they are not sure, they will most likely not call at all. Your address is optional, depending on your situation. In fact, you may want to have two business cards: one with just phone numbers for general distribution and one with an address and additional contact information for people you trust.

Printed Literature

With the advent of desktop publishing, it has become easy and economical to create (or have created) attractive flyers, posters, brochures, and other printed promotional materials. There are generic brochures and flyers available from several of the massage membership organizations and vendors, on which you can have your business name stamped or im-

printed. People like to have something to see, read, feel, and hold because, initially, massage is something new and possibly suspicious to them. A good brochure can be very effective when distributed to the employees of a firm for which you are about to begin providing seated massage. Flyers posted on company bulletin boards with your schedule and how to sign up can also be helpful.

For both your business card and printed literature, it is also important to consider the name of your business. It should describe what you do and be easily associated with you and your practice. Additionally, a business logo can make it easier for potential clients to remember and identify your business. If you are not artistic enough to create your own logo, consider having one professionally created. Although this can be expensive, it is well worth it once it is created, as it will yield you much publicity for a long time to come.

Internet

As part of an effective communication package, you should have an e-mail address. Basic e-mail service is inexpensive and sometimes free. Businesses and most people are communicating via e-mail nowadays. It is one more way for people to reach you and for you to reach them. Newsletters and advertising can now be sent to your client base virtually free compared to printed and mailed newsletters. Regular newsletters have been proven to generate appointments, especially when they provide helpful information along with your sales pitch.

As you develop your business, it is a wise idea to invest in a website. Even a simple website can be effective and convey information to interested potential clients. Free websites are available through some internet providers that can at least establish your presence on the net. A website can help project a professional image of your practice. As your business grows and you can afford a more sophisticated website, combine your e-mail with your website so your address becomes bill@billsmith.com or jane@citywidemassage.com. When people see your e-mail they know you have a website.

Websites can market gift certificates, holiday specials, and your availability (especially if you work out in the public at places such as airports and malls), as well as providing information and education. Eventually, you can add a shopping cart and sell gift certificates, appointments, and merchandise over the internet. There are many great books on internet marketing and on building websites. Take advantage of this effective yet inexpensive marketing tool.

Networking

Perhaps one of the most effective promotional strategies is simply networking with people or groups who are potential clients or who could refer you to potential clients. For example, becoming a donor to or patron of your local performing arts theater will likely gain you recognition and possible clients among the dancers, musicians, entertainers, and others who work there. They have strong loyalty toward those who support them. Furthermore, it will connect you with other donors who are also potential clients. They might recognize your name from the donor list or meet you at related social events, and thus be more likely to choose you for a massage. Sometimes you can even book appointments at social events sponsored by the organization to which you are a donor. Always keep your schedule book handy and try to keep in mind your availability for the next day or two. Support your community and it will support you.

Another effective way to network is to speak at "meet and eat" groups. These are groups, such as the Lions Club, that meet weekly or monthly to share a meal and to socialize. Such groups may be open to having you come and give a presentation on the benefits of massage. Find out who their program director is; he or she is usually always looking for guest speakers. These groups are usually composed of professional people who have the resources to afford your services, and thus are potential clients or could refer potential clients to you.

Often, networking and other word-of-mouth promotion can be more effective and more powerful than all the media advertising you can buy. Take advantage of this free advertising as much as possible. Below is a list of free promotional strategies.

- Network with healthcare providers, business owners, and other associates.
- Look for opportunities to introduce new acquaintances to seated massage and to your business.
- Volunteer your time at professional and charity events, gatherings, and organizations.
- Offer to give presentations on the benefits of massage at businesses and organizations.
- Give public demonstrations of seated massage at home shows, salons, spas, health clubs, fairs, health food stores, events, etc.
- Give sales demonstrations to potential business clients.

Learn to meet people and remember their names. Your effectiveness when networking depends on how you present yourself. Look and act professional. Learn to be prompt, courteous, compassionate, caring, and helpful. You can attract more flies with sugar than you can with vinegar.

Here is a great method to meet people in a way that makes them open to your message:

1. Say "Hi" or some other non-threatening phrase.
2. Ask them what they do or what brings them to this place.
3. Listen attentively and politely.
4. Eventually, most of them will ask, "What do you do?"
5. Now that you have their attention, explain what you do and how it can help them.

Advertising

In addition to the free promotional strategies discussed above, paid advertising can also help get the word out about your seated massage business. However, you need to be careful with advertising to make sure that you are getting a good return on your investment (at least a ratio of 5:1 return versus investment is recommended). Three good places for a massage therapist to advertise are your local phone book, newspapers and magazines, and the Internet.

Phone Book

In general, it is a good idea to advertise your business in the phone book white and yellow pages. If you list your business in the yellow pages, make sure that it appears under a heading that is simple and that will be logical to the average person looking for massage. For instance, "Massage" would be more likely to be referenced by a potential client than "Bodywork" or "Somatic Re-education." Even better would be "Massage-therapeutic" or "Massage-licensed," if those headings are available, to further specify the type of massage you offer.

In the white pages, besides listing your business under the business's name, it is also a good idea to list it under your own personal name, as many clients will more easily remember your name than the name of your business. In any case, make it as easy as possible for prospective clients to find you because if they cannot find you, you will lose their business.

Although advertising in the phone book has worked well for many therapists, it is not effective for everyone, so you should evaluate your market and advertising needs and determine whether it will work for you. In some cities, especially in unlicensed states, yellow page listings generate unwanted calls. Many therapists now only have a cell phone for their business, and thus are not listed in traditional phone books. If you choose not to be in the phone book, however, you will have to put more emphasis on other avenues of advertising to give your business exposure.

Newspapers and Magazines

Ads in newspapers and magazines can be effective. They are often expensive, so you must evaluate them carefully. Most newspapers will create ads for you. Magazines usually require you to have your ad made and brought to them. Unless you are a graphic artist, this becomes another expense on top of the ad space itself. Call the publication and ask to speak with an advertising or sales representative. He or she will arrange a meeting with you. You can usually get a better rate if you agree to run regular ads for a period of time. However, do not sign up for a long-term contract, as local print ads will usually draw the readership that is interested in your business in the first few months and then response will fall off. Also, there are penalties for canceling a contract.

Ads that offer a deal, a sale, a special offer, or a coupon seem to work best. For example, a coupon for 25% off on the first massage, a special rate for a "package" of four massages, or a discount on gift certificates have all worked successfully. Depending on how you structure your practice, you may be trying to reach businesses that want to bring you in to provide chair massage for their employees. In this case, advertise in specialized publications such as the Chamber of Commerce newsletter or some other "business-to-business" publication in your community. Offer some introductory rate or package deal, such as the first three businesses to sign up for three hours or more a week get a discount or a free hour per month. Offer free consultations or possibly a free demonstration. Always be sure to put an expiration date on coupons or special offers. It encourages people to respond quickly and prevents them from showing up with a coupon two years later.

Print advertising can bring excellent returns, but it can be a waste of money. Be careful not to overcommit yourself and be prepared to adjust or end the ad campaign if it is not working. It is wise to ask other therapists in your area what their experience with print ads has been.

Broadcast Media

Some therapists have had success with radio or television ads. These can be expensive to produce and run. They are probably too expensive for beginning therapists, but established practices may find them beneficial. They can be very effective around special times such as Mother's Day, Valentine's Day, Christmas, or special events in your community where you will be providing massage. Gift certificates are most commonly promoted for special days. The best way to get on television is to be noticed and interviewed at an event or to be selected as a human interest story. There is no sure way to accomplish this, but think about it and be creative.

Some cities have public access television stations on their cable systems that can allow you to produce a program for free or for very little expense, and you could become the host of your own television program on health and massage.

Publicity

Another way to gain the attention of your community is to appear regularly in the news in positive articles and stories. Press releases are one way to do this. Every time you go to a convention or take a seminar out of town, gain a certification, open a new location, receive an appointment to a position, or win an election, send a press release to your local newspaper, television, and radio stations. Sometimes they just do not have time or space for them, but on slow news days, you may become a headline. Media people are also potential clients, so it is good to network with them. If they see that your business is growing and that you are actively participating in your community, they may decide to do a human interest story on you, which can be some of the best publicity you can get.

When you write a press release, keep it brief and to the point—no more than one typewritten page. Put the most important information first and the details later. Be sure to include your name and phone number so that the reporter can call you if she needs to. Include a photo (digital or hardcopy), if possible, especially to newspapers.

PERMITS AND LICENSES

No matter what business entity you choose or who your target market is, there are some logistical matters that every massage business owner needs to address. One of these is obtaining all of the necessary permits and licenses for your business so that you comply with state, county, and municipal codes and ordinances. Be sure your business is legal before you begin to practice.

State Licenses and Permits

Most states now require a license to practice massage and bodywork. Seated massage *is* massage and *does* require a massage license. You *must* check with the state government regarding licensing requirements in the state in which you are practicing. Usually this is in the Department of Public Health or the Department of Professional Regulation. However, some states have unusual names for their licensing agencies.

You should also check with your state's Department of Revenue or whatever agency handles retail sales tax. Some states collect sales tax on massage services, whereas some do not. However, if you sell products of any kind you will most likely need to collect sales tax. State agencies are usually located at the state capitol.

County Licenses and Permits

County governments typically have their offices in the city or town that is the county seat. If you do not know where the country seat is, ask at the city offices. Some counties require licenses and permits and others do not. It is very common that counties require you to register your business name if you are using a DBA ("doing business as") name other than your own personal name.

Municipal Licenses and Permits

Check with the City Clerk's office or possibly the City Attorney's office in the city or cities you will be practicing in for information on business permits, occupational licenses, municipal licensing, required inspections, and zoning requirements. Some cities collect sales tax in addition to the state sales tax, so be sure to check on this. City government offices are usually at "City Hall."

It is absolutely essential that you check with all levels of government to be sure you are operating legally. If you are not operating legally, your insurance may not be valid; you may be subject to grievance and disciplinary action from your membership association or The National Certification Board

for Therapeutic Massage and Bodywork; and, most importantly, you could be arrested. Being arrested brings bad publicity to you and your business. Any legal hassle is an expensive and time-consuming event. Be a professional and do it right.

Be advised that it can take several months to get all of your licenses and permits. Plan ahead and allow for this time in your business plan. It has taken some therapists over six months to get a new license after moving from one licensed state to another state.

FINANCES

Another practical matter that you will face as a business owner is finances. Setting rates, establishing contracts, and accounting are all financial areas with which you should become familiar before starting your business.

Setting Rates

When working on individual clients who are paying for the massage themselves, therapists typically charge so much per minute of massage time. At the time of this writing, the average is $1.00 per minute. The client may specify how many minutes they desire, or agree to pay for however many minutes it takes to complete a specific routine.

The other common method is to have a flat rate for a set amount of time or a menu of services that offers specific routines or treatments, each for a flat rate. For example, a "Chair Massage" might be listed at $15.00, with the therapist working for however long he chooses. This could be a bit dangerous, as the amount of time spent for the price will not be consistent. If you massage someone for 20 minutes today and when he comes back tomorrow you only massage him for 10 minutes for the same price, the price per minute value becomes arbitrary. He may come back hoping for another 20-minute massage, but he may never come back because he felt cheated by the 10-minute session. However, floating the length of a massage works for some therapists.

A menu for chair massage might look like this:

THERAPEUTIC CHAIR MASSAGE:

5 minutes – $5
10 minutes – $10
15 minutes – $13
20 minutes – $15

It is not unusual for longer massages to be less money per minute, providing a sort of quantity discount as an incentive to the client to get more work done on them at once. However, you may decide to charge the same price per minute no matter how long the massage lasts.

These are just suggestions. You must decide what works for you. Prices in some markets are considerably higher and in some markets lower. Research what other therapists are charging in your market. Price your services comparable to others. Healthcare services are not best marketed through price wars. Do you want to trust your body to the cheapest therapist in town, or the best? Would you be suspicious of a dentist who advertises rates that are considerably less than everyone else's? Price your services in line with the market. Then you can provide specials, coupons, discounts, or other promotions. If you have superior training compared with the average therapist in your area or if you are doing specific therapeutic work, you should be able to charge more than the typical therapist who only does a relaxation routine. People are willing to pay more to get out of pain or to enhance their athletic ability than they are to just relax. Again, you can always run promotions, give discounts for advance payment of four massages if used in a month, etc.

Never forget that massage is a valuable service. No other profession does what massage therapists do. The public is very willing to pay for the benefits of massage. Do not feel guilty or hesitant to charge people for the unique services you provide. Do not overcharge for your market, either. Always strive to provide a fair exchange.

In addition to receiving direct payments from individual clients, seated massage therapists may also receive payment from businesses for services rendered. There are several ways such payment may be rendered, several of which are listed in Box 13-4.

The business could be a company, a college, a professional office, an event promoter, a person throwing a party, etc. When performing massage for employees of a business, some system needs to be put in place to schedule appointments, just as with individual clients. Sometimes the wellness department of the company does this. Sometimes it is up to the therapist to do the scheduling, which means some internal promotion and education should be done to create awareness that you are there and available, such as attractive flyers placed on the employee bulletin boards or distributed to each employee eligible for

---

Box 13-4

Payment Arrangements for Businesses

Several systems can be used to charge businesses for onsite massage; they are listed below:

- The business allows you to come to their site at specified times and work with their employees who desire your services. Their employees pay your fee directly to you.
- The business pays you a flat fee for being at their site for a specified amount of time. You do massage on however many or few of their workers take advantage of the service while you are there.
- The business pays you a flat fee per person, for each person whom you work on.
- The business pays you a flat fee per minute of massage performed.
- The business pays a percentage of each employee's massage, and the employee pays the remaining fee. This is like a co-payment system in insurance and is an excellent employee incentive to receive regular massage.

---

massage. Brief presentations by you at company safety or wellness meetings, including a demonstration, can be very effective. Demonstrate on an employee so that he can tell others how great seated massage is. Whatever financial, scheduling, and promotional arrangement you agree upon with a business, be sure to put it into writing—a contract—before performing the service.

Box 13-5

Gift Certificates

Gift certificates for massage are a very powerful way to reach new people. Be sure to let your clients and any businesses you provide massage for know that you have them available. Valentine's Day, Mother's Day, and Christmas are the most popular times to sell gift certificates. Make gift certificates highly visible during these times. However, they also make great birthday presents, excellent employee rewards, and prizes for contests. You can create your own or purchase pre-made ones from membership associations or massage supply vendors. Consider offering discounts for purchases of several at once.

Contracts

Ideally, you collect your payment from each client, preferably at the time of the massage. However, if you are being paid by a company to come and provide massage on-site or by an individual to come and do massage at a party or event, you may have to bill them for the services provided. Such an arrangement creates a debt owed to you by the organization or person you provided services for. This debt is known as **accounts receivable**. Before you agree to such arrangements, you should have the entire agreement in writing.

Your agreement should include the following:

1. What services you will provide, how often, for how long, where, and for what fees. Fees may be so much per person, so much per hour, so much per day, etc.
2. The name of the contact person to whom you should send invoices and statements.
3. The names of the financial officer or person to contact in case of a problem.
4. How often you will submit your billing: daily, weekly, monthly, quarterly.
5. When payment is due after your bill is submitted. Typically this is 10 or 30 days.
6. What rate of interest is due if payment is late.
7. The address to which the payment should be sent.
8. An expiration or renewal date and a cancellation clause.
9. Clearly defined obligations of both parties.

Contracts validate your agreement and make it very clear to all parties. They also provide you with legal back-up if collection becomes a problem.

Accounts receivable, sometimes called open accounts, require management. It is your obligation to be sure the person or business pays you on time. Do not let accounts get overdue. Send statements promptly at the first of each month, charge interest on any late balances, and enforce such interest charges. If you do not manage your accounts receivable in a timely manner and businesses pick up on this fact, they may delay payment or wait until you have contacted them several times to pay you. It is in your interest to enforce your open account agreements. It is the professional thing to do and other businesses will respect you for it.

Furthermore, it is also professional for you to pay others in a timely manner. Why should people pay you on time if you do not pay others on time? Timely payments help build your credit rating, whereas late payments rapidly destroy it.

As your business grows, you may decide to hire other therapists to work for you. You, as the business owner, would arrange the accounts and your staff would go out and perform the massages. Now you need a contract with both the account and with the therapist. The therapist may be your employee or an independent contractor, depending on your agreement with them (see "Employment Considerations" above). In the case of an independent contractor, the therapist should collect the money and pay you a percentage or flat fee. In the case of an employee, the therapist should collect the money and give it all to you, with you paying them later. In either case, you need a written agreement with them specifying this flow of cash. The agreement should specify each party's portion of the revenue, when payments are due to each, and penalties for late payment. All other terms of the agreement should be in writing as well. You may want to include non-compete clauses in such contracts so that the therapist doing the work will not be able to "steal" the account from you by going into business themselves in a few months. If you need help writing contracts, try computer programs such as *Family Lawyer*. It may be necessary to consult with an attorney, especially if you have unusual needs or circumstances.

In this day and age, it is totally inappropriate to do business with a verbal agreement and/or a handshake. Written contracts protect all parties involved.

Accounting

Accounting is financial record keeping, "a counting of the money." You *must* keep track of your money, your income, and expenses in an organized and timely manner. Taxes are mandatory and an obligation of a member of a society. However, you are not obligated to pay more than is required by law. To determine what you owe, you must be able to document your income and your expenses. While the primary tax filing is once a year, usually in April for most people, as a self-employed individual or a business with employees, you may have to pay quarterly estimates, monthly sales tax payments, payroll taxes, and other obligations. It is impossible to do so accurately without keeping timely and accurate books. Several systems were discussed in Chapter 5. Choose and implement one of them.

Accounting also allows you to know how your business is doing. Are you making any money or are you losing money? Are you doing better this year than last year? You cannot know if you do not keep track of your cash flow. If you have accounts receivable from clients, businesses, or possibly insurance companies, you must know exactly how much they owe you, what they have paid on their account, and when the balances are due. You can lose a lot of money quickly, find yourself in financial difficulty, or owe penalties and interest to the IRS and your creditors if you do not keep accurate and timely records. It is part of being honest and professional.

As a self-employed person, almost every possible expense related to your business can be expensed or deducted, thus saving you significantly on taxes. There are legal, creative ways to minimize your taxable income and to gain many benefits from your business. These are impossible to enjoy if you do not keep accurate financial records. Worse, should you be audited and you cannot prove your income and expenses, you could be liable for fines and possible tax fraud charges. You do not want to mess with the IRS.

It is highly recommended that you have a business tax professional figure your taxes each year and help you with other filings. If you cannot bring yourself to do your daily bookkeeping, hire a person or a service to do it for you and bring your records up to date at least once a month, preferably once a week.

MAINTAINING YOUR BUSINESS

Once you have successfully established your business, you face another challenge: maintaining it. Below are some tips on sustaining your business by finding a mentor, practicing professionalism, retaining clients, and getting referrals.

Mentors

As with all other areas of life, it is wise to seek out advice regarding your seated massage business from someone who is more experienced. If you are a beginning therapist, try to find a successful established therapist (maybe several) who will agree to serve as a mentor or advisor to you. This arrangement could be a formal program or a more casual relationship. Most successful therapists are secure in their success and are willing to help people who are just starting a career. If nothing else, schedule a massage with the person and pick his brain during the session. You probably need the massage, and you will learn a lot while getting it.

In the masterpiece of motivational books, *Think and Grow Rich,* author Napoleon Hill called such a group of advisors "The Master Mind Group." When soliciting advice and guidance, approach people who are successful and positive. You will be surprised how many people will be willing to help you without it becoming a formal consulting arrangement you have to pay for. Don't be a pest and always express your gratitude.

Another source of information is the Small Business Development Corporation. This is a division of the U.S. Small Business Association. It is a free, tax-funded service that helps small businesses develop business plans and get organized. They can be a valuable resource to you.

Professionalism

*T*he problem with the massage profession is there are too many amateurs in it.

KEN DUNCAN, Ad-Market Productions

Whether you are a part-time employee or the owner of a large massage business, one of your key objectives should be to conduct your practice with professionalism. Professionalism involves your appearance, your timeliness, your dependability, your demeanor, and your genuine concern for the people your work with and serve. Professionalism refers to the skill, competence, and character expected of a member of a highly trained profession.

One aspect of professionalism is accessibility. Your clients or potential employers should be able to reach you easily and promptly. In the case of prospective clients, their first call to you is the beginning of the client–therapist relationship. If you frustrate them at this initial level by being difficult to reach or by not returning calls promptly, you will probably lose them. They will think to themselves, "Next!" and try the ad below yours, the other card on their desk, or call a friend for a reference. It is critical that you be accessible.

Below are some tools and suggestions for making yourself accessible:
- Cell phone
- Numeric pager
- Answering service (a human voice is always best)
- Regular office hours
- After office hours and before office hours
- Call forwarding to your home or cell phone

- Answering service calls or pages you
- Returning all calls and messages promptly
- Website (keep it simple, quick to use, professional in appearance, clearly communicating your services and how they benefit potential clients/employers)
- E-mail (keep your address simple and easy to remember and associate with you)
- Returning e-mail promptly

Another critical aspect of professionalism is punctuality. Show up on time, ready to work. A 9:00 a.m. appointment does not mean you leave your house at 9:00 a.m. to go to it. It means you are at the appointment, ready to do massage at 9:00 a.m. Do not get there at 9:00 a.m. and then go to the bathroom, put on your makeup, then set up your chair, and finally be ready to work at 9:25 a.m. or even 9:05 a.m. While it is bad manners to show up excessively early, it is better to be five minutes early than five minutes late. Remember that being late is selfish and shows a lack of respect for other people's time.

Getting Referrals

As mentioned above, the best and least expensive advertisement is word-of-mouth referrals. Although some clients will naturally recommend you to their friends and family after enjoying a massage from you, most will not think to do so. Some assume you are busy and don't need any more clients. Most clients, especially regular ones, are delighted to help you and just need to be asked to help you. The list below offers some ways to create and /or increase your referrals from current clients.

- Do *really* good work on the client—know your stuff.
- Continue to learn and get better so that neither of you get bored.
- Teach the client about the techniques you are performing, about her anatomy, and about her posture. Become a health information resource for her.
- Communicate that you really care about helping the client.
- Ask! Yes, getting referrals from your satisfied clients is as easy as asking them to tell their friends and associates about you. Tell them you have openings and would like to help more people. Assure them you will always save an appointment for them! Some people do not refer because they fear you will get too busy to see them.

- Reward them: offer a discount on their next massage after each person they refer to you. Offer a free massage for three referrals. At least, send them a thank you card for each referral. Be sincerely grateful; really make them feel appreciated for helping you get more clients.

Getting Referrals from Other Providers

You can also increase your business by getting referrals from other providers. If you are working in a clinic setting or you want to do more specific therapeutic massage for complaints, injuries, and other conditions, you may want to reach out to other healthcare providers in your area. It is helpful but not necessary to have some background in the healthcare profession, such as nursing credentials, for example. More and more physicians are becoming open to massage. The way to get them to refer to you is to impress them with your skills and knowledge, your professionalism, and your dependability, and to ask!

To approach another healthcare professional to request referrals, first e-mail or mail some information about your practice to her. Wait a few days to allow her to receive it and review it and then call to schedule an appointment to see her and to give your presentation. Never just drop in to see healthcare professionals; they are busy and work by appointments. Schedule in advance so you can see them without intruding on their day. Also, remember to always be polite to secretaries and office managers, as they can make it easier for you to obtain an appointment with the health professional.

Booking Repeat Visits

The manner of the massage therapist is the most important attribute in a client's selection of their therapist, especially for return visits. It is the rapport you develop with the client; your professionalism, appearance, and "chairside manner" that brings them back for more.

LYNDA SOLIEN-WOLFE

Besides getting referrals to draw in new clients, you should also make every effort to retain current clients by booking repeat visits with them. You can accomplish this by explaining to the client the nature of his condition as you work on him and how massage can help improve this condition, both in the current and future massage sessions.

Explain what you are doing, why you are doing it, and how it can help him. It often takes several visits, especially when the sessions are short, to break the client's habits that contribute to his condition. Explain this to him. However, always be careful to focus on the client's needs when recommending future appointments, and not simply on your own need to have more business. Do not say, "Mr. Jones, I need to see you twice a week for quite awhile, how about every Tuesday and Thursday?" Instead, phrase it like this, "Mr. Jones, in order to effectively treat your condition, I recommend that you see me twice a week for at least three weeks. Then we will re-evaluate your condition and adjust your schedule. I will be back on Thursday—can you see me at this same time on that day?"

Know your schedule or have your book in sight when working. You should strive to have the next appointment booked by the time they get off the chair. Using the type of approach given above during the last few minutes of the client's current appointment, you can have him commit to his next appointment during the current one. When you have completed his treatment, write it in your book and give him a card. This can be very efficient.

Keep in touch with your clients through a newsletter, postcards, birthday cards, holiday cards, or an e-mail newsletter. You can target former clients who have not had an appointment for a while and offer them a special deal on a package of several massages, an office party, or a discount on their next appointment.

CASE STUDY

Employee versus Business Owner

You have started your own chair massage practice. Is growing slowly, but you are barely getting by. It is difficult to get out and promote your practice, make your appointments, and still have a life. Currently, you are doing 8 hours of massage per week at $60.00 per hour ($1.00 a minute). You are progressing toward your goals and you can see that your goals are attainable.

One day the owner of a very successful chair massage service in your city calls you and offers to hire you. She would take over your accounts, but let you to continue to service them. She would do all your scheduling and handle all the business aspects. You would just have to show up and do the work. You would have to provide your own transportation, equipment, supplies, and laundry for the uniforms, which she would supply. She tells you to expect to work 30–40 hours a week; however, there is no guarantee of any minimum or maximum amount of hours. She will pay you $25.00 per hour for doing massage. You would have to sign a 1-year contract with a 3-year non-compete clause.

1. What are the apparent pros and cons of each option?
2. Considering only the income, which option would be more profitable in the short term?
3. What do you see as the long-term implications of each option?
4. Will you be an employee or an independent contractor? Which would you prefer? Will the independent contractor agreement stand up in tax court if it is written according to the offer detailed above? How could you find out?

CASE STUDY

Launching Your New Chair Massage Business

You are ready to launch your on-site chair massage business. You want to develop accounts with professional offices such as lawyers, accountants, and insurance agents.

1. What would be a good way to meet such professional people? (Hint: What organizations might they belong to?)
2. Where could you find all the lawyers, accountants, and insurance agents in your area?
3. What forms of free or inexpensive advertising might reach this market?

SUMMARY

All the massage skills you have learned will not enable you to help people unless you can successfully plan, establish, and maintain your massage practice. Planning your massage career involves first determining your desires and creating a vision statement and a mission statement for your business. Then you can write goals with timelines to guide you in an organized manner to accomplish your desire.

Once you have a plan, you must decide on the best type of employment (employee versus self-employed) and business entity (if self-employed) to accomplish the plan. You may choose to be a sole proprietor, a general partnership, a "C" or "S" corporation, or a limited liability company, each of which has advantages and disadvantages, discussed earlier in the chapter.

If you choose to start your own business, you will need to market the services you offer to attract clients. The first step in marketing your business is to identify your market. Then, you may reach this market through a number of promotional and advertising strategies, including: business cards, networking, public demonstrations, speaking, giving programs, becoming involved in your community, websites, e-mail newsletters, press releases, printed literature, and paid advertising in newspapers, magazines, radio, and television. Remember, the best marketing is you getting out and meeting people and your clients recommending you to others.

In establishing your business, you must also address the practical matters of obtaining all state, county, and municipal licenses and certifications required of you and practicing ethical and efficient financial management, including setting of rates, creating contracts, and handling all accounting.

Finally, you must maintain your business through regular professional development, continuing education, mentors, professionalism, and retaining your clients through re-booking and regular communication. Always be grateful for the opportunity to serve a fellow human being through the medium of structured touch and always respect and treat each client as you would want to be treated.

REFERENCES

1. www.irs.gov
2. Allen CW, Hill CS, Kennedy D. *Inc. & Grow Rich!* Reno, NV: Sage International Inc.; 2000.
3. Field T, Ironson G, Scafidi F, et al. Massage Therapy reduces anxiety and enhances EEG pattern of alertness and math computations. *Int J Neurosci* 1996;86:197-205.

Client Charts

The forms included in this appendix are listed below:

1. Health Information Intake Form. (Reprinted with permission from Thompson DL. *Hands Heal: Communication, Documentation, and Insurance Billing for Manual Therapists*, 2nd ed. Baltimore, Lippincott Williams & Wilkins; 2002:227–228.)
2. SOAP Chart, with guidelines. (Reprinted with permission from Thompson DL. *Hands Heal: Communication, Documentation, and Insurance Billing for Manual Therapists*, 2nd ed. Baltimore, Lippincott, Williams & Wilkins; 2002:241.)
3. SOAP Chart, blank. (Reprinted with permission from Thompson DL. *Hands Heal: Communication, Documentation, and Insurance Billing for Manual Therapists*, 2nd ed. Baltimore: Lippincott, Williams & Wilkins; 2002:244.)
4. SOAP Chart, completed example. (Reprinted with permission from Thompson DL. *Hands Heal: Communication, Documentation, and Insurance Billing for Manual Therapists*, 2nd ed. Baltimore: Lippincott, Williams & Wilkins; 2002:277.)
5. Seated HxTxCx Chart. (Reprinted with permission from Thompson DL. *Hands Heal: Communication, Documentation, and Insurance Billing for Manual Therapists*, 2nd ed. Baltimore: Lippincott, Williams & Wilkins; 2002: 251–252.)

The health information form (Fig. A-1) is used as a client intake form for any client for whom you are going to be doing SOAP charting. This form is to be filled out by the client before his first massage. He can complete it once he arrives at your location, or it can be mailed to him to complete and bring with him.

Three S.O.A.P. charts are included: one version has guidelines to help you fill it in quickly and completely (Fig. A-2), one is mostly blank (Fig. A-3), and the other is a completed sample for your reference (Fig. A-4).

Finally, there is an HxTxCx chart. This is the chart you will probably use most of the time in your seated practice, especially when doing on-site work. It is a very complete form for seated massage. You may have your clients fill in a new form each time they come to you, or keep their files with you and use the back section for successive treatments. For regular clients, you may want to duplicate just the back side of the sample form onto both sides of an added page.

Provider Name _____   **HEALTH INFORMATION**

Patient Name _____ Date _____

Date of Injury_____ Insurance ID# _____

A. Patient Information

Address _____

City_____ State _____ Zip _____

Phone: Home _____

   Work _____ Cell/Pgr_____

Date of Birth_____

Employer _____

Occupation_____

Emergency Contact _____

Phone: Home _____

   Work _____ Cell/Pgr_____

Primary Health Care Provider

Name_____

Address _____

City/State/Zip_____

Phone: _____ Fax _____

I give my manual therapist permission to
consult with my referring health care provider
regarding my health and treatment.

Comments _____

Initials _____ Date _____

B. Current Health Information

List Health/Concerns Check all that apply

Primary _____
☐ mild ☐ moderate ☐ disabling
☐ constant ☐ intermittant
☐ symptoms ↑ w/activity   ☐ ↓ w/activity
☐ getting worse ☐ getting better ☐ no change
treatment received _____

Secondary _____
☐ mild ☐ moderate ☐ disabling
☐ constant ☐ intermittant
☐ symptoms ↑ w/activity   ☐ ↓ w/activity
☐ getting worse ☐ getting better ☐ no change
treatment received _____

Additional _____
☐ mild ☐ moderate ☐ disabling
☐ constant ☐ intermittant
☐ symptoms ↑ w/activity   ☐ ↓ w/activity
☐ getting worse ☐ getting better ☐ no change
treatment received _____

Have you ever received Manual Therapy
before? ☐ Y ☐ N Frequency? _____

List all conditions currently monitored by a
Health Care Provider _____

_____

_____

List the medications you took today
(include pain relievers and herbal remedies)

_____

_____

List all other medications taken in the last
3 months _____

_____

List Daily Activities

Work _____

_____

Home/Family _____

_____

Social/Recreational _____

Circle the activities affected by your condition,
☐ all of the above
Check other activities affected: ☐ sleep
☐ washing ☐ dressing ☐ fitness
How do you reduce stress? _____

_____

Pain? _____

_____

What are your goals for receiving Manual
Therapy?_____

_____

C. Health History

List and Explain. Include dates and treatment
received.
Surgeries _____

_____

Accidents _____

_____

Major Illnesses _____

_____

Figure A–1 Health information form.

Check All Current and Previous Conditions Please Explain **HEALTH INFORMATION** page 2

General

current	past		comments
☐	☐	headaches	_____
☐	☐	pain	_____
☐	☐	sleep disturbances	_____
☐	☐	fatigue	_____
☐	☐	infectious	
☐	☐	fever	_____
☐	☐	sinus	_____
☐	☐	other	_____

Skin Conditions

current	past		comments
☐	☐	rashes	_____
☐	☐	athlete's foot, warts	_____
☐	☐	other	_____

Allergies

current	past		comments
☐	☐	scents, oils, lotions	_____
☐	☐	detergents	_____
☐	☐	other	_____

Muscles and Joints

current	past		comments
☐	☐	rheumatoid arthritis	_____
☐	☐	osteoarthritis	_____
☐	☐	osteoporosis	_____
☐	☐	scoliosis	_____
☐	☐	broken bones	_____
☐	☐	spinal problems	_____
☐	☐	disk problems	_____
☐	☐	lupus	_____
☐	☐	TMJ, jaw pain	_____
☐	☐	spasms, cramps	
☐	☐	sprains, strains	
☐	☐	tendonitis, bursitis	
☐	☐	stiff or painful joints	_____
☐	☐	weak or sore muscles	_____
☐	☐	neck, shoulder, arm pain	_____
☐	☐	low back, hip, leg pain	
☐	☐	other	_____

Nervous System

current	past		comments
☐	☐	head injuries, concussions	_____
☐	☐	dizziness, ringing in the ears	_____
☐	☐	loss of memory, confusion	_____
☐	☐	numbness, tingling	_____
☐	☐	sciatica, shooting pain	_____
☐	☐	chronic pain	_____
☐	☐	depression	_____
☐	☐	other	_____

Respiratory, Cardiovascular

current	past		comments
☐	☐	heart disease	_____
☐	☐	blood clots	_____
☐	☐	stroke	_____
☐	☐	lymphadema	_____
☐	☐	high, low blood pressure	_____
☐	☐	irregular heart beat	_____
☐	☐	poor circulation	_____
☐	☐	swollen ankles	_____
☐	☐	varicose veins	_____
☐	☐	chest pain, shortness of breath	_____
☐	☐	asthma	_____

Digestive/Elimination System

current	past		comments
☐	☐	bowel dysfunction	_____
☐	☐	gas, bloating	_____
☐	☐	bladder/kidney dysfunction	_____
☐	☐	abdominal pain	_____
☐	☐	other	_____

Endocrine System

current	past		comments
☐	☐	thyroid dysfunction	_____
☐	☐	diabetes	_____

Reproductive System

current	past		comments
☐	☐	pregnancy	_____
☐	☐	painful, emotional menses	_____
☐	☐	fibrotic cysts	_____

Cancer/Tumors

current	past		comments
☐	☐	benign	_____
☐	☐	malignant	_____

Habits

current	past		comments
☐	☐	tobacco	_____
☐	☐	alcohol	_____
☐	☐	drugs	_____
☐	☐	coffee, soda	_____

Contract for Care

I promise to participate fully as a member of my health care team. I will make sound choices regarding my treatment plan based on the information provided by my manual therapist and other members of my health care team, and my experience of those suggestions. I agree to participate in the self care program we select. I promise to inform my practitioner any time I feel my well-being is threatened or compromised. I expect my manual therapist to provide safe and effective treatment.

Consent for Care

It is my choice to receive manual therapy, and I give my consent to receive treatment. I have reported all health conditions that I am aware of and will inform my practitioner of any changes in my health.

Signature _____ Date _____

Signature of parent or guardian _____ Date _____
(If patient is a minor)

Figure A–1 *Continued.*

Provider Name _____ **SOAP CHART**

Patient Name _____ Date _____

Date of Injury_____ Insurance ID# _____ Current Meds _____

S Focus for Today

    Symptoms: Location/Intensity/Frequency/Duration/Onset

    Activities of Daily Living: Aggravating/Relieving

O Findings: Visual/Palpable/Test Results

    Modalities: Applications/Locations

    Response to Treatment (see Δ)

A Prioritize Functional Limitations

    Goals: Long-term/Short-term

P Future Treatment/Frequency

    Homework/Self-care

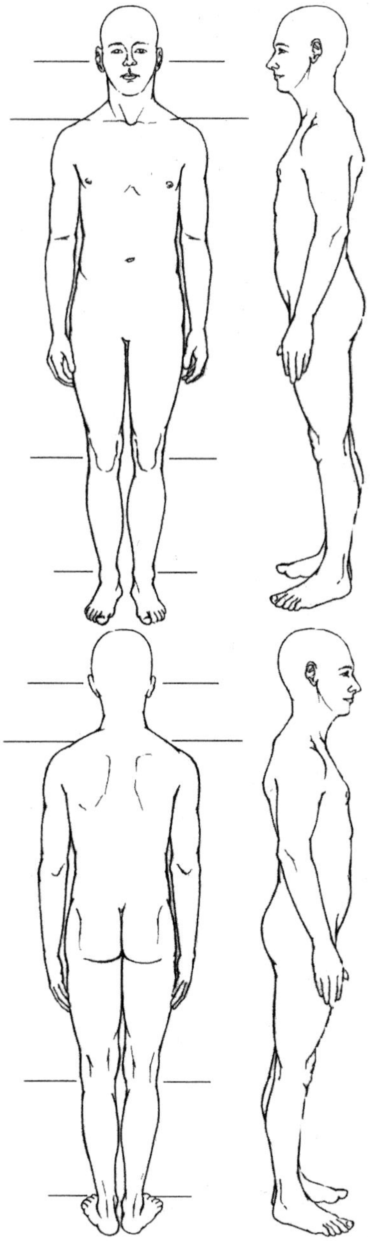

Provider Signature _____ Date _____

Legend:

℮ TP	● TeP	○ ⓟ	⋇ Infl	≡ HT	≈ SP
✕ Adh	≋ Numb	⟲ rot	╱ elev	⊶ Short	↔ Long

Figure A–2 SOAP chart with guidelines.

Provider Name _____ **SOAP CHART**

Patient Name _____ Date _____

Date of Injury_____ Insurance ID# _____ Current Meds _____

S

O

A

P

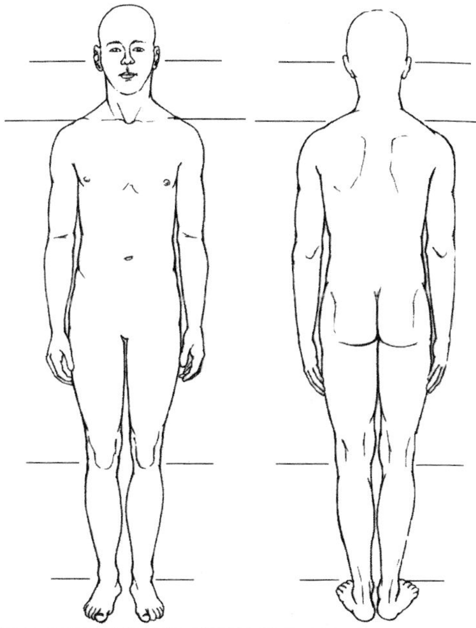

Provider Signature _____ Date _____

S

O

A

P

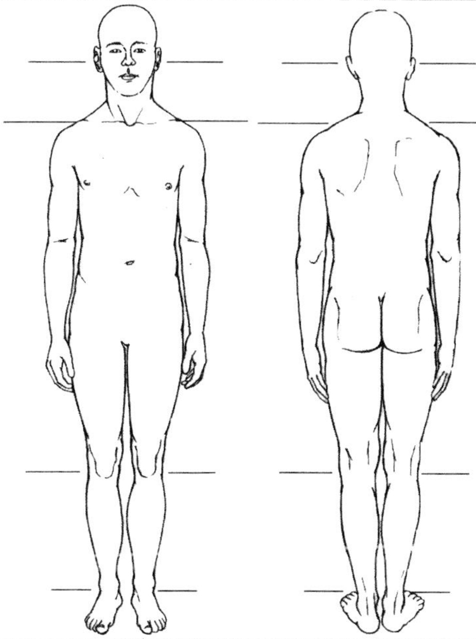

Provider Signature _____ Date _____

Legend:

℮ TP	● TeP	○ Ⓟ	✳ Infl	≡ HT	≈ SP
✕ Adh	≫ Numb	◯ rot	╱ elev	⊶ Short	↔ Long

Figure A–3 Blank SOAP chart.

HANDS HEAL

John Olson, LMP, GCFP
345 Moon River Rd. Ste. 6
Minnehaha, MN   55987
Tel   612 555 9889

SOAP CHART

Patient Name   *Darnel G. Washington*   Date *2-11-02*

Date of Injury *1-6-01*   Insurance ID# *123-45-6789*   Current Meds *Ø*

S   Focus for Today   ↓ *stiff back*

Symptoms: Location/Intensity/Frequency/Duration/Onset
Stiff T L cons, 4 da-bridge marathon 2-7—02
Δ WNL

Activities of Daily Living: Aggravating/Relieving
A: carrying GD ↑ 10 min, sit or garden ↑ 2 hrs
R: ex, stretch, rest

O   Findings: Visual/Palpable/Test Results
M weak c̄ sit Δ L
mvm't T vs hip
rib mob M ↓   BR L ↓ Δ N
       Δ L

Modalities: Applications/Locations
97140   Fl ribs T
60 min   CST — C, T, L trac c̄ unwinding

Response to Treatment (see Δ)

A   Prioritize Functional Limitations
has not regained prior functional status since
MVA 1-6-01 (see ADLS)

Goals: Long-term/Short-term
all goals have been reached within the limits of
current health condition

P   Future Treatment/Frequency
con't ATM classes 1x/mth, ↑ prn
released from care, ref. to P HCP

Homework/Self-care
BR ex ribroll ex c̄ ↑ sit
rest + ex ā stiff

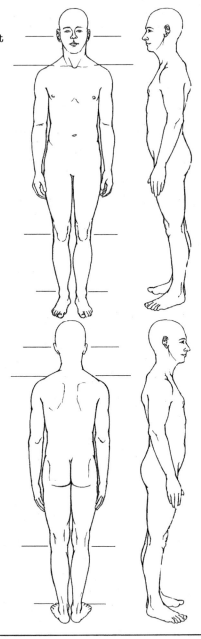

Provider Signature   *JO LMP, GCFP*   Date

Legend: ℮ TP   • TeP   ○ Ⓟ   ✳ Infl   ≡ HT   ≈ SP
              ✕ Adh   ≋ Numb   ◠ rot   ╱ elev   ⊢ Short   ↔ Long

Figure A–4   Completed SOAP chart.

Provider Name _____   **SEATED HxTxCx Chart**

Name _____ Date _____

Phone _____ Location _____

1. Are you currently experiencing any of the following? If yes, please explain.

   pain, tenderness   ☐ No ☐ Yes: _____   stiffness ☐ No ☐ Yes: _____
   numbness or tingling   ☐ No ☐ Yes: _____   swelling   ☐ No ☐ Yes: _____
   allergies   ☐ No ☐ Yes: _____

2. List all illnesses, injuries, and health concerns you have now or have had in the past 3 years. (Examples: arthritis, diabetes, car accident, pregnancy) _____
   _____

3. List medications and pain relievers taken today. _____
   _____

4. I have provided all my known medical information. I acknowledge that manual therapy is not a substitute for medical diagnosis and treatment. I give my consent to receive treatment.

   Signature _____ Date _____

   Tx: _____
   _____

   C: _____
   _____

initials _____

Figure A–5 HxTxCx chart.

SEATED HxTxCx

Name _____ Current Meds _____

Tx: _____   Tx: _____

C: _____   C: _____

date _____ initials _____   date _____ initials _____

Tx: _____   Tx: _____

C: _____   C: _____

date _____ initials _____   date _____ initials _____

Figure A–5 *Continued.*

Different Types of Referred Pain

Contributed by Ben Benjamin and Judith DeLany

Referred pain means that the site of injury is in one place and the person feels the pain in another place. An understanding of referred pain is critical when assessing an injury or pain problem. Without such knowledge the practitioner often ends up confused and treating the incorrect area. There are three types of pain referral that are often confused with one another. Referred pain within dermatomes from injured soft tissues such as muscles, ligaments, tendons, bursas and joints; radiating pain from direct pressure on nerves; and pain referred from trigger points. Let's take them one at a time.

ORTHOPEDIC MEDICINE MODEL OF REFERRED PAIN

Patterns of referred pain have been mapped and often run along specific pathways, known as dermatomes. These pathways are based on embryological tissue development. For example, when a person has a heart attack pain it is felt in the left arm and not necessarily in the chest at all. This phenomenon is due to the fact that the heart and various tissues in the left arm were made from the same piece of embryological material. This type of referred pain is understood in the context of four principles and primarily emanates from injuries to the neck, shoulder, back and hip areas.

The four principles of referred pain in the orthopedic medicine model are as follows

Distal Reference

Referred pain from soft tissue injuries is usually felt distally; this means out toward the periphery of the body. For example, pain may be referred from the neck or shoulder down to the wrist, but not from the elbow or wrist up to the neck.

Does Not Cross the Midline

The second rule is that pain does not cross the midline of the body. If a client has a pain in the right shoulder and says it travels across to the other shoulder, what is usually happening is that the person has another injury in the other shoulder, possibly by overusing it in compensation for the injured shoulder.

Distance of the Referral

The third rule of referred pain is that the distance a pain refers is directly proportional to the severity of the injury. A severe shoulder injury may refer pain down to the wrist, a mild one to the bottom of the deltoid muscle.

Referred Along the Dermatome

Patterns of referred pain have been mapped along specific embryologically determined pathways known as dermatomes. For example, if an injury in the shoulder affects a rotator cuff tendon, the pain will be referred to the arm in a C5 dermatome distribution. A similar referred pain can be caused by damage to other C5 structures in the shoulder, like the bursa. This is because these different parts of the shoulder refer pain to the very same dermatome or referred pain pathway. Other parts of the shoulder when injured may refer pain to different dermatomes.

RADIATING PAIN

If a nerve is compressed by a disc as it exits the intervertebral foramen, radiating pain may result. The pain is felt directly along the nerve pathway and weakens the specific muscles that are controlled by that nerve.

For example, if an injury in your shoulder affects a particular tendon, your pain may be referred to the arm area. A similar referred pain can also be caused by damage to other structures in the shoulder such as the joint capsule or the bursa. This is because these different parts of the shoulder refer pain to the very same dermatome or referred pain pathway. Other parts of the shoulder when injured may refer pain to different dermatomes. For example, pain referred from an injury to the acromio-clavicular joint refers pain to the chest. This joint's dermatome is different and includes the chest and scapula region on that side.

TRIGGER POINT MODEL OF REFERRED PAIN

The trigger point theory is quite different. A myofascial trigger point is an extremely hyperirritable point on a muscle associated with a sensitive nodule in a band of myofascial tissue. When palpated, the spot produces pain, tenderness, motor dysfunction, and other symptoms within a target zone that is usually removed from the location of the trigger point itself. Referred pain and tenderness appears in particular classic patterns that have been charted. Unlike other referred pain patterns, trigger points do sometimes cross the midline. The pain does not follow dermatomal pathways, and it can mimic the referred pain patterns of nerve root compression, zygapophyseal joints and viscera.

The target zones of trigger points are usually peripheral to the trigger point, sometimes central to the trigger point, and, more rarely (27%), the trigger point is located within the target zone of referral. In other words, if the practitioner is treating where the person is hurting and the cause is trigger points, he/she is "in the wrong spot" nearly 75% of the time! Practitioners who successfully address trigger points are often working in areas far removed from the painful region.

A trigger point is considered active if it produces pain when compressed, needled, etc. If palpation produces a pain pattern unfamiliar to the client, a latent trigger point may have been found. Signs that confirm the presence of a trigger point include: a local twitch response; altered sensation in the target zone; painful limit to a full range of motion; EMG evidence of spontaneous electrical activity; pain when the muscle is contracted; the muscle testing as weak; damp skin in that area; rough skin in that area; a "jump" sign when the area is palpated.

How a trigger point is treated is influenced by an understanding of its status. Is it a central trigger point or an attachment trigger point? Is it a key point or satellite point? Is it active or latent? After proper assessment, treatment options may include trigger point pressure release, muscles energy techniques, positional release, spray and stretch techniques, wet or dry needling, injection, or a number of other clinically proven therapeutic options.

SUGGESTED READINGS

1. Cyriax J. *Textbook of Orthopedic Medicine*, Volume 1. London: Bailliere Tindall; 1984.
2. Yates J. *A Physician' s Guide to Therapeutic Massage: Its Physiological Effects and Their Application to Treatment*. Vancouver, BC, Canada: Massage Therapists' Association of British Columbia, 1990.
3. Chaitow L, DeLany J. *Clinical Application of Neuromuscular Techniques*. Volume 1: The Upper Body. Edinburgh: Churchill Livingstone; 2000.
4. Chaitow L, DeLany J. *Clinical Application of Neuromuscular Techniques*. Volume 2: The Lower Body. Edinburgh: Churchill Livingstone; 2002.
5. Lewit K. *Manipulative Therapy in Rehabilitation of the Locomotor System*. Butterworth: London; 1985.
6. Simons D, Travell J, Simons L. *Myofascial Pain and Dysfunction: The Trigger Point Manual*. Volume 1: Upper Half of Body, 2nd ed. Baltimore: Williams and Wilkins; 1999.
7. Travell J, Simons D. *Myofascial Pain and Dysfunction: The Trigger Point Manual*. Volume 2: The Lower Extremities. Baltimore: Williams and Wilkins; 1992.

APPENDIX C

Pain

The most common reason people go to a health care provider is to gain relief from pain. What is pain? Pain is a psychological experience resulting from physical stimuli. Pain is an emotion, expressed as a feeling.

One of the best discussions of pain is found in an article entitled Basic Concepts in Pain Physiology, written by the staff of the American Medical Massage Association and published on their website, www.americanmedicalmassage.com. It is based on systematized pain terminology developed by the International Association for the Study of Pain. You should check it out.

There are four types of pain:
1. Neurological
2. Chemical
3. Emotional
4. Myofascial

Neurological pain is typically the result of nerve compression, nerve entrapment, disease, or degeneration. Examples of disease and degeneration would be neuropathy and multiple sclerosis. Compression or entrapment is pressure on a nerve from osseous or cartilaginous structures (bones, discs) causing pain that follows the distribution of the nerve being pinched. True sciatica is an example of this type of pain when caused by a protruding lumbar disc pressing against a nerve root. Pressure can also be placed on a nerve due to muscle spasm, overstretching or distortion of the fascia or scar tissue adhesions. True sciatica is also an example of this type of pain when caused by spasms in the gluteal muscles, usually the piriformis, entrapping the nerve as it passes through the muscle.

Adapted from an article by Gregory T. Lawton; originally published by the American Medical Massage Association on their website www.americanmedicalmassage.com. Used with permission.

Chemical pain is usually caused by proteolytic enzymes liberated from inflammatory or damaged cells. Chemicals that are released from the area of damaged or abnormal tissue lower the pain threshold and initiate nerve stimulation that the brain will interpret as pain (1). These chemicals include:
1. Bradykinin
2. Histamine
3. Prostaglandins
4. Substance P

Emotional pain is very real but very difficult to describe, as it varies greatly from one person to another. It is sometimes called psychogenic pain that is associated with psychological states (1).

Myofascial pain is also called soft tissue pain or somatic pain. It is primarily the result of muscle spasm or soft tissue strain. It takes two primary forms, ischemia and trigger point pain, both of which respond positively to massage therapy.

Ischemic tissues are blood deficient. They are painful upon palpation or when called upon to work (contract) or sometimes when called upon to move in any way. Ischemic tissue is likely to fatigue rapidly. Ischemic tissue in a small (localized) area is called a "tender point," abbreviated as TeP.

Trigger points are usually locally tender and also cause the person to feel sensations someplace other then the exact location of the trigger point. This is called referred pain. The referred pain from trigger points mimic many painful conditions like sciatica, headache, tendonitis, and carpal tunnel syndrome. Trigger point is abbreviated as TrP. (For more information on trigger points, see Appendix B.)

These factors can be put into two major categories of pain: mechanical pain and non-mechanical pain. Massage therapists can be very effective when the pain is mechanical in nature. Mechanical pain is alleviated or exacerbated by a specific posture or movement. If movement or position helps, soft tissue therapy is most likely indicated.

Non-mechanical pain is often constantly present and nothing makes it significantly better or worse. Spinal motions, in particular, do not correlate with the pain. Usually massage does not significantly reduce non-mechanical pain. This is a good sign the cause of pain may be visceral or pathological. Visceral problems with the esophagus, kidneys, gall bladder, intestinal tract, other organs and glands, tumors, and cancer can cause non-mechanical pain in the low back, for instance. It is in the interest of the patient to refer them to a physician for diagnosis if the pain seems to be non-mechanical. When in doubt, refer it out.

REFERENCES

1. International Association for the Study of Pain website. www.iasp-pain.org. Accessed January 27, 2004.

APPENDIX D

Inflammation

The term "inflammation" comes from the Latin words *inflammatio* and *inflammare,* meaning "to set on fire." It is defined as the condition into which tissues enter as a reaction to injury. The classical signs of inflammation are:

- Pain (dolor)
- Heat (color)
- Redness (rubor)
- Swelling (tumor)

Sometimes there is loss of function (*functio laesas*). Histologically, inflammation is characterized by hyperemia, stasis, changes in the blood and walls of the small vessels, and by various internal exudations. Acute inflammation is one in which the inflammatory processes are active.

If a body part has the suffix "-itis" attached to it, it means that that part is inflamed. Tendonitis means inflammation of a tendon. Bursitis means inflammation of a bursa. Arthritis means inflammation of an arthr- (a joint). If inflammation is present, the above symptoms will also be present. Massage should not be applied to inflamed tissue. However, massage may be applied above, below, or around the inflamed area to help reduce swelling and reduce muscle spasm. This will often bring some relief to the patient and will help the body complete its repair process faster.

Unfortunately, almost any painful soft tissue condition will be diagnosed as an inflammation, an "-itis." Tendonitis is the most common, especially near a joint, due to the prevalence of tendons near joints. Often there are no signs of inflammation present except for pain. This could well indicate a condition called "tendonosis," which refers to collagen degeneration, increased ground substance, and neovascularization in the absence of inflammatory cells (1). Because this diagnosis requires histopathologic tests, a better term is "tendonopathy," which refers to painful overuse tendon conditions without implying pathology. This term is appropriate in painful conditions where no inflammation is perceivable. Kahn et al (2000) found massage to be highly effective in cases of tendonosis (1). Therefore, if the patient brings a diagnosis of "itis," check for the telltale signs of inflammation—swelling, redness, and heat. If none of these is present, the inflammation may have resolved since the diagnosis was given or may not have ever been present. In this case, work around the pain and then directly over the area, starting lightly, yet never working hard enough to cause the patient discomfort. (See Chapter 9 for more information on appropriate working pressure.)

The inflammatory process is how the body heals itself. Sometimes the body gets so involved in healing itself that it causes a great deal of discomfort to the mind. The mind seeks relief. The two ways of relieving this discomfort are either to suppress the inflammatory response or assist it to rapid completion. Suppression is done with anti-inflammatory drugs which have very serious side effects like liver and kidney damage, digestive upset, and stomach damage, to name a few. The inflammatory response is a function of the immune system. Suppressing the inflammatory response for any period of time is also suppressing the immune system. Short-term use may be justified but long-term use poses serious risks.

The alternative is to support the body naturally and to assist it in completing the injury repair, after which the inflammatory process will end. Ice is a natural means of reducing the discomfort of the inflammatory process. There are many safe, effective, inexpensive over-the-counter homeopathic and herbal preparations which help the body get through the inflammatory stage efficiently. Some herbal tinctures, such as white willow root, are natural anti-inflammatories. Massage can help as well. Do not work on the actual damaged, inflamed tissue. Work above, below, or around the inflamed site. Relax the muscles of the area, particularly the ones directly associated with the injury. If the person has biceps tendonitis, work the biceps belly; just do not work the injury site of the tendon. In this case, massage takes the tension off the tendon (which improves blood flow to it), helps remove swelling, and reduces the spasm that is the result of the injury, thus reducing the painful ischemia around the injury site. Massage is also soothing to the injured patient and can help reduce stress and anxiety. In this case, massage is not treating the inflammation; it is treating the conditions of spasm and ischemia. If the inflammatory symptoms are reduced or go away completely, so much the better. Incredible results can be obtained by reducing muscle spasm-induced ischemia, eliminating trigger points, and restoring range of motion.

REFERENCES

1. Kahn KM, Cook JL, Taunton JE, Bonar F. Overuse tendinosis, not tendinitis. *Phys Sports Med* 2000;28(6):31–32.

Glossary

A

Absolute contraindication: a condition or circumstance that would make any massage a risk to the client.

Accounts receivable: money that is owed to you (your business) by another individual or business for goods or services provided by you. They are amounts you are to receive, usually due in 10 or 30 days from the date the service was provided.

Acetylcholine: a chemical normally present in many parts of the body, playing a role in vasodilation and in nerve impulse transmission from one nerve to another across the synaptic junction.

Angina (pectoris) pain: constricting pain, tingling, numbness, and ache radiating from the chest and down the arm, classically from myocardial ischemia (heart attack). However, "false angina" pain may arise from trigger points in the shoulder girdle, commonly the pectoralis major and minor, serratus anterior, and subclavius.

Anterior: the front of the body or toward the front, as in the ribs are anterior to the heart.

Antisepsis: prevention of infection; disinfection.

Areolar tissue: loose, irregularly arranged connective tissue that consists of collagenous and elastic fibers, a protein polysaccharide ground substance, and connective tissue cells including fibroblasts, macrophages, mast cells, and sometimes fat cells, plasma cells, leukocytes, and pigment cells.

Assessment: an evaluation of the client's condition based on objective and sometimes subjective findings.

ATP (adenosine 5′-triphosphate): a body chemical that is the primary source of energy (fuel) for the cell.

B

Biomechanics: the science concerned with the action of forces, internal or external, on the human body. In massage it concerns the forces placed on muscles and joints of the therapist while performing massage.

Body mechanics: the proper use of posture, movement and joint alignment to perform massage therapy efficiently and with minimum stress and trauma to the practitioner. The use of correct body mechanics reduces the chance of injury to the practitioner and improves the quality of touch to the recipient. Also called *biomechanics*.

Bracing massage: refreshing or invigorating massage, typically faster-paced.

Bursa: a sac lined with synovial membrane and fluid, usually formed in areas of friction where a tendon or muscle passes over a bone.

Bursitis: inflammation of a bursa, usually from too much pressure from the tendon passing over it or from overuse.

C

"C" corporation: the primary corporate structure that is used by most businesses and international companies.

Carpal tunnel syndrome: the most common nerve entrapment syndrome. It results from repetitive activity causing inflammatory swelling or hypertrophy in the carpal tunnel, which puts pressure on (entraps) the median nerve. Symptoms include pain, tingling, burning, prickling, and/or numbness, sometimes with sensory loss and wasting in the median distribution of the hand (part of thumb and first three fingers, along with proximal palm). Usually worse at night.

Compressive force: an action which results in the two sides of a joint being pushed together.

Concentric contraction: the shortening of a muscle during contraction; for example, a bicep curl.

Contraindication (kon′trah-in′di-ka′shun): any special symptom or circumstance that renders the use of a remedy or the carrying out of a procedure inadvisable, usually due to risk.

Coronal plane: the vertical plane that divides the body into anterior and posterior sections, running through the ankle, knee, hip, shoulder joints, and ear.

Corporation: a separate legal entity with perpetual life, governed by state law, which shields its investors (shareholder-owners) from personal liability, provides anonymity, gives tax advantages, and allows transfer of ownership through the sale of stock.

Cushion systems: a system of soft props to support the chest and face of someone who is receiving a seated massage.

D

Desktop systems: a face cradle with attachments that allow it to sit on the edge of a table or desk, providing face support during seated massage; may or may not include a chest support.

Diagnosis: the determination of the nature of disease or injury causing the client's complaint.

E

Eccentric contraction: the lengthening of a muscle during contraction; for example, slowly lowering a weight.

Endangerment points: relatively small, specific areas where massage could potentially cause harm.

Epicondyle: a projection or "knuckle" on a long bone near a joint, in this case the elbow, which has one on each side: lateral and medial.

Extensor: a muscle or a group of muscles that causes extension of a joint or joints. Extension causes a limb or the body to assume a more straight line, or causes the distance between the parts proximal and distal to the joint to increase. An extensor is the antagonist to the flexor.

F

Flexor: a muscle or a group of muscles which causes flexion of a joint or joints. Flexion is the bending of a joint, or the bending of the spine forward. A flexor is the antagonist to the extensor.

Fossa: a depression or indentation below the level surface of a bone or part.

G

General partnership: a business entity made up of a number of individuals known as "members." In insolvency there is no protection for the individual members of the partnership. The individual partners or members are fully liable for all the partnership debts and liabilities if the partnership cannot meet them. A partnership ends when one partner pulls out, dies, or becomes bankrupt.

Glenohumeral joint: the shoulder joint.

Glenoid fossa: the hollow in the head of the scapula that receives the head of the humerus to make the shoulder joint.

H

Herberden's nodes: little hard knobs about the size of a pea, near the distal joint. They are painful at first but become pain-free, usually remaining for life.

Histamine: a powerful dilator of the capillaries.

Horizontal plane: a plane that runs through the body, parallel to the horizon (level) when in the anatomical position, that divides the body into upper and lower halves or sections. Also known as the transverse plane.

Hyperemia: an excess of blood or increased circulation in tissue, increasing oxygen and nutrient delivery and improving waste removal.

Hypertonic: a state of excessive muscle tonus (hypertonus) which causes discomfort, restricts range of motion, and wastes body energy.

I

Independent contractor: a business or individual who makes a contractual agreement (preferably in writing) to provide services, usually involving labor, to another business, but does not become an employee of that business.

Inhibition: a signal from the nervous system telling a muscle to relax.

Innervation: a signal from the nervous system telling a muscle to contract.

Ischemic: lacking blood in a part or tissue as a result of functional constriction of blood vessels. Ischemic tissue is tender upon palpation and fatigues easily.

Isometric: a muscle contraction with no movement of the involved body parts; force development at constant length.

J

Joint and several liability: implies that all members of a partnership are liable for the partnership debts in full or in part individually, usually dependent on their ability to pay. Thus a creditor or creditors can first "go after" the member with the most assets, then other members, and so on until all debts are satisfied or until all partners are made bankrupt.

Joint: the point of union, more or less movable, between two or more bones. There are three types of joints, each with several divisions. See an anatomy text for details.

K

Kinetic chain: the line of structures that work together to support a particular movement; in the case of the hand, the kinetic chain would include the forearm, elbow, humerus, shoulder joint, clavicle, ribs, and neck.

L

Lamina groove: the trough or gutter-like space formed between the spinous process and the transverse process of each vertebra (except C-1). The deep and some superficial paraspinal muscles lie in this groove.

Lateral epicondylitis: an injury to the extensor tendons of the forearm at or near their attachment on the lateral epicondyle of the humerus. Often called "tennis elbow."

Ligament: a specialized form of fascia that connects two or more bones, thus holding a joint together. An injury to a ligament is called a "sprain."

Limited Liability Company (LLC): a relatively new business entity that combines the limited liability of a corporation with the pass-through income flow of a partnership. In some states, LLCs may apply for "S" corporation status. Good for individuals or a few owners, LLCs can provide an alternative to the professional corporation.

M

Marketing: presenting products or services to potential customers in such a way as to make them eager to buy.

Massage chair: a specially designed chair which supports the entire body during a seated massage while allowing a massage therapist access to most body areas.

Mechanical pain: pain associated with movement or a particular position.

Medial epicondylitis: an injury to the flexor tendons of the forearm at or near their attachment on the medial epicondyle of the humerus. Often called "golfer's elbow." In young baseball players, often called "Little League elbow."

Median nerve: a major nerve of the forearm, passing through the carpal tunnel and innervating part of the thumb and first three fingers. Entrapment of this nerve at the wrist is called carpal tunnel syndrome.

Microbe: any very minute organism, including both microscopic and ultramicroscopic organisms (spirochetes, bacteria, rickettsiae, and viruses).

Microorganism: a microscopic organism (plant or animal).

Mid-sagittal plane: the vertical plane that divides the body into left and right halves. Also called the median plane.

Military neck: when the cervical spine loses its natural lordotic curve and the vertebra are in a straight line, usually at an anterior angle, presenting a straight neck, head-forward posture.

Mission statement: a statement of purpose and function for your business.

Muscular dysfunction: an abnormal state of a muscle, most commonly resulting in local discomfort and restricted elongation, but sometimes also involving trigger points and referred pain. Hyper-tonicity and the resulting ischemia is the most common muscle dysfunction. Cramps, contractures, or the inability to respond are the most severe dysfunctions.

N

Nerve compression: pressure placed on a nerve by bone or cartilaginous structures, compromising the nerve's function and usually causing pain. Nerves may also be compressed by muscles as they pass through them, when the muscle is in spasm. Also called nerve entrapment.

Neuropathy: a disease or disorder, sometimes degenerative, that affects the nervous system.

Non-mechanical pain: pain that is relatively constant and not significantly affected by movement or positions.

Normal range of motion: the amount of movement, usually measured in degrees, that a healthy joint should be able to perform without pain or injury.

O

OSHA: Occupational Safety and Health Administration of the U.S. Department of Labor; responsible for establishing and enforcing safety and health standards in the workplace.

P

Paradigm: a pattern or model for something, especially one that forms the basis of a methodology or theory.

Parasympathetic response: the response by the parasympathetic division of the autonomic nervous system, which conserves body resources and brings about body calmness; generally antagonistic to the sympathetic division.

Partial contraindication: a condition or circumstance that allows massage but restricts it from a particular area or prohibits a particular technique. Also known as local contraindications.

Pathogen: any virus, microorganism, or other substance causing disease.

Personal services corporation: also called a professional corporation, is an IRS designation placed on a "C" corporation formed by a professional in the field of healthcare, veterinary services, law, engineering, architecture, accounting, performing arts, or consulting that taxes all income at 35%. This is not a desirable entity. Alternatives to this are the "S" corporation and the LLC.

Plantarflex: extension of the ankle, to point the foot and toes.

Posterior: the back of the body or toward the back; for example, the scapula is *posterior* to the ribs.

Postural distortion: lack of alignment on the midsagittal, coronal, and horizontal planes of a person when standing erect and relaxed in the anatomical position; for example, head anterior, high or low shoulder, internally rotated shoulders or arms.

R

Reciprocal: something that is mutual or done in return; in this application, the neurological communication mechanism between opposing pairs of muscles signaling contraction (innervation) in the agonist while signaling relaxation (inhibition) in the antagonist.

Referral: the act or process of referring somebody to somebody else, especially sending a client to consult with a medical practitioner.

Referred pain: pain or sensation experienced in an area different from the source of the sensation; for example, pain felt in the forearm coming from injury to the shoulder joint.

Relaxation routine: a sequence of massage techniques assembled to be a general, non-specific treatment that will relax and sedate the client but not address any specific complaint, condition, or injury. A relaxation routine is designed to create a systemic parasympathetic response as opposed to a localized relaxation.

Repetitive-strain injuries: involve tendon, muscle, joint, and nerve damage resulting from the body being subjected to direct pressure, vibration, or repetitive movements for prolonged periods. Also called cumulative trauma disorders.

S

"S" corporation: a "C" corporation that has filed IRS form 2553 applying for "S" election with the IRS. An "S" corporation becomes a pass-through entity to the owners (shareholders), who are limited in number. It can be an alternative to the personal services corporation for professionals such as massage therapists.

Sanitation: use of measures designed to promote health and prevent disease; development and establishment of conditions in the environment favorable to health.

Sanitize: to clean something thoroughly by disinfecting or sterilizing it.

Shareholders: owners of a corporation, who own (hold) shares of stock, which are ownership units. The shareholders can write and adopt resolutions that direct how the corporation operates. Usually one share gives its holder one vote. One person can own all the stock in a corporation, or many people may own shares. The shares can be freely bought and sold.

Shearing forces: a force or strain that pressures a joint to move across its axis instead of on or around it. This abnormal movement or pressure, when coupled with compressive force, is destructive to joint capsules.

Soft tissue: body connective tissues other than osseous (bone), cartilaginous, and visceral; in massage, usually considered to be skin, fascia, muscle, tendon, ligament, and sometimes periosteum.

Sole proprietorship: a simple business entity (structure) in which your personal assets and liabilities and your business' assets and liabilities are one and the same, even if you use a business name. Unless you set up a formal structure, you will be considered a sole proprietorship if you are self-employed.

Spasm: an involuntary contraction of one or more muscle groups, which cannot be stopped by voluntary relaxation, ranging from increased tension causing discomfort and restricted movement to cramps causing pain and sudden, uncontrolled movement or distortion.

Sterilize: to destroy all microorganisms in or about an object.

Sternum pad: an accessory for a massage chair that provides additional comfort for women with large breasts and people with large abdomens.

Stimulus: any agent, act, or influence that produces a functional or tropic reaction in a receptor or a tissue.

Subluxation: an incomplete or partial dislocation of a joint; contact between joint surfaces remains, but not in the ideal or correct position. Correction is typically achieved through a thrusting manipulation (adjustment) by a chiropractor

Sympathetic response: the response by the sympathetic division of the autonomic nervous system that spends body resources and prepares the body for emergency situations; it is the "fight or flight" response to perceived stress or threats.

T

Tendon: a specialized form of fascia that connects the contractile part of a muscle to its attachment site, usually a bone. An injury to a tendon (or a muscle) is called a "strain."

Tendonitis: an inflammation of a tendon, a tendon capsule, or a tendon sheath.

Therapeutic routine: a massage routine that has the goal of reducing a specific soft tissue complaint by examination and treatment.

Thoracic outlet syndrome: compression of blood vessels and nerves of the brachial plexus at any point between the neck and the armpit, most commonly between the 1st rib and the clavicle or under the pectoralis minor, causing discomfort, compromised function, and often swelling.

Tonus: a state of continuous, partial contraction of muscle tissue, creating a normal, continuous tension by virtue of which the parts are kept in shape, alert, and ready to response to stimulus. Excessive tonus (hypertonus) causes discomfort, restricts range of motion, and wastes body energy.

Travel bag: a fabric case used to protect massage equipment during travel and storage.

Trigger point: a small, isolated area or spot of abnormal physiology in soft tissue that, when palpated or stressed, is locally tender and causes referred pain or sensation to an area remote (distant) from itself. Sometimes abbreviated TrP.

Tubercle: a slight elevation or nodule on a bone providing an attachment site for a muscle.

V

Vasodilation: the widening or opening of a blood vessel.

Vision statement: a statement of your preferred future, based on your desires.

W

Whiplash: an imprecise term for a cervical acceleration–de-acceleration injury resulting from sudden and violent hyperextension and hyperflexion of the head and neck, as in a car wreck or fall. Such injuries include fractures, subluxations, sprains, strains, and even concussions.

Index